LACTOSE DIGESTION

LACTOSE DIGESTION

CLINICAL AND NUTRITIONAL

IMPLICATIONS

DAVID M. PAIGE, M.D., M.P.H.

THEODORE M. BAYLESS, M.D.

EDITORS

THE JOHNS HOPKINS UNIVERSITY PRESS

BALTIMORE AND LONDON

This book has been brought to publication through the generous assistance
of the Shadow Medical Research Foundation, Inc.
1330 Beacon Street
Brookline, Massachusetts 02146

The Johns Hopkins University Press, Baltimore, Maryland 21218
The Johns Hopkins Press Ltd., London

Library of Congress Cataloging in Publication Data
Main entry under title:
Lactose digestion.
Includes index.
1. Lactose intolerance.   2. Lactose intolerance in children.
3. Lactose intolerance—Diet therapy.   I. Paige, David M.   II. Bayless, Theodore M.
[DNLM: 1. Lactose—Metabolism.   2. Lactose intolerance.   QU 83 L151]
RC632.L33L3   616.3'998   81-1537
ISBN 0-8018-2647-0   AACR2

To Nancy, Tara, Danny, Jaye, Jeff, Andy, and Neal
and to Donald A. Cornely, teacher, adviser, and friend

CONTRIBUTORS

D. H. ALPERS, M.D., Professor of Medicine, Washington University, St. Louis, Missouri.

LEWIS A. BARNESS, M.D., Professor and Chairman, Department of Pediatrics, University of South Florida College of Medicine, Tampa, Florida.

RONALD G. BARR, M.A., M.D.C.M., F.R.C.P.(C), Assistant Professor of Pediatrics, McGill University–Montreal Children's Hospital Research Institute, Montreal, Quebec, Canada.

THEODORE M. BAYLESS, M.D., Professor of Medicine, The Johns Hopkins University School of Medicine, Baltimore, Maryland.

JOHN H. BOND, M.D., Chief, Gastroenterology Section, Minneapolis Veterans Administration Medical Center, Minneapolis, Minnesota.

KENNETH H. BROWN, M.D., Assistant Professor of Pediatrics, The Johns Hopkins University School of Medicine, Baltimore, Maryland.

JOGINDER G. CHOPRA, M.D., F.A.A.P., M.P.H., Special Assistant for Medical Affairs, Bureau of Foods, U.S. Food and Drug Administration, Washington, D.C.

BEVERLY B. FINK, B.S.N., R.N., Pediatrics, The Johns Hopkins University School of Medicine, Baltimore, Maryland.

CUTBERTO GARZA, M.D., PH.D., Assistant Professor of Pediatrics, Baylor College of Medicine, Houston, Texas.

DAVID G. GUY, PH.D., Principal Clinical Coordinator, Mead Johnson Nutritional Division, Mead Johnson Laboratories, Evansville, Indiana.

ROBERT H. HERMAN, M.D., Chief of Division of Surgery, Letterman Army Institute of Research, San Francisco, California.

V. H. HOLSINGER, PH.D., Research Chemist, Eastern Regional Research Center, Agricultural Research, Science and Education Administration, U.S. Department of Agriculture, Philadelphia, Pennsylvania.

JOHN D. JOHNSON, M.D., Associate Professor of Pediatrics, University of New Mexico School of Medicine, Albuquerque, New Mexico.

ROBERT S. KATZ, PH.D., Assistant Director of Nutrition Research, National Dairy Council, Rosemont, Illinois.

ALAN E. KLIGERMAN, Senior Partner, SugarLo Company, Pleasantville, New Jersey.

NORMAN KRETCHMER, M.D., PH.D., Director, National Institute of Child Health and Human Development, National Institutes of Health, Bethesda, Maryland.

JOSEPH LEICHTER, PH.D., Associate Professor of Human Nutrition, School of Home Economics, The University of British Columbia, Vancouver, British Columbia, Canada.

MICHAEL D. LEVITT, M.D., Associate Chief of Staff for Research, Minneapolis Veterans Administration Medical Center, Minneapolis, Minnesota.

FIMA LIFSHITZ, M.D., Professor of Pediatrics, Cornell University Medical College, New York, New York; Associate Director of the Department of Pediatrics, Chief of the Division of Endocrinology, Metabolism and Nutrition, and Chief of Pediatric Research, North Shore University Hospital, Manhasset, New York.

WILLIAM C. MACLEAN, JR., M.D., Associate Professor of Pediatrics and Chief of the Pediatric Gastroenterology and Nutrition Unit, The Johns Hopkins University School of Medicine, Baltimore, Maryland.

ALBERT D. NEWCOMER, M.D., Professor of Medicine, Division of Gastroenterology and Internal Medicine, Mayo Clinic and Mayo Foundation, Rochester, Minnesota.

DAVID M. PAIGE, M.D., M.P.H., Professor of Maternal and Child Health, The Johns Hopkins School of Hygiene and Public Health, and Pediatrics, The Johns Hopkins University School of Medicine, Baltimore, Maryland.

SIDNEY F. PHILLIPS, M.D., Professor of Medicine, Mayo Medical School and Director, Gastroenterology Unit, Mayo Clinic, Rochester, Minnesota.

ARTHUR G. RAND, JR., PH.D., Professor of Food Science and Nutrition, University of Rhode Island, Kingston, Rhode Island.

FREDERICK J. SIMOONS, PH.D., Professor of Geography, University of California, Davis, California.

NOEL W. SOLOMONS, M.D., Associate Professor of Clinical Nutrition, Massachusetts Institute of Technology, Cambridge, Massachusetts; Affiliated Investigator, Division of Human Nutrition and Biology, Institute of Nutrition of Central America and Panama, Guatemala.

L. S. STEPHENSON, PH.D., Assistant Professor, Division of Nutritional Sciences, Cornell University, Ithaca, New York.

JOHN B. WATKINS, M.D., Chief of the Division of Gastroenterology and Nutrition, Children's Hospital of Philadelphia and Associate Professor of Pediatrics, University of Pennsylvania School of Medicine, Philadelphia, Pennsylvania.

JACK D. WELSH, M.D., Professor of Medicine, The University of Oklahoma Health Sciences Center, Oklahoma City, Oklahoma.

CONTENTS

I. INTRODUCTION

II. GENETIC, GEOGRAPHIC, AND HISTORIC CONSIDERATIONS

III. PHYSIOPATHOLOGIC CONSIDERATIONS

VII. DEVELOPMENT OF LOW-LACTOSE PRODUCTS

TABLES

⚜

FIGURES

PREFACE

Lactose, the carbohydrate found in milk and milk products, is broadly consumed in its natural form and in a variety of manufactured and processed products. The adequacy of lactose digestion and absorption, therefore, has important implications for research scientists, health professionals, and policy planners.

Few scientific areas of interest have forged such strong interdependence among investigators from different disciplines as has the study of lactose. Discoveries by biochemists have influenced nutritionists and clinicians, who in turn have prompted additional study by cultural anthropologists, who have stimulated further questions about the nutritional implications of dietary practice and milk drinking. A review of the literature on lactose reveals over 1,000 scientific papers published in the past ten years. This high level of interest and scientific inquiry is testimony to the impact and importance of the differences in lactose digestion that exist in various population groups.

The clinical and nutritional significance of lactose intolerance spans the entire human life cycle, from an understanding of the evolving lactase patterns in utero, to the infant with chronic diarrhea, to the black adolescent unable to digest completely the lactose in a glass of milk, up to the elderly individual for whom the calcium in milk is a vital nutrient. Differences in digestive capacity at different age periods are being investigated, as is the quantity of lactose one can consume without interference with nutrient absorption. The use of milk and of foods containing lactose has been at the center of concern for scientists, nutritionists, health professionals, and policy planners.

Lactose Digestion: Clinical and Nutritional Implications brings together in one volume the full spectrum of research findings in the field. The book begins by addressing the evolution of differences in lactose digestion among various populations genetically programmed for declining levels of lactase activity. Autosomal recessive inheritance of low levels of lactase activity is proposed and defended. As one considers the fetal changes in disaccharidase activity and the postweaning fall in lactase activity that occurs in most populations, the need for more information on the control of gene expression of lactase activity will become apparent to the reader.

The physiology of lactose digestion then is explored in terms of current knowledge of enzyme production, hydrolysis, and absorption. There is a series of interrelated physiologic events affecting the amount of undigested sugar and fluid that the small intestine and subsequently the colon must metabolize or reabsorb. A balance of these factors tends to prevent symptoms when the stomach, small intestine, and colon can compensate for the increased solute load, but abdominal discomfort or diarrhea occur when these small intestinal and colonic physiologic mechanisms are loaded beyond their capacity. The role of the colonic flora in metabolizing unabsorbed sugar and the importance of colonic salvage of unabsorbed carbohydrate will be an important area for continuing research.

Diagnostic and screening techniques for lactose tolerance are presented next, together with evaluations of their relative accuracy and utility. Breath hydrogen excretion as a measure of unabsorbed carbohydrate reaching the colon and its bacterial flora occupies a central position in many investigative programs described in this section.

Clinical and nutritional consequences of lactose digestion in adults are examined in relation to malabsorption, intolerance, milk rejection, symptoms and their recognition. Estimates of how frequently milk intolerance will be a clinically significant problem in adults vary with the nature of associated gastrointestinal disorders and the format of the individual studies.

The prevalence of lactose malabsorption in children is considered along with an evolving pattern of symptom production and shifting milk-drinking practices. The use of milk in federal programs targeted to young children seemed to be an important and reasonable nutritional practice, but symptomatic milk intolerance has been a problem in some older children and teenagers presenting with abdominal pain. Acquired lactose intolerance secondary to infectious gastroenteritis and malnutrition poses some important questions concerning proper feeding regimens for infants and children following acute intestinal insults.

The focus then shifts to the responses of milk biochemists, industry, and government in meeting the need for lactose-reduced or lactose-free products among consumers who wish to drink milk and milk-based products but are lactose intolerant. In this section, as throughout the volume, the nutritional implications of lactose intolerance for the clinician, the dairy industry, and the public health professional are considered. As a reference resource for the interested professional this volume contains citations to a majority of the scientific literature published on lactose digestion.

Despite recent advances in our understanding of lactose digestion, much remains to be learned. The Conference on Lactose Digestion, held at The Johns Hopkins University in December 1979 and sponsored by the Shadow Medical Research Foundation, brought together sixty investigators in an attempt to integrate current knowledge and to consider new directions of inquiry. The editors are grateful to the Shadow Medical Research Foundation, Dr. Irwin Sizer, Consultant in Resource Development, Professor Emeritus of Biochemistry, and Dean Emeritus of the Massachusetts Institute of Technology, and Mr. Harry Miller, foundation directors, for their efforts in organizing the conference and for their support in the publication of this volume. The foundation continues to support basic research, clinical applications, and education in the field of lactose intolerance in the hope that technological advances will lead to a resolution of the problem of lactose indigestion.

Progress to date, as documented in this volume, is only the threshold to the acquisition of greater knowledge in the field of lactose digestion. Armed with additional substantive information, decisions that affect the health and well-being of large population groups can be made more rationally.

Finally, the editors are grateful to The Johns Hopkins University Press and Mr. Anders Richter for their support and guidance in the preparation of this volume. We wish specifically to thank Ms. Judie Zubin for her invaluable editorial assistance, Mr. Daniel Hungerford and Ms. Lenora Davis for their dedicated research assistance, and Dr. E. David Mellits for his important contributions to our research effort.

We note with sorrow the death of our friend and colleague Robert H. Herman.

I

INTRODUCTION

CHAPTER 1

THE SIGNIFICANCE
OF LACTOSE INTOLERANCE
AN OVERVIEW

Norman Kretchmer

Milk is the major food of newborn mammals, but most human adults cannot digest it because they lack sufficient quantities of lactase, the enzyme that breaks down lactose, or milk sugar. Adults of all animal species other than man also lack the enzyme. The study of lactose malabsorption has encompassed an approach broader than the confines of medicine and biology, and has stimulated input from the areas of history, sociology, geography, and anthropology. The amazing new insights emanating from these social science disciplines are responsible for the development of a new perspective on lactose malabsorption. As a result of these studies, we have come to realize that the ability to digest lactose is a phenomenon peculiar to most northern European and white American ethnic groups, while the majority of human adults in the world are nondigesters of lactose. Consequently, in dealing with the topic of lactose digestion, it seems reasonable to shift the emphasis from clinical intolerance to tolerance, i.e., to focus on the ability to digest lactose rather than on the much more usual phenomenon encountered in all mammals—an inability to digest lactose, along with its accompanying symptomatology, after early childhood.

To trace the developments leading to the shift in emphasis from intolerance to tolerance, an historical approach will be utilized. Intolerance to milk was described first by the early pediatricians Czerny, Finkelstein, and Jacobi (1901), who emphasized an association between infantile diarrhea and carbohydrate in-

3

gestion. At the turn of the century, these findings, along with problems of diarrhea encountered by veterinarians, stimulated the great biochemist Lafayette B. Mendel to study lactose digestion. His efforts culminated with the publication in the *American Journal of Physiology* of a series of nine papers concerned with the biochemistry of development. The section on lactase described lactase activity in the calf as elevated during the neonatal period and greatly diminished in the adult (Mendel 1907). Studies on a number of mammals, including the rat, rabbit, mouse, cat, dog, guinea pig, and the human, have confirmed Mendel's concept and have shown that the general shape of the developmental curve for intestinal lactase activity is similar in most mammals. Maximal activity is observed in the perinatal period followed by a decrease in activity, with the lowest values reached after weaning. The only difference in pattern among the mammals studied was the time at which lactase activity reached a maximum; this seems to depend on the state of maturity of the species studied at the time of birth (Johnson et al. 1974).

The decrease in intestinal lactase activity at the time of weaning in most mammals occurs almost simultaneously with diminished lactose ingestion. This observation has stimulated speculation regarding the possibility that lactase activity is adaptively regulated by the concentration of dietary lactose (Johnson et al. 1974), i.e., persistence of lactase can be induced by continuation of milk in the diet after weaning. But earlier, investigation of this hypothesis using rabbits and rats had led Plimmer (1906–07) to conclude that adaptation of lactase activity to the presence of lactose in the diet does not occur. In spite of these elegant experiments, the controversy regarding the "adaptability" of intestinal lactase continues to this day.

In his presidential address to the American Pediatric Society in 1921, John Howland postulated that milk intolerance encountered in infants and children often is due to some deficit in the "ferments" (enzymes) necessary for the hydrolysis of lactose (Howland 1921). For almost forty years thereafter, the investigation of lactose intolerance went into obscurity until the publication of Durand's (1958) and Holzel's (1959) classic papers, describing case studies of lactose intolerance in children. These publications were significant because they reawakened interest in a problem of which pediatricians had been aware for a long time. Time and effort still are devoted to this problem in order to assess whether or not lactose malabsorption produces clinical symptoms.

Since Mendel's description of the developmental aspects of the enzyme lactase in the early 1900s (Mendel 1907), there have been numerous studies. There still remain unanswered some very critical questions. Of paramount importance is the following: what factors are responsible for the appearance and disappearance of lactase activity? These changes are obviously genetically controlled; however, they may be stimulated by environmental factors, hormones, or substrates produced via other pathways. Further elucidation of the factors responsible for the appearance and disappearance of lactase activity would serve as a major contribution to the field of developmental biology, where studies of such phenomena (what turns a molecule "on" and "off") are common investigative foci. In addition, the changes in activity during development observed with lactase also are encountered with the intestinal peptidases; hence, the knowledge reaped from studies of lactase could be extrapolated to other systems.

It is only within the past 10,000 years that milk has served as a dietary constituent beyond infancy and into adulthood. In those societies in which breast feeding is the established mode of infant nutrition, the lactose in milk serves as the major source of carbohydrate in the diet until approximately age two. In the Western world, milk is a major dietary constituent throughout life; in many other parts of the world, milk never is utilized as a foodstuff once weaning has been completed (Johnson et al. 1974). These socioeconomic and cultural factors (dairying versus nondairying), along with heredity, are related to the incidence of tolerance versus intolerance of lactose.

In contrast to congenital intolerance, secondary intolerance is that form accompanying numerous intestinal disorders and other disease states. The rapid disappearance of lactase in secondary intolerance and its slow reappearance, even after severe diarrhea, have raised the question of how this enzyme is topographically situated on the brush border of the epithelial cells of the small intestine. We now have a reasonable conception of how sucrase is positioned on the membrane. Recent studies have shown that sucrase exists in an enzymatically inactive form in the crypt cells of the human intestine and is converted to an enzymatically active form as the crypt cells migrate to the villus (Johnson et al. 1974). Perhaps this possibility or some variation of it should be considered in evaluating how lactase is stationed on the membrane. This information would provide a valuable contribution in the field of membrane biology.

The most fascinating findings emanating from lactose studies are in the field of comparative biology, where exceptions to the general developmental pattern of lactase activity have been found. The usual developmental pattern of lactase can be described by a curve with maximal activity in the perinatal period, followed by a decrease in activity, with the lowest values at the time of weaning. Exceptions to this pattern are the California sea lion and other Pacific pinnipeds, which have no lactose in their milk and no lactase activity in the small intestine, even in the newborn period. When fed lactose, these animals develop severe fermentative diarrhea (Johnson et al. 1974).

The work on the Pinnipedia of both the Atlantic and Pacific basins has contributed information that has been instrumental in expanding knowledge of the taxonomy of these organisms. The animals of the Pacific and of the Atlantic probably represent two different phyla; the animals of the Pacific apparently are derived from an ancient type of bear, whereas the seals, sea lions, and walruses in the Atlantic presumably are derived from a land otter.

Based on the erroneous assumption that elevated lactase activity in the adult intestine is normal in humans, man also was considered an exception to the developmental pattern of lactase until the studies of Cuatrecasas et al. (1965) and Bayless and Rosensweig (1966) recognized the existence of striking ethnic or racial differences in the incidence of primary adult lactose malabsorption. In the next few years, it was revealed that such differences occur in other countries. These observations led to Simoons's "geographic" or "culture-historical" hypothesis (Simoons 1970). It is likely, he argued, that some human groups developed low prevalences of lactose malabsorption because of selective pressures over a long historical period that favored the adult lactose absorber under particular ecological conditions, e.g., living in a dairy-oriented culture.

Superimposed upon the culture-historical hypothesis, the principles of genetics and evolution help to explain the emergence of the aberrant phenomenon of lactose tolerance. Darwin and other evolutionists before him have referred to food as a major factor in selective pressures. The lactose story is most effective in illustrating how a certain food, by indirectly favoring the survival of those able to digest that substance, can influence the evolutionary processes of man.

Given that the ability to digest lactose results from a mutation responsible for the production of intestinal lactase in the adult, it is reasonable to assume that the increased activity in human adult lactose digesters is evidence of a mutation that has persisted as a result of some selective advantage. This selection process probably was initiated about 10,000 years ago with the inception of dairying, according to Cavalli-Sforza (1973). The selective advantage would be exercised in an environment characterized by the consumption of large amounts of milk and milk products in lactose-rich forms. In such a dairying culture, lactose absorbers would enjoy greater health and vigor, multiply better, and fare more successfully in general. Along with "survival of the fittest," there would be perpetuation of the "fittest," for lactose digesters transmit their tolerance as a dominant characteristic. Persistence of this genetic mutation in an environment where milk is prevalent and highly utilized provides an explanation for the emergence of that abnormal group that can tolerate lactose (Johnson et al. 1974).

It is difficult to find another cogent illustration in the biology of foods that has had such an impact on human development. Celiac disease may be another example, but its investigation is complicated by the inability, at present, to isolate the genetics of wheat and barley from the genetics of man.

Aside from the fascinating areas of study discussed above, some practical considerations deserve attention as well: the question of policy regarding milk use. Lactose digestion has an important influence in the development of a suitable policy regarding the use of milk and dairy products by the lactose malabsorber and by ethnic or racial groups, in the United States and abroad, among whom high rates of malabsorption prevail. Milk has tremendous economic, nutritional, and emotional significance in Western culture, a culture strongly committed to the concept that milk is an ideal food. Any attempts to regulate its distribution or the advertising claims of the industry are bound to be met with strong resistance, as was shown in the case of the Federal Trade Commission versus the California Milk Producers Advisory Board. This case exemplifies the confusion involved in the question of lactose tolerance versus intolerance. When the case was brought to court, the judge decided that lactose intolerance was not sufficiently significant to place a ban on the California milk producers' advertising campaign, advocating "Everybody needs milk." The judge decided that there was insufficient evidence to indicate that lactose intolerance was a significant clinical threat to the health of individuals (*Federal Trade Commission* v. *California Milk Producers Advisory Board*).

So, in a legal sense, lactose intolerance was not deemed significant. However, lactose intolerance is a normal physiological condition, shared by every adult animal except for certain ethnic and racial groups in man, most of whom are located in the United States or in northern parts of Western Europe. It is lactose tolerance rather than lactose intolerance, as initially assumed, that is most significant. The ability to digest lactose is the abnormal state, while lactose intolerance is the usual, normal condition in the human adult world population. This concept ensues from the multidisciplinary approach to the lactose/lactase problem. The approach has resulted in enormous contributions to the disciplines of history, anthropology, comparative biology, membrane biology, geography, evolution, genetics, nutrition, medicine, and development.

REFERENCES

Bayless TM, Rosensweig NS: A racial difference in the incidence of lactase deficiency: A survey of milk tolerance and lactase deficiency in healthy males. *JAMA* 197:968-72, 1966.

Cavalli-Sforza LL: Analytic review: Some current problems of human population genetics. *Am J Hum Genet* 25:82-104, 1973.

Cuatrecasas P, Lockwood DH, Caldwell JR: Lactase deficiency in the adult. *Lancet* 1:14-18, 1965.

Durand P: Lactosuria idiopathica in una paziente cond diarrea cronica et acidosi. *Minerva Pediatr* 10:706-11, 1958.

Federal Trade Commission v. California Milk Producers Advisory Board, Federal Trade Commission 8988, Commission Order dated 21 September 1979.

Holzel A, Schwartz V, Sutcliffe KW: Defective lactose absorption causing malnutrition in infancy. *Lancet* 1:1126-28, 1959.

Howland J: Prolonged intolerance of carbohydrates. *Trans Am Pediatr Soc* 33:11-19, 1921.

Jacobi A: Milk-sugar in infant feeding. *Trans Am Pediatr Soc* 13:150-60, 1901.

Johnson JD, Kretchmer N, Simoons FJ: Lactose malabsorption: Its biology and history. In *Advances in Pediatrics,* vol. 21, I Schulman (ed). Chicago: Yearbook Medical Publishers, 1974, pp 197-237.

Mendel LB, Mitchell PH: Chemical studies on growth: I. The inverting enzymes of the alimentary tract, especially in the embryo. *Am J Physiol* 20:81-96, 1907.

Plimmer RHA: On the presence of lactase in the intestine of animals and on the adaptation of the intestine to lactose. *J Physiol* (Lond) 35:20-31, 1906-07.

Simoons FJ: Primary adult lactose intolerance and the milking habit: A problem in biological and cultural interrelations: II. A culture historical hypothesis. *Am J Dig Dis* 15:695-710, 1970.

II

GENETIC, GEOGRAPHIC, AND HISTORIC
CONSIDERATIONS

CHAPTER 2

THE REGIONAL AND ETHNIC
DISTRIBUTION OF LACTOSE MALABSORPTION
ADAPTIVE AND GENETIC HYPOTHESES

John D. Johnson

It has been known since the work of Lafayette B. Mendel in 1907 that lactase is present in the intestine of the infant mammal, but that its activity is greatly diminished in the adult (Mendel and Mitchell 1907). Since that time more detailed analyses of the developmental pattern of lactase activity have been made. Figure 2.1 shows intestinal lactase in the rat during development. Lactase activity appears late in gestation, reaches a peak at 2 to 3 days following birth, remains high until weaning begins at about 14 days, then falls rapidly to the low level of activity characteristic of the adult animal by 21 days of age, the time of complete weaning. Similar patterns of activity are seen in the pig, calf, rabbit, cat, and dog (table 2.1).

DEVELOPMENTAL PATTERN OF INTESTINAL LACTASE
ACTIVITY IN HUMANS

Original studies of lactase in human small intestine in the early 1960s indicated that high activity persisted into adulthood, suggesting that man was an exception to this general developmental pattern. More recent studies have shown that high lactase activity persists into adulthood only in a minority of human ethnic groups (and perhaps in some species of nonhuman primates). Two of the original reports of low lactase activity in adults came from studies in Baltimore and showed a

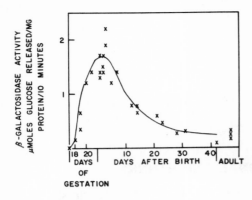

FIGURE 2.1. β-galactosidase activity (substrate lactose, pH 5.0) in homogenates from the intestine of the developing rat. Source: Doell and Kretchmer 1962, reprinted with permission.

significantly higher prevalence of lactose absorbers in white American adults than in American blacks (Cuatrecasas et al. 1965, Bayless and Rosensweig 1966). Working in Uganda, Cook and Kajubi (1966) reported that most African adults had low intestinal lactase activity, whereas those with an Hamitic ancestry had high lactase activity.

Subsequently, numerous studies of lactose absorption and malabsorption have been performed in many different ethnic groups. Table 2.2 indicates that the world's peoples among whom lactose malabsorption is common as adults—most Africans and Asians as well as Arabs, Jews, and the Eskimos and Indians from North and South America—far outnumber the groups among whom lactose absorption is found with high frequency in adults (e.g., most northern Europeans, and a few isolated tribes from Africa and India).

Thus, the developmental pattern of lactase activity in the intestine is, for most humans, like that in other mammals. Auricchio et al. (1965) and others subsequently have shown that although lactase is detectable as early as the third month of gestation in the human, it continues to increase throughout gestation, reaching a maximum only at term.

Antonowicz and Lebenthal (1977) found that human fetuses at 26 to 34 weeks gestation have lactase activity only 30% of that present in full-term infants,

TABLE 2.1
Lactase activity of the intestine in relation to the suckling phase of growth

Phase	Units of activity per gram of material						
	Rat	Pig	Calf	Rabbit	Guinea Pig	Cat	Dog
At birth	18.0	18.0	50.0	14.0	5.0	4.0	6.0
At end of suckling period	2.0	2.0	11.0	5.0	4.0	—	—
Adult	2.0	~1.0	~0.2	0.3	4.0	0.5	0.7

Source: Adapted from Blaxter 1961.

TABLE 2.2

Differences in lactose malabsorption among the world's peoples (adults)

I. Groups among whom malabsorption predominates (60% to 100% malabsorbers)
   A. Near East and Mediterranean: Arabs, Jews, Greek Cypriots, southern Italians
   B. Asia: Thais, Indonesians, Chinese, Koreans
   C. Africa: South Nigerian peoples, Hausa, Bantu
   D. North and South America: Eskimos, Canadian and U.S. Indians, Chami Indians
II. Groups among whom absorption predominates (2% to 30% malabsorbers)
   A. Europe: Danes, Finns, Germans, French, Dutch, Poles, Czechs, North Italians
   B. Africa: Hima, Tussi, Nomadic Fulani
   C. India: Punjab and New Delhi areas

Source: Adapted from Johnson et al. 1974.

whereas the other disaccharidases, sucrase and maltase, reach 70% of term activity during this same gestational period. Subsequently, in those populations in which lactose malabsorption is characteristic of the adult, lactase activity, as reflected by the results of lactose loading tests, declines during infancy and childhood so that lactose malabsorption is seen in the majority of individuals from 2 to 5 years of age in certain populations, such as the Pima Indians (fig. 2.2). In other populations, such as American blacks and Finns, the proportion of lactose malabsorption increases into the teenage years.

Lactose absorption in adults, therefore, is an *unusual* situation that deserves attention and explanation. Two major hypotheses have been put forward to explain the regional and ethnic distribution of lactose absorption and malabsorption in adults. Based on the observation that lactase activity decreases at the time of weaning in most mammals, Bolin, Davis, and co-workers from Australia have advocated the hypothesis that lactase activity is regulated adaptively by the concentration of lactose in the diet (Bolin et al. 1971, Bolin and Davis 1972). According to this thesis, group differences in malabsorption derive from con-

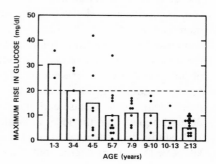

FIGURE 2.2. Results of lactose-loading tests in various age groups of full-blooded Pima Indians. Chart shows maximum elevation of blood glucose above fasting levels (bars represent means). Source: Johnson et al. 1977, reprinted with permission.

trasts in the consumption of milk and milk products after weaning. Should the individual at weaning continue to consume such products, lactose would induce lactase activity and this would continue at the high level typical of infancy. The other major hypothesis is that lactose absorption and malabsorption in adults is genetically determined.

It is of historical interest that the two early papers from Johns Hopkins describing the high incidence of lactose malabsorption among American blacks took different sides of this argument. Cuatrecasas and co-workers (1965) were struck by the correlation of lactose malabsorption and dietary milk deprivation, and of loss of symptoms with prolonged lactose intake. They suggested that lactase may be an adaptive enzyme, but did not rule out a genetic polymorphism. On the other hand, Bayless and Rosensweig (1966) stated that the marked racial differences in incidence of lactase deficiency strongly suggest that the level of the enzyme is genetically controlled. Evidence for and against the induction or adaptive hypothesis is considered below.

INDUCTION OR ADAPTIVE HYPOTHESIS

Experimental Animal Studies. In 1906, Plimmer presented experimental results in rats and rabbits suggesting that lactase activity does *not* adapt to the presence of lactose in the diet (Plimmer 1906–07). Heilskov (1951) showed that feeding rabbits a diet rich in lactose from birth until 15 weeks of age did not influence the normal postnatal decline in intestinal lactase activity. Similar results, with slight modifications in experimental design, have continued to appear in the more recent literature.

Elegant experiments by Ferguson and collaborators have shown that changes in lactase activity in mice during development are intrinsically determined (Ferguson et al. 1973). These workers implanted isografts of fetal mouse intestine into adult mice and found that lactase activity in the isografts—which were *never* exposed to food—followed a pattern identical to that seen in the intestine of developing animals.

In contrast to these studies, several investigators have reported increased lactase activity in adult rats after 5 to 10 weeks of very high lactose intake (Girardet et al. 1964, Cain et al. 1969, Bolin et al. 1969, Bolin et al. 1971). Although the increases in activity were statistically significant in these studies, the high concentration of lactose fed in some studies was unphysiologic and the magnitude of the increases was small compared to the profound changes in lactase activity that occur around the time of weaning. Thus, a 100% increase in lactase activity after lactose feeding may be statistically significant, but may have little meaning nutritionally if the lactase activity of the newborn of the same species is 10- to 30-fold higher than the level in adult animals.

A study by Lebenthal et al. (1973) illustrates that lactase activity may be adaptive to a minor degree, but that this adaptation is quantitatively small when compared to normal developmental changes in enzyme activity. In this study, rat pups were nursed beyond the usual time of weaning and compared to controls. Prolonged nursing did not prevent the usual decline in lactase observed during development, but did result in slightly higher specific activity of the enzyme between 18 and 26 days of age. On the basis of other experiments, these authors suggested that the presence of lactose may, by a process of substrate stabilization, protect the enzyme from degradation.

There are also some hormonal influences on lactase activity. Thyroid hormone appears to be necessary for the normal postnatal decline in intestinal lactase activity, but its mechanism of action has not been elucidated. Yeh and Moog (1974) have shown that lactase does not decline in rats hypophysectomized at 6 days of age, and that treatment with thyroxine lowers activity to control levels at 24 days.

Human Studies.   No studies in man have demonstrated lactase "adaptability" clearly. Removal of lactose from the diet for 2 months does not decrease lactase activity in adults (Knudsen et al. 1968). Cautrecasas and co-workers (1965) fed seven subjects with low intestinal lactase activity 150 g lactose daily for up to 45 days without any changes in jejunal lactase activity. Nigerian medical students were fed up to 50 g lactose daily for 6 months but remained unable to digest lactose with lactose loading tests (Kretchmer 1971). Gilat et al. (1972) in Israel fed more than 1 liter of milk per day for 6 to 14 months to 10 adults with low intestinal lactase activity, but found no change in jejunal lactase activity. Finally, almost all Thai children develop lactose malabsorption by age 4 years even if nursing is prolonged or regular milk consumption continues following weaning (Keusch et al. 1969). In summary, evidence for *major* adaptive changes in intestinal lactase activity, particularly in man, is not available.

THE GENETIC HYPOTHESIS

Two lines of evidence support the genetic hypothesis: the prevalences of lactose absorption/malabsorption in racially mixed populations, and direct evidence from family studies in diverse ethnic groups. These are discussed separately below.

Racially Mixed Populations.   If lactose absorption/malabsorption is determined genetically, the distribution of absorbers and malabsorbers among the offspring of parents belonging to populations with markedly differing prevalences of lactose absorption and malabsorption may test the genetic hypothesis. There are now many such studies. Bayless and co-workers (1969) proposed that intestinal lactase deficiency was inherited as an autosomal recessive trait based on their observation that 70% of the American black population were lactose malabsorbers, and 8% of American whites were lactose malabsorbers. Assuming that the population of coastal West Africa, from which American blacks were derived, was 100% malabsorbers and that American blacks had a 30% Western European gene admixture, the observed incidence of lactose malabsorbers in the American black population fit well with the expectation.

Kretchmer, Ransome-Kuti, and co-investigators (1971) reported that the Yoruba and Ibo tribes of coastal Nigeria, from which many American blacks originally derived, in fact did consist of almost 100% malabsorbers, fulfilling one of Bayless's assumptions. Subsequently Ransome-Kuti et al. (1975) reported that almost 60% of individuals of Yoruba-European mixture were lactose absorbers.

Studies of American Indians reveal similar results. Newcomer and others (1977) have studied lactose absorption in the Chippewa Indians in Minnesota and found that the greater the percentage of Indian blood the higher the percentage of lactose malabsorbers. In subjects with less than 50% Indian blood, 33% were lactose malabsorbers, whereas in those with greater than 84% Indian blood, 97% were malabsorbers. In studies of lactose absorption among southwestern Indian tribes around Phoenix, Arizona, lactose malabsorption was found in 92% of full-blooded Indians representing 15 different tribes (mostly Apache, Hopi, Pima, and Papago), but among Indians with known European grandparents or great-grandparents lactose malabsorption was present in only 50% (Johnson et al. 1978). In a more detailed study of the Pima tribe, 95% of full-blooded persons over 4 years of age were lactose malabsorbers, compared to 76% of those who were 1/8 Anglo and 39% of those who were 1/4 or 1/2 Anglo (table 2.3).

In all such studies to date, lower prevalences of lactose malabsorption have been found in mixed persons than in full-blooded persons from native groups characterized by a high prevalence of lactose malabsorption.

Family Studies. More direct evidence for the genetic hypothesis is provided by family studies examining the segregation of lactose absorbers and malabsorbers. Although isolated individual family pedigrees were reported beginning in the late 1960s, reports of large numbers of families have appeared only in the recent

TABLE 2.3
Lactose absorption/malabsorption correlated with degree of Indian blood

Indian blood	No. of absorbers	No. of malabsorbers	Percentage malabsorbers
Full-blooded Indians	3	59	95
Mixed Anglo-Indian			
1/16 Anglo	0	2	100
1/8 Anglo	5	16	76
1/4 or 1/2 Anglo	11	7	39
Total mixed	16	25	61

Source: Johnson et al. 1977, reprinted with permission.

literature. Sahi et al. (1973) reported a large family study from Finland. From a population survey, they selected 11 probands with lactose malabsorption and studied most of the descendents of the grandparents of these probands. Formal genetic analysis of the sibships in which at least one sibling had lactose malabsorption was consistent with inheritance of lactose malabsorption as an autosomal recessive trait. Furthermore, using the assumptions that penetrance of lactose malabsorption is complete and is controlled by a single recessive autosomal gene, they could calculate the frequency of the lactose malabsorption gene in their community and, with this gene frequency, calculate expected lactose malabsorption frequencies among different relatives of the probands. The calculated and observed frequencies for various relatives were quite close.

Ransome-Kuti et al. (1975) studied families in which progeny emanated from marriages between proper Yoruba from Nigeria and northern Europeans (fig. 2.3). When both parents were lactose malabsorbers, all the progeny were lactose malabsorbers. However, in matings between lactose absorbers and lactose malabsorbers, both types of progeny were found.

Similar results were found in a family study of Pima Indians on the Gila River Reservation (Johnson et al. 1977). Figure 2.4 shows pedigrees from five families in this study. As with the Nigerian study, when one parent was a lactose absorber and the other a lactose malabsorber, progeny of both types were found with equal frequency. When both parents were lactose malabsorbers, 49 of the 51 progeny from 13 such families were lactose malabsorbers, as determined by the lactose loading test. When one parent was a malabsorber and the other an absorber, half the 18 progeny from 4 families were absorbers and half malabsorbers. In one family in which both parents were lactose absorbers, both types of progeny were observed.

These data are consistent with the hypothesis that lactose absorption, the uncommon trait or phenotype on a world-wide basis, is inherited as a completely

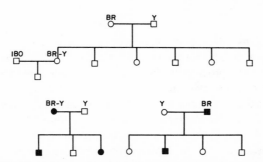

FIGURE 2.3. Pedigrees of three families in Lagos, Nigeria. □ and ○ indicate male and female lactose malabsorbers, ■ and ● indicate individuals who are lactose absorbers. Yoruba (Y), British (BR), Ibo or first-generation crosses of these ethnic groups (e. g., BR-Y) are indicated in the figure. Adapted from Ransome-Kuti et al. 1975, reprinted with permission.

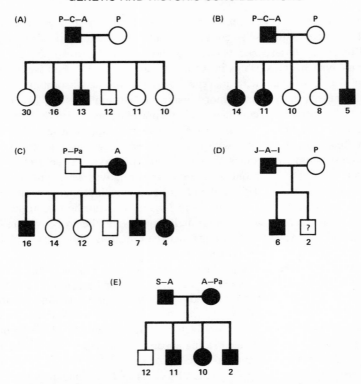

FIGURE 2.4. Pedigrees of five families on the Gila River Reservation. □
and ○, male and female lactose malabsorbers; ■ and ●, subjects who are
lactose absorbers. Number beneath offspring symbol gives subject's age;
letters above parent symbol give ethnic background, in order of greatest
genetic contribution: P, Pima; Pa, Papago; C, Crow; A, Anglo; J, German-
Jewish; I, Indian, unknown tribe; S, Sioux. Source: Johnson et al. 1977,
reprinted with permission.

penetrant autosomal dominant characteristic. Table 2.4 summarizes family
studies of lactose malabsorption published up to 1977, and compares the expected frequencies of progeny to those observed, assuming that lactose absorption is a completely penetrant dominant characteristic. The expected values are
based on the further assumption that all lactose absorbers in these studies are
heterozygotes. While this clearly is not the case, the groups from which the data
are derived for the most part have a high prevalence of lactose malabsorption so
that the gene frequency for lactose absorption will be low and the incidence of
homozygotes for lactose absorption low.

The observed values are quite close to those expected for this mode of inheritance. The major discrepancy consists of the 12 progeny from a total of 220
(5.5%) who were classified as lactose absorbers and both of whose parents were

TABLE 2.4
Summary of family studies of inheritance of lactose malabsorption (LM)

Matings	No. of families	No. of progeny	Progeny with LM	Observed proportion of LM	Expected proportion of LM‡
1a* × 1a	10	31	8	0.26	0.25
1a × 1m⁺	60	196	101	0.515	0.50
1m × 1m	76	220	208	0.945	1.00

Source: Johnson et al. 1977, reprinted with permission.
*1a = lactose absorber.
†1m = lactose malabsorber.
‡Expected proportions of LM are the theoretical Mendelian proportions assuming lactose absorption is inherited as a completely penetrant autosomal dominant trait with all lactose absorbers in these studies assumed to be heterozygotes.

classified as lactose malabsorbers (there should be none). Three of these could be persons with slight delays in onset of lactose malabsorption, for example, one was a 5-year-old lactose absorber from the study in Pima Indians. Potential reasons for misclassification of the other nine subjects include falsely high glucose values following the lactose loading test, a phenomenon encountered in 7% of subjects with lactase deficiency in one study (Welsh 1970); progeny of a union in which one parent has secondary or acquired lactose malabsorption, who otherwise would be a primary absorber; and nonpaternity. These discrepancies are not of enough magnitude to discount the proposed mode of inheritance. It is also noteworthy that the accumulated family pedigree studies are derived from several different ethnic groups, including West Africans, Mexican Americans, Israeli Jews, and American Indians and that each individual study, as well as the combined results, generally support this mode of inheritance.

If one accepts this genetic hypothesis, several additional questions arise. For example, what selective advantage(s) have existed to favor the perpetuation of the lactose absorber and has there been enough time since the proposed mutation for the differences in the prevalence of lactose malabsorption which currently exist to have evolved? Simoons addresses these questions in chapter 3. Another unanswered question relates to the molecular nature of the mutation that has resulted in persistence of higher lactase levels in some groups of adults.

One possibility is that a molecular structural difference exists between intestinal lactases from absorbers versus malabsorbers. However, Asp et al. (1971) and Lebenthal et al. (1974) showed that residual lactase in lactose malabsorbers has the same chromatographic characteristics, kinetic properties, and pH dependency as the enzyme from adults with high activity. Freiburghaus and co-workers (1976) subjected solubilized intestinal brush border proteins to gel electrophoresis and identified a protein fraction with lactase activity and electrophetic mobility both in adults with lactose malabsorption and in infants with congenital lactase deficiency which was identical to that of lactase from adults with high lactase activity. Although this is a powerful tool for the separation of proteins and enzymes, a discrete alteration in the structure of lactase might not change the size or charge characteristics of the protein, so that this question is not totally settled.

A second and attractive possibility is that a mutation in a regulatory gene might explain the persistence of high lactase activity in lactose absorbers, with incomplete repression of lactase synthesis in adult lactose absorbers. This mechanism might be analogous to the switch-off in production of hemoglobin gamma chains during the first year of life. Before a final genetic mechanism can be established, intestinal lactase must be isolated in pure form and further characterized.

SUMMARY

Intestinal lactase activity is normally high during the suckling period in nonhuman mammalians, then decreases to low levels following weaning. Although original studies in human adults of northern European origin suggested that homo sapiens was an exception to this pattern of mammalian development, subsequent work has shown that most groups of human adults have low intestinal lactase activity and, in fact, do conform to the usual mammalian ontogenetic pattern.

Two major hypotheses have been advanced to explain the regional and ethnic distribution of lactose malabsorption in adults that have been observed: (1) the adaptive or induction hypothesis, which postulates that lactase activity is regulated by the concentration of lactose in the diet; and (2) the genetic hypothesis, which postulates that the level of intestinal lactase activity in the postweanling human is a heritable characteristic. Little evidence supports the adaptive hypothesis, especially in man; the genetic hypothesis has gained support by several recent studies of the prevalences of lactose absorption/malabsorption in racially mixed populations, and, more directly, from family pedigrees in diverse ethnic groups, including Finns, West Africans, and American Indians.

The family studies suggest that lactose absorption in the human adult, the unusual "phenotype" on a world-wide basis, is inherited as a completely penetrant autosomal dominant characteristic. Adaptive regulation of lactase activity may occur to a small degree, at least in animals, but only over a relatively narrow, genetically determined range.

REFERENCES

Antonowicz I, Lebenthal E: Developmental pattern of small intestinal enterokinase and disaccharidase activities in the human fetus. *Gastoenterology* 72:1299–1303, 1977.

Asp NG, Berg NO, Dahlqvist A, Jussila J, Salmi H: The activity of three different small intestinal β-galactosidases in adults with and without lactase deficiency. *Scand J Gastroenterol* 6:755–62, 1971.

Aurricchio S, Rubino A, Mürset G: Intestinal glycosidase activities in the human embryo, fetus, and newborn. *Pediatrics* 35:944–54, 1965.

Bayless TM, Christopher NL, Boyer SH: Autosomal recessive inheritance of intestinal lactase deficiency: Evidence from ethnic differences. *J Clin Invest* 48:6a, 1969.

Bayless TM, Rosensweig NS: A racial difference in the incidence of lactase deficiency: A survey of milk tolerance and lactase deficiency in healthy males. *JAMA* 197:968-72, 1966.

Blaxter KL: Lactation and the growth of the young. In *Milk: The Mammary Gland and Its Secretion*, vol. 2, SK Kow, AT Cowie (eds). New York: Academic Press, 1961, p 329.

Bolin TD, Davis AE: Primary lactase deficiency: Genetic or acquired? *Gastroenterology* 62:355-56, 1972.

Bolin TD, McKern A, Davis AE: The effect of diet on lactase activity in the rat. *Gastroenterology* 60:432-37, 1971.

Bolin TD, Pirola RC, Davis AE: Adaptation of intestinal lactase in the rat. *Gastroenterology* 57:406-09, 1969.

Cain GD, Moore P, Patterson M, McElveen MA: The stimulation of lactase by feeding lactose. *Scand J Gastroenterol* 4:545-50, 1969.

Cook GC, Kajubi SK: Tribal incidence of lactase deficiency in Uganda. *Lancet* 1:725-30, 1966.

Cuatrecasas P, Lockwood DH, Caldwell JR: Lactase deficiency in the adult. *Lancet* 1:14-18, 1965.

Doell RG, Kretchmer N: Studies of small intestine during development: I. Distribution and activity of β-galactosidase. *Biochim Biophys Acta* 62:353-62, 1962.

Ferguson A, Gerskowitch VP, Russell RI: Pre- and postweanling disaccharidase patterns in isografts of fetal mouse intestine. *Gastroenterology* 64:294-97, 1973.

Freiburghaus AU, Schmitz J, Schindler M, Rotthauwe HW, Kuitunen P, Launiala K. Hadorn B: Protein patterns of brush-border fragments in congenital lactose malabsorption and in specific hypolactasia of the adult. *N Engl J Med* 294:1030-32, 1976.

Gilat T, Russo S, Gelman-Malachi E, Aldor TAM: Lactase in man: A nonadaptable enzyme. *Gastroenterology* 62:1125-27, 1972.

Girardet P, Richterich R, Antener I: Adaptation de la lactase intestinale á l'administration de lactose chez le rat adulte. *Helv Physiol Pharmacol Acta* 22:7-14, 1964.

Heilskov NSC: Studies on animal lactase: II. Distribution in some of the glands of the digestive tract. *Acta Physiol Scand* 24:84-89, 1951.

Johnson JD, Kretchmer N, Simoons FJ: Lactose malabsorption: Its biology and history. In *Advances in Pediatrics*, vol. 21, I Schulman (ed). Chicago: Yearbook Medical Publishers, 1974, pp 197-237.

Johnson JD, Simoons FJ, Hurwitz R, Grange A, Mitchell CH, Sinatra FR, Sunshine P, Robertson WV, Bennett PH, Kretchmer N: Lactose malabsorption among the Pima Indians of Arizona. *Gastroenterology* 73:1299-1304, 1977.

Johnson JD, Simoons FJ, Hurwitz R, Grange A, Sinatra FR, Sunshine P, Robertson WV, Bennett, PH, Kretchmer N: Lactose malabsorption among adult Indians of the Great Basin and American Southwest. *Am J Clin Nutr* 31:381-87, 1978.

Keusch GT, Troncale FJ, Miller LH, Promadhat V, Anderson PR: Acquired lactose malabsorption in Thai children. *Pediatrics* 43:540-45, 1969.

Knudsen KB, Welsh JD, Kronenberg RS, Vanderveen JE, Heidelbaugh ND: Effect of a nonlactose diet on human intestinal disaccharidase activity. *Am J Dig Dis* 13:593-97, 1968.

Kretchmer N: Memorial lecture: Lactose and lactase—a historical perspective. *Gastroenterology* 61:805-13, 1971.

Kretchmer N, Ransome-Kuti O, Hurwitz R, Dungy C, Alakija W: Intestinal absorption of lactose in Nigerian ethnic groups. *Lancet* 2:392-95, 1971.

Lebenthal E, Sunshine P, Kretchmer N: Effect of prolonged nursing on the activity of intestinal lactase in rats. *Gastroenterology* 64:1136-41, 1973.

Lebenthal E, Tsuboi K, Kretchmer N: Characterization of human intestinal lactase and hetero-β-galactosidases of infants and adults. *Gastroenterology* 67:1107-13, 1974.

Mendel LB, Mitchell PH: Chemical studies on growth: I. The inverting enzymes of the alimentary tract, especially in the embryo. *Am J Physiol* 20:81-96, 1907.

Newcomer AD, Thomas PJ, McGill DB, Hofmann AF: Lactase deficiency: A common genetic trait of the American Indian. *Gastroenterology* 72:234–37, 1977.

Plimmer RHA: On the presence of lactase in the intestine of animals and on the adaptation of the intestine to lactose. *J Physiol* (Lond) 35:20–31, 1906–07.

Ransome-Kuti O, Kretchmer N, Johnson JD, Gribble JT: A genetic study of lactose digestion in Nigerian families. *Gastroenterology* 68:431–36, 1975.

Sahi T, Isokoski M, Jussila J, Launiala K, Pyörälä K: Recessive inheritance of adult-type lactose malabsorption. *Lancet* 2:823–26, 1973.

Welsh JD: Isolated lactase deficiency in humans: Report on 100 patients. *Medicine* (Baltimore) 49:257–77, 1970.

Yeh K, Moog F: Intestinal lactase activity in the suckling rat: Influence of hypophysectomy and thyroidectomy. *Science* 182:77–79, 1974.

CHAPTER 3

GEOGRAPHIC PATTERNS OF
PRIMARY ADULT LACTOSE MALABSORPTION
A FURTHER INTERPRETATION OF EVIDENCE
FOR THE OLD WORLD

Frederick J. Simoons

In this chapter is presented the geographic evidence, old and new, mainly from Eurasia and Africa, as it bears on the culture-historical hypothesis I first advanced in 1969 and 1970 to explain ethnic and racial differences in prevalence of primary adult lactose malabsorption (hereafter "primary adult lactose malabsorption" is referred to as "lactose malabsorption") around the world. The concentration here is on the evidence for Eurasia and Africa, the Old World, because that region is so critical in the early history of milk use and dairying, and because evidence for the New World (Simoons 1978) continues to fit the hypothesis quite well.

It was medical research in the mid- and late 1960s, much of it done at The Johns Hopkins Medical School, that first brought on an awareness that striking ethnic and racial differences exist in prevalence of lactose malabsorption among normal, healthy adults. Dr. John Johnson (chapter 2) convincingly demonstrates that those ethnic or racial differences in lactose malabsorption have a genetic basis. As a geographer long interested in the history of dairying, I was led quite early to the further question of whether the group differences in question were related to the history of milk use.

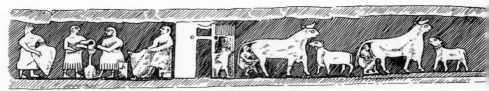

FIGURE 3.1. Milking scene from Al'Ubaid, Mesopotamia (after H. R. Hall and C. Leonard Woolley). Source: Simoons 1971, reprinted with the permission of the American Geographical Society.

THE CULTURE-HISTORICAL PERSPECTIVE

One should recognize that in the hunting and gathering stage, which prevailed among all human groups until very recent times in human evolution, there were no domesticated herd animals to be milked. The first herd animal kept by humans, sheep, seems to have been domesticated about 9000 B.C. Yet in the initial period following domestication, though herd animals were used for meat and perhaps certain other purposes, they seem not to have been milked. Earliest convincing evidence (figs. 3.1 to 3.3) that humans milked domesticated animals dates to about 4000–3000 B.C., in northern Africa and Southwest Asia (Simoons 1971). Following that time, dairying spread across Eurasia and into sub-Saharan Africa. Dairying was not, however, adopted by all groups in Asia and Africa who had suitable herd animals. Even as late as A.D. 1500, the beginning of the great European overseas expansion, there were sizeable areas occupied by non-

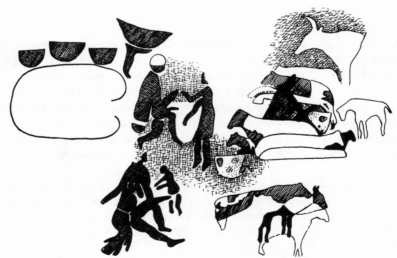

FIGURE 3.2. Possible milking scene from Sahara Neolithic (after F. Mori and G. Forni). Source: Simoons 1971, reprinted with the permission of the American Geographical Society.

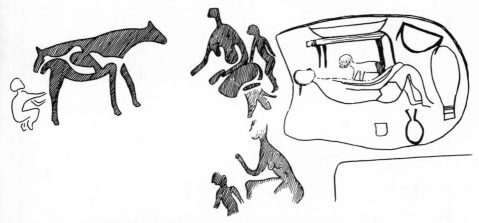

FIGURE 3.3. Possible milking scene from Sahara Neolithic (after H. Lhote).
Source: Simoons 1971, reprinted with the permission of the American Geographical Society.

milking groups. In Africa (fig. 3.4) the zone of nonmilking centered on the Congo Basin but extended beyond to cover about one-third of the continent (Simoons 1954). In Asia (fig. 3.5) the zone of nonmilking covered the bulk of the eastern and southeastern portions of the continent, including Burma, Thailand, Malaya, Vietnam, China, and Korea as well as the islands to the east (Simoons 1970b). Moreover, dairying remained unknown in the Pacific region and in the Americas in pre-European times. In those days the nonmilking peoples of Asia, Africa, and the Americas consumed mother's milk as infants, but normally ingested no milk after weaning, for animal milk was not part of their diet.

Geographers, anthropologists, and others long had speculated on the reasons for the failure of dairying to spread to all peoples in Eurasia and Africa (fig. 3.6) who had herd animals (Simoons 1973). Many scholars have focused on environmental and ecologic barriers to the spread of dairying. In Africa, for example, the presence of tsetse-borne sleeping sickness was seen as excluding pastoral groups from the moist savannah and rain forest regions of West Africa and the Congo, thus keeping such groups from introducing there the practices of dairying and milk use. In China, others suggested, dairying was unsuited to the intensive agricultural system that prevailed. And in Southeast Asia, animal disease and the low nutritional quality of tropical grasses were invoked. Other scholars looked less to environmental/ecological barriers than to human ones. They noted that native nonmilking groups, when questioned by early European travelers, objected to the practice of milking as unnatural manipulation of an animal's udder. The nonmilker in Asia also looked on milking as wrong because it violated the ahimsa (nonviolence) concept, stealing, as it were, from the young animal to

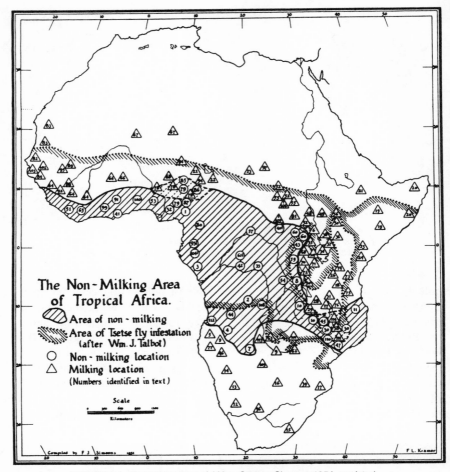

The Non-Milking Area
of Tropical Africa.
⬭ Area of non-milking
⬓ Area of Tsetse fly infestation
(after Wm. J. Talbot)
○ Non-milking location
△ Milking location
(Numbers identified in text)

Scale

Kilometers

FIGURE 3.4. Nonmilking area of Africa. Source: Simoons 1954, reprinted
with permission.

whom the milk rightfully belonged. As a final human barrier some observers
pointed to what seemed to be psychosomatic symptoms (stomach gas, cramps,
diarrhea, nausea, and vomiting) reported by some nonmilkers when they were
pressed into drinking milk. The collection of cultural views against milking
and milk use—the "nonmilking attitude"—was held to be as real a barrier to the
spread of milk use as were environmental/ecological factors.

It is unlikely, in retrospect, that the symptoms reported by nonmilkers when
they consumed milk were solely psychosomatic in origin. Instead, they may have
been those of lactase deficiency, brought on in lactose malabsorbers when they
consumed more than their threshold amount of milk. On first reading the medical

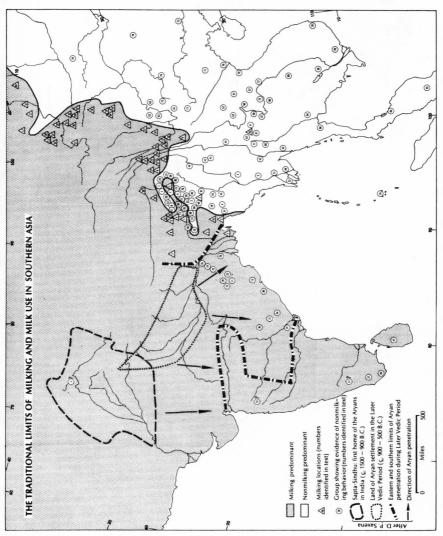

FIGURE 3.5. Traditional limits of milking and milk use in southern Asia. Source: Simoons 1970b, reprinted with permission.

THE TRADITIONAL LIMITS OF MILKING AND MILK USE IN SOUTHERN ASIA

Milking predominant

Nonmilking predominant

△ Milking locations (numbers identified in text)

Ⓡ Group showing evidence of nonmilking behavior (numbers identified in text)

Sapta-Sindhu: first home of the Aryans in India (c. 1500 – 900 B.C.)

Land of Aryan settlement in the Later Vedic Period (c. 900 – 500 B.C.)

Eastern and southern limits of Aryan penetration during Later Vedic Period

Direction of Aryan penetration

After D. P. Saxena

0   Miles   500

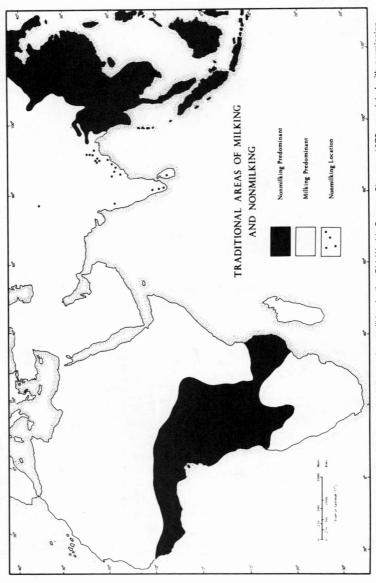

TRADITIONAL AREAS OF MILKING
AND NONMILKING

Nonmilking Predominant

Milking Predominant

Nonmilking Location

FIGURE 3.6. Traditional areas of milking and nonmilking in the Old World. Source: Simoons 1970a, reprinted with permission.

28

research on lactose malabsorption, in the late 1960s, the question was raised in my mind of what the links might be between group differences in prevalence of lactose malabsorption and contrasts, over a long historical period, in consumption of lactose-rich forms of milk. This was the question that first drew me into a literature survey.

It was striking that adults of all groups whose origins lay in the traditional zone of nonmilking were predominantly malabsorbers, usually from 70% to 100% of the individuals tested. Also striking was the fact that the peoples with low prevalences of lactose malabsorption (northwest Europeans and certain East African pastoral groups) came from a long tradition of consuming milk, much of it in lactose-rich forms. This suggested the geographic or culture-historical hypothesis. By that hypothesis, in the hunting and gathering stage, human groups everywhere were like most other land mammals in their patterns of lactase activity. That is, in the normal individual lactase activity would drop at weaning to low levels, which prevailed throughout life. With the beginning of dairying, however, significant changes occurred in the diets of many human groups. In some of these, moreover, there may have been a selective advantage for those aberrant individuals who experienced high levels of intestinal lactase throughout life. That advantage would have occurred only in certain situations: where milk was a specially critical part of the diet, where the group was under dietary stress, and where people did not process all their milk into low-lactose products such as aged cheese. Under those conditions, most likely to occur among pastoral groups, such aberrant individuals would drink more milk, would benefit more nutritionally as a result, and would enjoy increased prospects of survival, well-being, and of bearing progeny and supporting them. In a classical Mendelian way, then, the condition of high intestinal lactase activity throughout life would come to be typical of such a group.

QUESTIONS AND ALTERNATIVE SUGGESTIONS

Several important questions have been raised with respect to the culture-historical hypothesis. One is whether, given equal access to milk, lactose absorbers indeed would consume significantly more than malabsorbers. Without higher milk consumption, the early absorber might not enjoy the general nutritional advantage hypothesized. Even if one assumes that the early lactose absorber did enjoy such a selective advantage over others, one may question whether it was a general nutritional advantage, as in the hypothesis, or a specific advantage relating, for example, to a particular nutrient.

A third question is whether the sizeable differences in prevalence of lactose malabsorption among present-day ethnic groups could have evolved in the historical period since humans first practiced dairying and consumed milk. The evidence bearing on those questions was considered in a recent article (Simoons 1978). New evidence has come to light since then, and the whole matter needs to be re-evaluated. Here, however, the emphasis is on the geography of primary adult lactose malabsorption, and it is appropriate to comment only briefly on the three questions cited above.

With respect to the third question, there does indeed seem to have been sufficient time available since the origin of dairying for the development of presently observed differences in prevalence of lactose malabsorption among human groups. Estimates have been made that selection intensities of 1% or 2% to 3% would have been required, and that such intensities are not unusual (Heston and Gottesman 1973, Cavalli-Sforza 1973).

Turning to the first question, whether a general nutritional advantage may have occurred under the conditions hypothesized, one reaches the conclusion that some malabsorbers, in recognition of the distress milk brings on, do reduce their consumption of it. It also suggests that some malabsorbers, especially those with very low levels of intestinal lactase, may reject milk altogether. Even when a malabsorber does not reduce milk consumption, however, there remains the possibility that the increased intestinal motility he usually experiences, reduces absorption of other nutrients, thereby placing him at a nutritional disadvantage. Research completed through 1978, however, did not establish the manner and degree to which such increased intestinal motility might be detrimental to the individual.

While the culture-historical hypothesis postulates a general nutritional advantage, specific selective advantages are suggested by Flatz and Rotthauwe (1973) and Cook and Al-Torki (1975). Flatz and Rotthauwe, who since have elaborated their hypothesis (Flatz 1976, Flatz and Rotthauwe 1977, Flatz, personal communication), see their hypothesis as complementary to the culture-historical one. They believe it likely that a general selective advantage was enjoyed by lactose absorbers in various Old World milk-using populations, in Europe and elsewhere. They also hypothesize that in Northern Europe a powerful additional selective pressure favored lactose absorbers. They base their views on research by others showing that in humans hydrolysis of dietary lactose, like vitamin D, enhances calcium absorption. Early Northern Europe, their argument goes, was a cloudy region with ultraviolet radiation insufficient to produce an adequate amount of vitamin D in humans. Poverty-struck adults, moreover, frequently experienced dietary shortages of vitamin D, which could lead to late rickets or osteomalacia. These, in turn, contributed to morbidity and, in women, to pelvic deformation and reduced ability to bear offspring. Adult lactose absorbers among these early Europeans, however, were better able to absorb calcium, thereby enjoying a specific selective advantage. This advantage, in the opinion of Flatz and Rotthauwe, was a major contributor to the widespread present-day high prevalences of adult lactose absorption among northern Europeans (fig. 3.7).

Cook and Al-Torki (1975) suggest that Arabia is the likely place where "persistence of intestinal lactase into adult life originated" (fig. 3.8), and that the gene for such persistence was spread by peoples migrating to Africa and—more

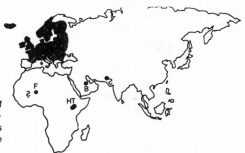

FIGURE 3.7. Populations with a frequency of the "persistence of lactase activity" gene (F = Fulani, B = Bedouins, HT = "Hamitic" groups of East Africa). Source: Flatz and Rotthauwe 1977, reprinted with permission.

conjecturally—to Northern Europe (Cook 1978). The high prevalences of adult lactose absorption in the Bedouin Arabs may have developed, according to Cook and Al-Torki, because of a selective advantage "associated with the fluid and calorie content of camels' milk, which is important for survival in desert nomads." They add that "in severe gastrointestinal infections active absorption of monosaccharides is coupled with water absorption," and that it is possible, in a group whose diet was mainly milk, that adult lactose absorbers could better "have survived epidemics such as cholera." Whatever the merits of their hypothesis as related to survival advantages, it is hard to imagine that the high prevalences of adult lactose absorption found in the vast area from India to Northern Europe and far into Africa would all derive from a single source, Arabia.

To this writer it seems unlikely that present-day high prevalences of lactose absorption among human groups originated in just one region and spread out from there. It also seems unlikely that high prevalences of lactose absorption derive from a single selective advantage that prevailed everywhere through history. Thus, it appears that whatever specific advantages the lactose absorber may

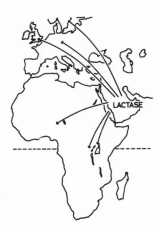

FIGURE 3.8. Map of Africa and Europe showing the possible route of dispersal for the persistence of lactase activity gene from an original focus in the Arabian peninsula. Source: Cook 1978, reprinted with permission.

have had at a particular time and place, there also existed a general nutritional advantage, and that this was basic.

RECENT GEOGRAPHIC FINDINGS AND THE HYPOTHESIS

The Importance of India. I have long held the view that significant regional and ethnic differences in primary adult lactose malabsorption must exist in the Indian subcontinent (Simoons 1970a). Dairying likely was introduced to India from the northwest, perhaps by the Indo-European Aryans about 1500 B.C., and peoples of the northwest consume significantly more milk and milk products than peoples of the south and east. The practice of dairying spread across India from the northwest, yet three thousand years later, in A.D. 1500, India remained on the border between the zones of milking and nonmilking (Simoons 1970b), with many nonmilking groups on the eastern borderlands and some in the south as well. By the culture-historical hypothesis, one would expect the southern and eastern groups, who at best became milk users in quite recent historical times, to have high prevalences of lactose malabsorption. One also would expect that peoples in the west and northwest of the Indian subcontinent, who have consumed milk in abundance and in lactose-rich forms since antiquity, would have significantly lower prevalences.

Unfortunately only one of the early studies of lactose malabsorption among groups of Indian origin identified the subjects' ethnic affiliations or place of birth (Murthy and Haworth 1970). In that one study, however, nine adults born in Punjab were found to have a prevalence of lactose malabsorption of only 33%. A second study, carried out in the New Delhi area (Gupta et al. 1970, 1971), moreover, found a prevalence of lactose malabsorption among 70 individuals (not identified as to origins) to be 27%. Both percentages were notably lower than the all-India average (53%). They were also in keeping with what the culture-historical hypothesis led one to expect, but were, at best, suggestive. Now, however, there are several new studies that cast light on the problem, providing enough information for a crude mapping (fig. 3.9) of the pattern of high and low prevalences of lactose malabsorption in South Asia. In the west and northwest of the Indian subcontinent, which includes the first home of the Aryans in India (from circa 1500 to 900 B.C.), low prevalences of lactose malabsorption are typical today, from 0% to 15% of the persons tested. The groups represented are Baloochis, Sindhis, Pathans (Rab and Baseer 1976), Kashmiris (Malik et al. 1977), and Punjabis (Murthy and Haworth 1970, Rab and Baseer 1976, Tandon et al. 1977). Prevalences of lactose malabsorption increase in India with distance from the first Aryan homeland: 27% in the New Delhi area (Gupta et al. 1970, 1971); 35% in a group of women mostly from Madhya Pradesh, eastern Uttar Pradesh, Bihar, and Orissa (Tandon et al. 1977); 58% in Bombay (Desai et al. 1967, 1970); 61% in Hyderabad in south central India (Reddy and Pershad

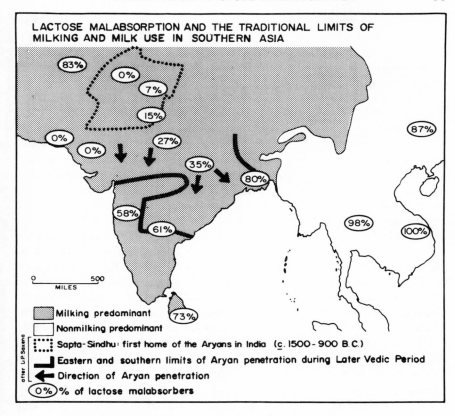

FIGURE 3.9. Percentage of lactose malabsorbers in southern Asia.
Adapted in part from Simoons 1970b, map 3.

1972); 100% of Indians randomly selected from four south Indian provinces (Swaminathan et al. 1970, Swaminathan, personal communication); 73% of Sinhalese and 71% of Tamils in Ceylon (Senewiratne et al. 1977); and 80% in Bangladeshi children over 3 years of age (Brown et al. 1979). All of the above fits with the culture-historical hypothesis. Moreover, when one passes over the traditional eastern boundary of milking and into the zone of nonmilking, percentages of malabsorption are generally higher: 98% of several groups of Thais tested in their homeland (Troncale et al. 1967, Flatz et al. 1969, Flatz and Saengudom 1969, Keusch et al. 1969, Flatz and Rotthauwe 1971, Varavithya et al. 1976); 87% of various groups of Chinese tested in Singapore, Taiwan, Australia, and the United States (Bolin and Davis 1969, 1970; Calloway et al. 1969; Bryant et al. 1970; Sung and Shih 1972; Chua and Seah 1973); and 100% of a group of Vietnamese tested in the United States (Anh et al. 1977). Similar high prevalences of lactose malabsorption are found in all other lands of Southeast and East Asia (Simoons 1978), as expected in a traditional zone of nonmilking.

If one were to undertake further work in India, or with Indians abroad, one should obtain a sample of the Indian peoples originating within the eastern zone of nonmilking. The Naga and Chin are the most numerous peoples there, but other nonmilking groups are found in the Khasi and Jaintia Hills, in the Chota Nagpur region, and some even in peninsular India (Simoons 1970b). These groups would be expected to have high prevalences of lactose malabsorption. Also critical are other groups in India's northwest who would be expected to have low prevalences, such as the Gujars of the Punjab (by tradition cattle herders with an abundance of milk available) and other peoples of pastoral tradition, such as the Ahirs, and the Gaddis of the Dhauladhar Range. Of interest, too, would be a broader study of the Hindu and Sikh population of the lowland Punjab, and of the populations of other areas of western India, such as Rajasthan.

Of particular interest is the prevalance of lactose malabsorption among the relatively unmixed Dravidian peoples of south India. At present, there is no convincing evidence that the people of the Indus Valley Civilization (circa 2500 to 1700 B.C.), now known to be Dravidian, milked their cattle, water buffalo, or other domesticated animals. It seems likely that dairying was introduced to the Dravidians only after the Aryan invasion mentioned earlier. If this were so, one would expect south Indian Dravidians to have prevalences of malabsorption significantly higher than the Indo-Europeans of northern India. The Toda of the Nilgiris, however, may be an exception, a Dravidian people whose dairy traditions closely resemble those of early Mesopotamia (2000 B.C. or earlier) and who may have practiced dairying since antiquity. It would not be surprising, therefore, if the Toda differ from the general Dravidian population in having significantly lower prevalences of malabsorption.

The Indo-European Problem. Of special interest are the patterns of lactose malabsorption that exist beyond India in other members of the Indo-European language family, whose original homeland is presumed by many to lie somewhere in the grasslands from the Ukraine to Turkestan. It is from that homeland that Indo-European groups are believed to have pushed out, to the west and southwest across Europe and to the south and southeast into Anatolia, Iran, and India. I had early raised the possibility—because of the common view that the Indo-Europeans were pastoralists when they first rose to prominence—that selection for lactose malabsorption may have begun in their ancestral homeland. That possibility seems strengthened by the clear evidence of low prevalences not only among Indo-Europeans in Western Europe but also among those in Pakistan and northwest India. But what of the vast intervening zone stretching thousands of miles across Eurasia? What is the evidence there?

When I first sketched the geography of lactose malabsorption, there were virtually no studies in that intervening zone, but, since then, several studies have added to our knowledge and raised intriguing questions. Extending the western European belt of low prevalences of lactose malabsorption have been studies in Eastern Europe, or among persons of eastern European origin. Poles studied in Canada had a 29% prevalence of lactose malabsorption (6 of 21 adults) (Leichter 1972). Groups of Czechs in Canada, Bohemia, and Moravia had an overall prevalence of 8% (3 of 37 adults) (Leichter 1972, Madzarovova-Noheljlova 1969). And a low prevalence—15% (38 of 248 adults)—also was found recently in a large test conducted in Leningrad; 88% of the group tested were of Russian nationality (Valenkevich 1977, Valenkevich, personal communication).

There also have been studies in Eastern Europe involving non-Indo-European peoples, the Estonians, Finns, and Lapps, all of whom belong to the Finno-Ugric section of the Uralic language family. There is a single study of Estonians, by Villako et al. (Valenkevich, personal communication), which found 28% of a group of adults to be malabsorbers. Because one of the earlier studies in Finland, in the small Finnish rural community of Pornainen, had been criticized as not representative of all Finns, a new study was completed involving 156 Finnish-speaking students aged 21 to 30 years (Sahi 1974, 1978; Sahi unpublished observations). Each had three or more Finnish-speaking grandparents, and the student group was chosen to represent the nation as a whole. The prevalence of lactose malabsorption among the students was 17%, identical with that of the Pornainen adults. Also tested in the study were 91 Swedish-speaking students, each with three or more Swedish-speaking grandparents. The Swedish-speaking students had a significantly lower prevalence of lactose malabsorption (8%). That prevalence, however, is far higher than the less than 1% reported for adults in Sweden (Dahlqvist and Lindquist 1971). Sahi (1974, 1978; Sahi unpublished data) suggests that the higher prevalence of lactose malabsorption among the Swedes in Finland derives from the fact that they are a mixed Swedish/Finnish population. The Finns, too, are to varying degrees a mixed people, and it is interesting that Sahi, in mapping prevalence of lactose malabsorption by county, found hints of regional contrasts among Finns that may reflect differences in genetic background.

The third ethnic group studied in Finland, the Lapps (Sahi, unpublished observations 1975; Dahlqvist and Lindquist 1971; Sahi et al. 1976), are reindeer-herding people of the arctic tundra and forest regions of Scandinavia and Russia. Though all Lapp groups today are milk drinkers, there are suggestions that they first took up the practice of milking recently, perhaps only in the last several centuries, following Scandinavian example (Itkonen 1948). Thus it is understandable that adults of all Lapp subgroups have higher prevalences of lactose malabsorption, from 25% to 60%, than do Swedes and Finns.

One only hopes that similar studies will be done in the Soviet Union, for that area constitutes a critical gap in the geographic knowledge of lactose malabsorption among Indo-Europeans. What of the Ukrainians, the Indo-European peoples of the Caucasus area, the Kurds, and what of Iran and Afghanistan?

Until recently only a single Iranian seems to have been tested for lactose malabsorption, by Graham Neale in Britain (Neale, personal communication). That person, like other subjects of Near Eastern origin in Neale's test, was a malabsorber. A recent study done in Teheran (Sadre and Karbasi 1979) found 86% of a group in Iranian adults (18 of 21 subjects) to be lactose malabsorbers. The subjects were not identified as to region of birth or linguistic affiliations, but one assumes that most were speakers of Fārsī, the Persian language proper, and were settled folk from rural and urban areas. One wonders whether such high prevalences occur among Iran's other ethnic groups, especially peoples of nomadic tradition such as the Qashkai and Bakhtiari.

Of equal importance is the recent study that found high prevalences of lactose malabsorption among various ethnic groups in Afghanistan: 82% of Tajiks (65 of 79 subjects), 79% of Pashtuns (56 of 71 subjects), 87% of Pasha-i (52 of 60 subjects), 100% of Uzbeks (16 of 16 subjects), 80% of Hazara (8 of 10 subjects), and 76% of a mixed urban group (26 of 34 persons) (Rahimi et al. 1976). The Uzbek are Turkic in speech. Other groups (Hazara, Tajik, Pashtun, Pasha-i) are Indo-European. Results for one of the above groups, the Pashtun, however, differed strikingly with results obtained by Rab and Baseer (1976), who found no lactose malabsorption among 15 Pathan (Pashtun) subjects tested in Pakistan. Because of this and because Afghanistan is on the fringe of the Indo-European distribution, an unusual meeting place of races and language families, one should be cautious in interpretation. Anthropologist Robert Canfield has noted, for example, that the Hazara are a mixed people with strong Mongol physical affinities; that their traditional language, though Persianized, contains many Mongol words; and that there are further Mongol resemblances in the Hazara kinship system (Canfield 1978). Similarly the Tajik were described by anthropologist Louis Dupree (1978) as "a classic example of miscegenation." Though basically of Mediterranean type (Caucasian), "Tajik groups exhibit increasing Mongoloid characteristics as one moves north from Kabul into Badakhshan and Soviet Central Asia. The resulting genetic admixtures have produced Tajik with red or blond hair, blue or mixed eye color combinations, in association with high cheekbones and epicanthic eyefolds."

If, in the Teheran study cited, the subjects were indeed Fārsī speakers, Indo-Europeans, there would seem to be, in both Iran and Afghanistan, a situation like that of southern Italy and Greece, where Indo-Europeans also have high prevalences of lactose malabsorption. In Italy and Greece, failure to consume abundant lactose-rich dairy products into adulthood, and racial mixing with earlier Mediterranean groups have been suggested as the principal contributing factors (Simoons 1978). The Iranian investigators, Sadre and Karbasi (1979), indicate that such interbreeding has been common in Iran as well, that though "the Iranians were originally of Indo-European stock," invading peoples through history have made contributions to the Iranian gene pool. This, say Sadre and Karbasi, may explain why the glucose curve of Iranians given the blood sugar test for lactose malabsorption, resembles that of Chinese and Indians rather than that of other "Caucasians" (Northern Europeans). One might add that, as with the Aryans in India, the Iranians were preceded in their land by non-Indo-European groups, most notably the Elamites, with whom they must have inter-bred as well.

What is especially needed now is study in the southern belt of Indo-Europeans, from India to the Mediterranean, as to their traditional patterns of milk use, including lactose content of dairy products, and the nature and extent of ethnic and racial intermixture.

Southwest Asia and North Africa. My review published in 1978 included 14 studies that found high prevalences of lactose malabsorption (average 72%) among 716 subjects, mostly settled people, of Southwest Asian and North African origin: Jews in Israel and abroad; and Arabs in or from Iraq, Syria, Saudi Arabia, Jordan, Israel, Egypt, Tunisia, and Morocco. Since then I have located additional studies that found similar high prevalences of lactose malabsorption: 78% (108 of 138 subjects) of one group of Lebanese students, mostly 16 to 26 years of age (Loiselet and Jarjouhi 1974); 78% (58 of 74 subjects) of another group of healthy Lebanese volunteers with ages ranging from 17 to 43 years. (Nasrallah 1979); 80% (20 of 25 subjects) of a group of Egyptian children 9 to 12 years of age (Gabr et al. 1977); and 78% of a group of 55 adults (aged 20 to 70 years), without digestive complaints, from the Maghreb (Morocco, Algeria, Tunisia) (O'Morain et al. 1978). The new studies confirm the existence of high preva-lences of malabsorption in the Near East among groups of settled tradition who as adults generally consume small quantities of milk products, much of it in fermented forms that are low in lactose content.

In a 1973 review of the literature, I had suggested that certain Arab nomad groups, for example the Bedouin of Saudi Arabia, might prove to have notably lower prevalences of lactose malabsorption than the settled Arabs studied up to that time (Simoons 1973). That suggestion was based on the antiquity of dairying in that region, on the importance of dairy products in the diet of various nomads of Arabia, and on the report that Yemeni Jews had lower prevalences of such lactose malabsorption (44%) than did Jews of other communities studied in Israel (62% to 85%) (Gilat et al. 1970). It appeared that the Yemen Jews, who lived in a mountain homeland surrounded by Arab pastoral folk, had been influenced genetically by those Arabs. Shortly afterward there appeared a study of 40 Syrian Arab adults (18 to 39 years of age) that included 3 Bedouins, the first to be identified in any study of lactose malabsorption (El-Schallah et al. 1973). Two of the 3 (67%), however, proved to be malabsorbers. Though this was a lower prevalence than that for the remainder of the study group (36 of 37, or 99%, were malabsorbers), it did little to support my suggestion. Since then, however, Cook and Al-Torki (1975) have strongly confirmed the existence of low prevalences of lactose malabsorption in various Arab groups in Saudi Arabia, a land in which nomads have constituted a higher proportion of the population than in other Arab countries. These researchers found only 2 in 14 Bedouins (14%) to be malabsorbers; 1 in 8 urban Saudi Arabs (13%); and 2 in 8 (25%) Yemen Arabs.

Another finding of Cook and Al-Torki is that the "Khadiry," a group of mixed ethnic origins, depart strongly from other Saudi Arabs studied. Of the Khadiry tested (5 of them had clear African traits), 78% (7 of 9 subjects) were malabsorbers, a percentage approaching those reported for various African agricultural peoples. African slaves had been taken to the Arabian peninsula since pre-Christian times, and in certain places there are even entire villages of people who are strikingly African in appearance. One suspects that the African component has contributed to notable differences in prevalence of lactose malabsorption from place to place in Arabia and that these will become clear in future studies.

Sub-Saharan Africa.   Some of the most important early studies bearing on the culture-historical hypothesis were done in sub-Saharan Africa, especially those of G. C. Cook and co-workers in Uganda (Cook 1967, Cook and Dahlqvist 1968, Cook and Howells 1968, Cook and Kajubi 1966, Cook et al. 1967) and Norman Kretchmer and co-workers in Nigeria (Kretchmer 1971, 1972; Kretchmer and Ransome-Kuti 1970; Kretchmer et al. 1971; Ransome-Kuti et al. 1972, 1975). Both Uganda and Nigeria are critical locations in terms of the history of dairying in Africa. Nigeria straddles the boundary between the traditional zones of milking and nonmilking (Simoons 1954). The peoples of northern Nigeria were milk users, most notably the Fulani, a group of pastoral tradition who consumed milk in large quantities and in lactose-rich forms. Though it is a matter of controversy, some ethnologists hold the Fulani to be descendants of early Saharan pastoralists who practiced milking since perhaps 4000 B.C. and possibly earlier (Simoons 1971). The peoples of southern Nigeria, such as the Yoruba, lived in the zone of nonmilking and until European contact they normally consumed no milk after weaning. One would expect the Yoruba and other south Nigerians to be predominantly lactose malabsorbers as adults, and the Fulani to be absorbers. This is what Kretchmer and his colleagues established (1971): 98% of Yoruba tested were found to be lactose malabsorbers, compared to only 22% of nomadic Fulani. Subsequent work in West Africa has mainly started to fill in the map. Other south Nigerians also have been found to have high prevalences of lactose malabsorption, from 75% to 100% of the groups involved (Olatunbosun and Adadevoh 1971, Elliott et al. 1973). In Ghana, a 73% incidence of lactose malabsorption was found in a group of 100 children (ages 2 to 6 years) (White and Latham 1973), and for older children and adults the percentage is probably even higher. Like southern Nigeria, most of Ghana was in the traditional zone of nonmilking (Simoons 1954).

Uganda lies fully within the East African zone of milking, but that region has experienced migrations and intermingling of peoples of quite different traditions of milk use. The early people of East Africa were hunters and gatherers, whether

Negroid or Bushmanoid. Certain of them survive even today, and—though they have not yet been tested—one would expect lactose malabsorption to be typical of unmixed adults. Moving into the territory of the hunters and gatherers and settling there in early times were agricultural groups of three quite different traditions (Ehret 1974): Southern Cushites, seed cultivators and keepers of livestock, who seem to have pushed southward from Ethiopia at least by 2000 B.C. (Ehret 1979); Central Sudanic peoples, believed initially to have been grain farmers and livestock herders, who moved south from the Sudan through the lacustrine region in the first millennium B.C. (Ehret 1973); and the Bantu, planters who emerged from the Congo forests somewhat later, possibly as early as 400 to 300 B.C., and who pushed eastward to join, displace, or absorb the East African groups who preceded them. Since the ancestors of the East African Bantu seem to have left the Congo zone of nonmilking quite late, they would be expected to be predominantly malabsorbers. This is the first thing that Cook established. Adults of Bantu agricultural tribes of Uganda and nearby areas were found to have prevalences of lactose malabsorption from 96% to 100%.

Some scholars have viewed the Hima, Tussi, and certain other East African pastoralists as descended from the ancient herding peoples of the Sahara mentioned previously. If so, or if they come from a long tradition of consuming milk in lactose-rich forms, one might expect them to have quite low prevalences of lactose malabsorption. This is what Cook found: prevalences from 0% to 17% among the Hima and Tussi, and intermediate prevalences, from 33% to 38%, among mixed groups (Iru, Hutu) (Cook and Kajubi 1966, Cook and Dahlqvist 1968). Cook also found, however, a much higher prevalence of lactose malabsorption, 44% (4 of 9 subjects), in a group of adult "Nilotes or Nilo-Hamites" studied in Uganda.

Confirming the first of Cook's findings, additional Bantu groups, in East Africa and elsewhere, have been found to have high prevalences of lactose malabsorption. One study (Elliott et al. 1973) found a 98% prevalence of lactose malabsorption (57 of 58 subjects) among Bantu of various tribes from the Cameroons and Congo, center of the African zone of nonmilking. Another (Cox and Elliott 1974) found a 96% prevalence (27 of 28 subjects) among the Shi, a Bantu people of the Lake Kivu area in the Congo. Still other studies found high prevalences among Bantu groups in East Africa: 92% (117 of 127 subjects) in a group of Tanzania Bantu children (ages 5 to 14 years) (Jackson and Latham 1978), and 73% (52 of 71 subjects) in children (ages 5 to 15) tested in Kenya, the overwhelming majority from Bantu agricultural tribes (Kikuyu, Kamba) (Pieters and Van Rens 1973). Bantu adults in Zambia (Cook et al. 1973), like Bantu studied earlier in South Africa (Jersky and Kinsley 1967), also have been found to be primarily malabsorbers (90% and over). Though the Zambia Bantu are milk users today, their ancestors derive from the nonmilking zone to the north and likely did not take up dairying until well into the first millennium A.D.

Later studies also have confirmed another of Cook's early findings (Cook and

Kajubi 1966, Cook and Dahlqvist 1968), of a very low prevalence of lactose malabsorption (12%, or 2 of 17 subjects) among the Tussi and intermediate prevalences among the Hutu, a mixed people. In one study (Elliott et al. 1973), of 15 Tussi pastoralists tested in the Congo, none were malabsorbers. In another, of 27 Tussi tested in Rwanda (Cox and Elliott 1974), only 2 (8%) were malabsorbers, whereas 21 of 36 Hutu (58%) were.

I had expected (Simoons 1970a) Cook's initial finding of a moderate 44% prevalence of lactose malabsorption among a group of "Nilotes or Nilo-Hamites" in Uganda to be followed by findings of low prevalences among other Nilotic groups. The bases for this expectation were several. One was the widely held view that the Hima and Tussi, who had been found to have low prevalences of lactose malabsorption, are descended from Nilotic pastoralists. Also of relevance was the strongly pastoral element and importance of milk among many Nilotic groups and the presumed antiquity of dairying among them. Instead of low prevalences, however, intermediate to high prevalences of lactose malabsorption have been found among the few other Nilotic peoples tested so far. Elliott et al. (1973) found 6 adult Sudanese Nilotics (5 Dinka, 1 Alur) tested in Zaïre all to be malabsorbers. The Alur live primarily by agriculture, but the Dinka are mainly pastoral. Still more recently, Jackson and Latham (1978, 1979) found high prevalences of lactose malabsorption among the Nilotic Masai: 62% (13 of 21 subjects) of a group of children (ages 5 to 14 years) tested in Tanzania. This prevalence, it is true, was much less than those found in Bantu groups, but is surprisingly high in view of the pastoral way of life typical of the Masai.

Where such variable prevalences of lactose malabsorption (44% to 100%) have been found in related peoples in other parts of the world (as among Mestizos in Latin America), there have been strong presumptions of different degrees of interbreeding among absorber and malabsorber populations. With respect to Nilotics, one should note first that considerable differences of opinion exist as to Nilotic history and relations with other linguistic groups (Ehret 1971). Anthropologist George P. Murdock (1959) calls the Masai and many other Eastern and Southern Nilotics "Cushiticized Nilotes," because of strong cultural and linguistic borrowings and presumed interbreeding with agricultural Cushites.* Cushites, according to Christopher Ehret (1979), did possess cattle, sheep, and goats and used milk before the Southern Cushitic migration into East Africa. One suspects, however, that milk was not a critical item in the diet of early East African Cushites and, if this is correct, they would be expected to have had high prevalences of lactose malabsorption. Also of note is the process of "Masai-ization" alluded to by various writers, under which Bantu become Masai. Exten-

---

*Recent archeological excavations (Lynch and Robbins 1979) have uncovered remains dating from the first millennium A.D. that the excavators believe to be those of Eastern Nilotics, the group to which the Masai belong, in their original homeland near Lake Turkana in northwest Kenya. This was not far from earlier sites believed to be Cushitic. The presumed Eastern Nilotics had a fishing-pastoral economy (sheep, goats, common cattle).

sive interbreeding with malabsorber Cushites or Bantu might be sufficient to account for the relatively high prevalence of lactose malabsorption among the Masai. There is also, however, the question of the recency of dairying among them. Murdock (1959) suggests further that at the time the Bantu pushed into East Africa, the East African Nilotics "seem to have been a relatively backward agricultural people occupying only a fraction of their present territory." Within a few centuries, Murdock suggests, these Nilotic peoples "had developed a full-fledged pastoral complex." If so, dairy products would have become important to them quite recently.

But what of the Sudanese Nilotics who also seem to have high prevalences of lactose malabsorption? And what of the Hima and Tussi with their very low prevalences? The Hima and Tussi speak Bantu languages today, but are widely held to be descended from Nilotic pastoralists. Do they in fact have a different ancestry? Ehret (1968) has argued, on the basis of linguistic evidence, that the ancient people who introduced livestock and milking to southern Africa spoke Central Sudanic languages. May the Hima and Tussi be descended from ancient Central Sudanic migrants to East Africa?

Present-day Central Sudanic groups are found far to the north, in an east-west belt along the Sahara-Sudan borderlands east of Lake Chad and on the Sudan-Congo fringe to the southeast. With the exception of certain peoples who lost their cattle and sheep on migrating into tsetse-infested forest lands, all Central Sudanic groups today are milk users. One can only speculate on how long their ancestors may have possessed livestock and milked them. A recent archeologic excavation at Kadero (Krzyzaniak 1978), north of Khartoum and beyond the present-day Central Sudanic language distribution, found a cereal cultivating, herding, food-gathering people living there late in the fourth millennium B.C. The Kadero people possessed cattle, sheep, goats, and dogs, with cattle of great importance and "possibly milked." If so, it lends credence to the view that Central Sudanic groups could have adopted dairying quite early.

Whatever the truth may be, it is to historical investigation that one must look in seeking explanations of the striking differences in prevalence of lactose malabsorption that seem to exist among pastoral groups in the Sudan and East Africa. This writer suggests that the low prevalences of lactose malabsorption among Hima and Tussi indicate a long history of pastoralism, milk-use, and little intermixture with malabsorber groups, whereas the variable prevalences among Nilotic groups (in Uganda and among the Dinka and Masai) result either from the recency of a strongly pastoral way of life among them, from extensive interbreeding with malabsorber populations, or both.

The prevalences of lactose malabsorption among pastoral groups in northeast Africa remain a mystery. One study (Habte et al. 1973) found 90% of a group of 58 older children (7 to 13 years of age) in highland Ethiopia and Eritrea to be lactose malabsorbers. Those children were mainly Semitic Amhara and Tigre, highland farming peoples rather than pastoralists, and they can be classified with settled Arabs and with Jews with respect to prevalence of lactose malabsorption. One can only guess what prevalences of lactose malabsorption may be among pastoral groups in lowland northeast Africa (Somali, Afar, and others) and in the Sahara and areas to the north—along the route by which dairying and milk use spread southward.*

One problem raised in earlier reviews was that of Bushmen and Hottentots in southern Africa, and of the Pygmies of the Congo and adjacent areas. The Bushmen, who number perhaps 55,000, are among the small number of hunting and gathering peoples surviving in Africa. Today the Bushmen live mainly in South-West Africa and Botswana. Traditionally they had no domesticated herd animals, and thus no opportunity for dairying or consumption of milk after weaning. The Hottentots, members of the same race (Bushmanoid) and language family (Khoisan) as the Bushmen, were pastoralists who kept common cattle, sheep, and goats as milk animals. At least some Hottentot groups consumed milk fresh (Kroll 1928). Though the ancestry of the Hottentots remains controversial, they seem to have lived far to the north in East Africa in the tenth century A.D. and to have been pushed southward by the advancing Bantu. Some scholars also contend that the Hottentots have an intermixture with Caucasoid "Hamites" from the north. In any case, if the Hottentots consumed lactose-rich types of milk for a long historical period, they would, by the culture-historical hypothesis, be expected to have developed a significantly lower prevalence of lactose malabsorption than both their Bushmen relatives and Bantu neighbors. Thus, the first studies of such lactose malabsorption among Bushmen and Hottentots are of considerable interest. They were done in part collaboratively by investigators from the University of the Witwatersrand and Cambridge University (Jenkins et al. 1974, Nurse and Jenkins 1974). Two Bushmen groups were studied, the !Kung of Tsumkwe in South-West Africa and the ≠huâ of southern Botswana, as well as one Hottentot group, the Nama of Keetmanshoop, South-West Africa. Neither Bushman group ever was known to keep cattle or drink milk, but some

---

*Since the above was written, results of an important new study, by Gebhard Flatz and colleagues in the Republic of Sudan, have been communicated to me (Flatz, personal communication). That study included a total of 563 adults drawn from ethnic groups from various parts of the country. Of 6 Beja tested, all were lactose absorbers, which would seem sharply to separate these pastoralists from malabsorber farming groups to their north and south (Egypt, Ethiopia) and to place them, with their Afro-Asiatic relatives the Bedouin of Arabia, among the world's absorber populations. Nomads of the northern desert of the Sudan in general had a prevalence of lactose malabsorption of 38%; this, moreover, was lower than the 52% found among the Baggara, those Negroid cattle-herding Arab pastoralists of the central Sudan; and the latter, in turn, was lower than the 61% prevalence of lactose malabsorption found among Nilotics, whose homeland is in the southern Sudan. What we seem to be dealing with is a general increase in prevalence of lactose malabsorption among pastoral groups from north to south in the Sudan and beyond to the Masai. This makes sense in terms of what is known of the spread of dairying southward. Remaining a mystery, however, are the Hima and Tussi, those East African pastoralists with very low prevalences of lactose malabsorption. One suspects that the latter two pastoral groups, like the Fulani of west Africa, have histories quite different from that of the Masai, that they have a pastoral tradition reaching far back in history, possibly to the Neolithic pastoralists of the Sahara.

≠huâ live as serfs of the Kgalagadi, a cattle-keeping Tswana Bantu people who drink milk fresh and soured. The Nama studied have few common cattle at present, though they have many goats and consume fresh and soured goat milk. Of 25 unrelated ≠huâ Bushmen (including 22 adults and 3 children about 10 years of age), 23 were malabsorbers, or 92%; and of 40 !Kung, 39 were malabsorbers, or 98%. By contrast the Nama, who belong to the largest surviving Hottentot group in Africa, had a significantly lower prevalence of lactose malabsorption: only 9 of 18 adults (50%) proved to be malabsorbers (Jenkins, personal communication). These results are fully in keeping with the culture-historical hypothesis, as is the fact that Hottentots have a significantly lower prevalence of lactose malabsorption than Bantus in South Africa and Zambia (where prevalences of malabsorption are 90% or more).

Somewhat puzzling, however, is more recent data gathered by the Witwatersrand investigators on the Rehoboth Basters (Jenkins, personal communication), a genetically mixed people believed to be 50% Caucasoid and 50% Hottentot (Nurse 1975). The group turned out to have a prevalence of lactose malabsorption of 65% (13 of 20 subjects), higher than expected. One may raise various questions about these results, but one must acknowledge that these investigators have pioneered research in an extremely important area, one well suited for using differences in prevalance of lactose malabsorption as genetic markers, as Cook (1969) did in East Africa.

As for the Pygmies, traditionally hunters and gatherers subservient to, and to a degree interbreeding with, Bantu and other full-statured Negroes, there is now a first study, by Cox and Elliott (1974). It involved 22 Twa Pygmies (ages 15 to 58) of Rwanda, of whom 17 (77%) were malabsorbers. If these were pure-bred Pygmies, one would expect higher prevalences of lactose malabsorption. One suspects that a degree of interbreeding with other groups, the agricultural Hutu and pastoral Tussi, accounts for the 23% of absorbers among them.

PROSPECT

This chapter has been concerned primarily with geographic evidence from the Old World as it bears on the culture-historical hypothesis of primary adult lactose malabsorption. Since 1970, when that hypothesis first was advanced, there have been many studies which from a geographic point of view bear on its validity (fig. 3.10). It remains true that all groups studied whose origins are in the traditional zones of nonmilking—in Africa, Southeast and East Asia, New Guinea, and the Americas—have been found to have high prevalences of lactose malabsorption (Simoons 1978). The sample now available includes a broad range of peoples, some of hunting and gathering and others of agricultural tradition. It is also true that all groups with a millennia-long tradition of consuming milk in quantity and in lactose-rich forms have been found to have low prevalences of such malabsorption. Their unmixed descendants maintain the ancestral preva-

A: Hunting and gathering peoples (N = 287; with LM, 247; prevalence of LM, 86%)

B: Agricultural peoples from the traditional zones of nonmilking and their relatively un-mixed overseas descendants (N = 1,311; with LM, 1,186; prevalence of LM, 90%)

    In North and South America (N = 167; with LM, 162; prevalence of LM, 97%)
    In sub-Saharan Africa (N = 311; with LM, 270; prevalence of LM, 87%)
    In Southeast and East Asia (N = 829; with LM, 750; prevalence of LM, 90%)
    In the Pacific region (N = 20; with LM, 20; prevalence of LM, 100%)

C: Agricultural peoples whose ancestry lies in the traditional zones of nonmilking but who migrated into an adjacent zone, to become milk users at a relatively recent date (N = 226; with LM, 199; prevalence of LM, 88%)

D: Peoples, including some of pastoral tradition, who have consumed large amounts of milk and lactose-rich dairy products for a long historical period and have lived under condi-tions of dietary stress (also their relatively unmixed overseas descendants) (N = 3,489; with LM, 376; prevalence of LM, 11%)

    In Africa and the Near East (N = 101; with LM, 10; prevalence of LM, 10%)
    Europeans and their overseas descendants (N = 3,269; with LM, 344; prevalence of LM, 11%)
    In India and Pakistan (N = 119; with LM, 22; prevalence of LM, 18%)

E: Peoples who have used milk since antiquity but who do not meet conditions of strong selective pressures against LM (N = 716; with LM, 514; prevalence of LM, 72%)

FIGURE 3.10. Prevalence of primary adult lactose malabsorption (LM) among ethnic or racial groups.

lences of lactose malabsorption regardless of whether they remain in the original homeland or have migrated abroad. Should an absorber people interbreed with a malabsorber group, moreover, their prevalences of malabsorption have been found to be intermediate between the two parental groups. Though the evidence fits the hypothesis in general terms and in many specific cases, there have been surprises—as with the Nilotic peoples—that test the hypothesis. When one looks further into the specific cases, however, one finds gaps: in historical and present-day knowledge of milk use, including lactose content of dairy products consumed; and in our understanding of ethnic or racial origins and interbreeding. In such cases, prevalences of lactose malabsorption can serve as genetic markers to aid in historical reconstruction and to stimulate more careful research by anthropologists, geographers, and historians.

REFERENCES

Anh NT, Thuc TK, Welsh JD: Lactose malabsorption in adult Vietnamese. *Am J Clin Nutr* 30:468–69, 1977.

Bolin TD, Davis AE: Asian lactose intolerance and its relation to intake of lactose. *Nature* 222:382–83, 1969.

Bolin TD, Davis AE: Lactose intolerance in Australian-born Chinese. *Aust Ann Med* 19:40–41, 1970.

Brown KH, Parry L, Khatun M, Ahmed MG: Lactose malabsorption in Bangladeshi village children: Relation with age, history of recent diarrhea, nutritional status, and breast feeding. *Am J Clin Nutr* 32:1962-69, 1979.

Bryant GD, Chu YK, Lovitt R: Incidence and aetiology of lactose intolerance. *Med J Aust* 1:1285-88, 1970.

Calloway DH, Murphy EL, Bauer D: Determination of lactose intolerance by breath analysis. *Am J Dig Dis* 14:811-15, 1969.

Canfield RL: Hazara. In *Muslim Peoples: A World Ethnographic Survey*, RV Weekes (ed). Westport, Conn.: Greenwood Press, 1978, pp 163-67.

Cavalli-Sforza LL: Analytic review: Some current problems of human population genetics. *Am J Hum Genet* 25:82-104, 1973.

Chua KL, Seah CS: Lactose intolerance: Hereditary or acquired? Effect of prolonged milk feeding. *Singapore Med J* 14:29-33, 1973.

Cook GC: Lactase activity in newborn and infant Baganda. *Br Med J* 1:527-30, 1967.

Cook GC: Lactase deficiency: A probable ethnological marker in East Africa. *Man* 4:265-67, 1969.

Cook GC: Did persistence of intestinal lactase into adult life originate on the Arabian peninsula? *Man* 13:418-27, 1978.

Cook GC, Al-Torki MT: High intestinal lactase concentrations in adult Arabs in Saudi Arabia. *Br Med J* 3:135-36, 1975.

Cook GC, Asp NG, Dahlqvist A: Activities of brush border lactase, acid β-galactosidase, and hetero-β-galactosidase in the jejunum of the Zambian African. *Gastroenterology* 64:405-10, 1973.

Cook GC, Dahlqvist A: Jejunal hetero-β-galactosidase activities in Ugandans with lactase deficiency. *Gastroenterology* 55:328-32, 1968.

Cook GC, Howells GR: Lactosuria in the African with lactase deficiency. *Am J Dig Dis* 13:634-37, 1968.

Cook GC, Kajubi SK: Tribal incidence of lactase deficiency in Uganda. *Lancet* 1:725-30, 1966.

Cook GC, Lakin A, Whitehead RG: Absorption of lactose and its digestion products in the normal and malnourished Ugandan. *Gut* 8:622-27, 1967.

Cox JA, Elliott FG: Primary adult lactose intolerance in the Kivu Lake area: Rwanda and the Bushi. *Am J Dig Dis* 19:714-23, 1974.

Dahlqvist A, Lindquist B: Lactose intolerance and protein malnutrition. *Acta Paediatr Scand* 60:488-94, 1971.

Desai HG, Chitre AV, Parekh DV, Jeejeebhoy KN: Intestinal disaccharidases in tropical sprue. *Gastroenterology* 53:375-80, 1967.

Desai, HG, Gupte UV, Pradhan AG, Thakkar KD, Antia FP: Incidence of lactase deficiency in control subjects from India: Role of hereditary factors. *Indian J Med Sci* 24:729-36, 1970.

Dupree L: Tajik. In *Muslim Peoples: A World Ethnographic Survey*, RV Weekes (ed). Westport, Conn.: Greenwood Press, 1978, pp 389-95.

Ehret C: Sheep and Central Sudanic peoples in southern Africa. *J Afr History* 9:213-21, 1968.

Ehret C: *Southern Nilotic History*. Evanston, Ill.: Northwestern University Press, 1971.

Ehret C: Patterns of Bantu and Central Sudanic settlement in central and southern Africa (ca. 1000 B.C.-500 A.D.). *Transafrican J History* 3:1-71, 1973.

Ehret C: Agricultural history in central and southern Africa ca. 1000 B.C. to A.D. 500. *Transafrican J History* 4:1-25, 1974.

Ehret C: On the antiquity of agriculture in Ethiopia. *J Afr History* 20:161-77, 1979.

Elliott FG, Cox J, Nyomba BL: Intolerance au lactose chez l'adulte en Afrique Centrale. *Ann Soc Belg Med Trop* 53:113-32, 1973.

El-Schallah MO, Rotthauwe HW, Flatz G: Laktose-Intoleranz in der arabischen Bevölkerung. *Med Welt* 24:1376-77, 1973.

Flatz G: Lactose tolerance: Genetics, anthropology, and natural selection. In *Excerpta Medica*

International Congress Series no 411: Human Genetics (Proceedings of the Fifth International Congress of Human Genetics, Mexico City, 10-15 October 1976), pp 386-96.

Flatz G, Rotthauwe HW: Evidence against nutritional adaption of tolerance to lactose. *Humangenetik* 13:118-25, 1971.

Flatz G, Rotthauwe HW: Lactose nutrition and natural selection. *Lancet* 2:76-77, 1973.

Flatz G, Rotthauwe HW: The human lactase polymorphism: Physiology and genetics of lactose absorption and malabsorption. In *Progress in Medical Genetics, NS, II*, AG Steinberg, AG Bearn, AG Motulsky, B Childs (eds). Philadelphia: Saunders, 1977, pp 205-49.

Flatz G, Saengudom C: Lactose tolerance in Asians: A family study. *Nature* 224:915-16, 1969.

Flatz G, Saengudom C, Sanguanbhokhai T: Lactose intolerance in Thailand. *Nature* 221:758-59, 1969.

Gabr M, El-Beheiry F, Soliman AA, El-Mahdi M, El-Mougy M, El-Akkad N: Lactose tolerance in normal Egyptian infants and children and in protein calorie nutrition. *Gaz Egypt Paediatr Assoc* 26:27-33, 1977.

Gilat T, Kuhn R, Gelman E, Mizrahy O: Lactase deficiency in Jewish communities in Israel. *Am J Dig Dis* 15:895-904, 1970.

Gupta PS, Misra RC, Ramachandran KA, Chuttani HK: Lactose intolerance in adults. *J Assoc Physicians India* 18:765-68, 1970.

Gupta PS, Misra RC, Ramachandran KA, Sarin GS, Chuttani HK: Intestinal disaccharidases activity in normal adult population in tropics. *J Trop Med Hyg* 74:225-29, 1971.

Habte D, Sterky G, Hjalmarsson B: Lactose malabsorption in Ethiopian children. *Acta Paediatr Scand* 62:649-54, 1973.

Heston LL, Gottesman II: The evolution of lactose tolerance. In *Summary of the Conference on Lactose and Milk Intolerance*, II Gottesman, LL Heston (eds). Washington, D.C.: Office of Child Development, US Dept of Health, Education and Welfare, 1973, pp 29-30.

Itkonen TI: Suomen Lappalaiset vuoteen 1945. [The Lapps in Finland up to 1945], vol 1. Porvoo, Helsinki: Werner Söderström Osakeyhtiö, 1948. Translated from the Finnish for the Human Relations Area Files by Eeva K. Minn.

Jackson RT, Latham MC: Lactose and milk intolerance in Tanzania. *East Afr Med J* 55:298-302, 1978.

Jackson RT, Latham MC: Lactose malabsorption among Masai children of East Africa. *Am J Clin Nutr* 32:779-82, 1979.

Jenkins T, Lehmann H, Nurse GT: Public health and genetic constitution of the San('Bushmen'): Carbohydrate metabolism and acetylator status of the !Kung of Tsumkwe in the north-western Kalahari. *Br Med J* 2:23-26, 1974.

Jersky J, Kinsley RH: Lactase deficiency in the South African Bantu. *S Afr Med J* 41:1194-96, 1967.

Keusch GT, Troncale FJ, Thavaramara B, Prinyanont P, Anderson PR, Bhamarapravathi N: Lactase deficiency in Thailand: Effect of prolonged lactose feeding. *Am J Clin Nutr* 22:638-41, 1969.

Kretchmer N: Memorial lecture: Lactose and lactase—a historical perspective. *Gastroenterology* 61:805-13, 1971.

Kretchmer N: Lactose and lactase. *Sci Am* 227:70-78, 1972.

Kretchmer N, Ransome-Kuti O: Lactose intolerance: An international problem. *Proc Inst Med Chic* 28:213-17, 1970.

Kretchmer N, Ransome-Kuti O, Hurwitz R, Dungy C, Alakija W: Intestinal absorption of lactose in Nigerian ethnic groups. *Lancet* 2:392-95, 1971.

Kroll H: Die Haustiere der Bantu. *Z Ethnologie* 60:177-290, 1928.

Krzyzaniak L: New light on early food-production in the central Sudan. *J Afr History* 19:159-72, 1978.

Leichter J: Lactose tolerance in a Slavic population. *Am J Dig Dis* 17:73-76, 1972.

Loiselet J, Jarjouhi L: L'intolérance au lactose chez l'aculte libanais. *J Med Liban* 27:339-50, 1974.

Lynch BM, Robbins LH: Cushitic and Nilotic prehistory: New archaeological evidence from north-west Kenya. *J Afr History* 20:319-28, 1979.

Madzarovova-Noheljlova J: Activity of intestinal disaccharidases. *Rev Czech Med* 15:212-34, 1969.

Malik GM, Khuroo MS, Ahmed SZ: Incidence of lactase intolerance in Kashmir. *J Assoc Physicians India* 25:623-25, 1977.

Murdock GP: *Africa: Its Peoples and Their Culture History*. New York: McGraw-Hill, 1959.

Murthy MS, Haworth JC: Intestinal lactase deficiency among East Indians. *Am J Gastroenterol* 53:246-51, 1970.

Nasrallah SM: Lactose intolerance in the Lebanese population and in 'Mediterranean lymphoma.' *Am J Clin Nutr* 32:1994-96, 1979.

Nurse GT: The origins of the northern Cape Griqua. ISMA paper No. 34. Johannesburg: Institute for the Study of Man in Africa, 1975.

Nurse GT, Jenkins T: Lactose intolerance in San populations. *Br Med J* 2:728, 1974.

Olatunbosun DA, Adadevoh BK: Lactase deficiency in Nigerians. *Am J Dig Dis* 16:909-14, 1971.

O'Morain C, Loubiere M, Rampal P, Sudaka P, Delmont J: Étude comparative de l'insuffisance en lactase de deux populations adultes différentes (55 Niçois et 55 Maghrebins). *Acta Gastroenterol Belg* 41:56-63, 1978.

Pieters JJL, Van Rens R: Lactose malabsorption and milk tolerance in Kenyan school-age children. *Trop Geogr Med* 25:365-71, 1973.

Rab SM, Baseer A: High intestinal lactase concentration in adult Pakistanis. *Br Med J* 1:436-37, 1976.

Rahimi AG, Delbruck H, Haeckel R, Goedde HW, Flatz G: Persistence of high intestinal lactase activity (lactose tolerance) in Afghanistan. *Hum Genet* 34:57-62, 1976.

Ransome-Kuti O, Kretchmer N, Johnson J, Gribble JT: Family studies of lactose intolerance in Nigerian ethnic groups. *Pediatr Res* 6:359, 1972.

Ransome-Kuti O, Kretchmer N, Johnson JD, Gribble JT: A genetic study of lactose digestion in Nigerian families. *Gastroenterology* 68:431-46, 1975.

Reddy V, Pershad J: Lactase deficiency in Indians. *Am J Clin Nutr* 25:114-19, 1972.

Sadre M, Karbasi K: Lactose intolerance in Iran. *Am J Clin Nutr* 32:1948-54, 1979.

Sahi T: Lactose malabsorption in Finnish-speaking and Swedish-speaking populations in Finland. *Scand J Gastroenterol* 9:303-08, 1974.

Sahi T: Intestinal lactase polymorphisms and dairy foods. *Hum Genet* suppl 1:115-23, 1978.

Sahi T, Eriksson AW, Isokoski M, Kirjarinta M: Isolated adult-type lactose malabsorption in Finnish Lapps. In *Circumpolar Health: Proceedings of the 3rd International Symposium on Circumpolar Health, Yellowknife, Northwest Territories 1974*, RJ Shepherd, S Itoh (eds). Toronto: University of Toronto Press, 1976, pp 145-49.

Senewiratne B, Thambipillai S, Perera H: Intestinal lactase deficiency in Ceylon (Sri Lanka). *Gastroenterology* 72:1257-59, 1977.

Simoons FJ: The non-milking area of Africa. *Anthropos* 49:58-66, 1954.

Simoons FJ: Primary adult lactose intolerance and the milking habit: A problem in biological and cultural interrelations. II. A culture historical hypothesis. *Am J Dig Dis* 15:695-710, 1970a.

Simoons FJ: The traditional limits of milking and milk use in southern Asia. *Anthropos* 65:547-93, 1970b.

Simoons FJ: The antiquity of dairying in Asia and Africa. *Geog Rev* 61:431-39, 1971.

Simoons FJ: The determinants of dairying and milk use in the Old World: Ecological, physiological, and cultural. *Ecol Food Nutr* 2:83-90, 1973.

Simoons FJ: The geographic hypothesis and lactose malabsorption: A weighing of the evidence. *Am J Dig Dis* 23:963-80, 1978.

Sung JL, Shih PL: The jejunal disaccharidase activity and lactose intolerance of Chinese adults. *Asian J Med* 8:149-51, 1972.

Swaminathan N, Mathan VI, Baker SJ, Radhakrishnan AN: Disaccharidase levels in jejunal biopsy specimens from American and South Indian control subjects and patients with tropical sprue. *Clin Chim Acta* 30:707-12, 1970.

Tandon RK, Goel U, Mukherjee SN, Pandey SC, Lal K: Lactose intolerance during pregnancy in different Indian communities. *Indian J Med Res* 66:33-38, 1977.

Troncale FJ, Keusch GT, Miller LH, Olson RA, Buchanan RD: Normal absorption in Thai subjects with non-specific jejunal abnormalities. *Br Med J* 4:578-80, 1967.

Valenkevich LN: Activity of lactase and the syndrome of milk intolerance. *Klin Med* (Mosk) 55:66-70, 1977.

Varavithya W, Valyasevi A, Manu P, Kittikool J: Lactose malabsorption in Thai infants and children: Effect of prolonged milk feeding. *Southeast Asian J Trop Med Public Health* 7:591-95, 1976.

White EO, Latham MC: Lactose and milk intolerance in Ghanaian nursery school children. *J Nutr* 103:xviii, 1973.

III

PHYSIOPATHOLOGIC
CONSIDERATIONS

CHAPTER 4

LACTOSE MALABSORPTION

AND GASTROINTESTINAL FUNCTION

EFFECTS ON GASTROINTESTINAL TRANSIT AND

THE ABSORPTION OF OTHER NUTRIENTS

Sidney F. Phillips

The purpose of this chapter is to give perspective to the range of pathophysiological consequences that accompany malabsorption of lactose. These consequences will be considered in more detail in subsequent chapters, and the present material should be considered as an overview of the subject.

LACTOSE MALABSORPTION—A VARIABLE BALANCE

Man is a complex organism and it is therefore not surprising that activities so fundamental to life and health as the absorption of nutrients are complex, integrated functions, involving many steps. However, prime attention often is directed more towards the results than to the component steps. Thus, something apparently as simple as a glucose tolerance test involves numerous steps, including gastric emptying, mucosal uptake, and metabolism of absorbed glucose. So it is with lactose malabsorption. The level of intestinal lactase is only one of several important factors, any one of which has rate-limiting potential, in determining the symptomatic consequences and pathophysiology of lactose ingestion.

Figure 4.1 shows this concept as a simple balance diagram. Several factors tend to reduce the consequences of lactose ingestion in susceptible individuals:

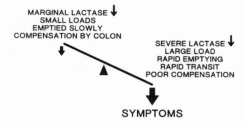

MARGINAL LACTASE ↓
SMALL LOADS
EMPTIED SLOWLY
COMPENSATION BY COLON

SEVERE LACTASE ↓
LARGE LOAD
RAPID EMPTYING
RAPID TRANSIT
POOR COMPENSATION

SYMPTOMS

FIGURE 4.1. Scheme showing some factors that tend to minimize (left side) or maximize (right side) the symptomatic response to ingestion of lactose in hypolactasia.

(1) minimal deficiencies of mucosal lactase; (2) small oral loads of lactose; and (3) slow emptying from stomach to small intestine. Thus, the small bowel faces a theoretical overload that covers a full spectrum of severity. Further, with regard to the symptoms resulting from lactose malabsorption, the role of the colon is key. Figure 4.1 indicates simply that "compensation" by the colon may be adequate or poor. Even here, another integrated activity must be considered. Many of the symptoms of lactose malabsorption are attributable to the actions of bacterial enzymes on carbohydrate. Thus, the nature and number of the fecal flora, the degree to which they hydrolyze unabsorbed lactose, and the ability of the colonic mucosa to deal with the end products (gases and volatile fatty acids) all are important potential contributors to the degree of compensation that can be achieved.

LACTOSE AND GASTRIC EMPTYING

Although the hypothesis has not been tested by specific experiments, it is probable that gastric emptying influences the nature of any symptoms that may develop. Thus, for any given oral load of lactose the small intestine should deal more easily with sugar that empties slowly, as a steady stimulus, than with a large bolus. A further point concerns the possible effects of lactose maldigestion per se on the rate of gastric emptying.

Pirk and Skala (1972) used an x-ray technique to show that milk containing lactose emptied from the stomachs of subjects with lactase deficiency more slowly than did lactose-free milk. On the other hand, Welsh and Hall (1977) showed that lactase-deficient subjects emptied lactose faster than they emptied equivalent loads of glucose. In normal subjects, glucose and lactose emptied at the same rate. The latter results are anticipated, since gastric emptying is thought to be modified by duodenal osmo-receptors that are located interior to the brush border. In other words, healthy subjects should respond to the osmotic force of disaccharides as if they were monosaccharides, whereas lactase-deficient subjects should "see" lactose only as a disaccharide. In hypolactasia, lactose will have a lesser osmotic potential and be a correspondingly reduced stimulus to the slowing of gastric emptying.

The possibility remains, therefore, that meals containing lactose might empty rapidly in hypolactasia, and one might speculate that rapid emptying might play a role in the development of symptoms. The area probably deserves further study. After gastric surgery, when gastric emptying of liquids is rapid, lactose malabsorption is said to be "unmasked" (Bank et al. 1966, Gudmand-Høyer 1969).

LACTOSE AS AN OSMOTIC FORCE IN THE SMALL BOWEL

This first major consequence of lactose malabsorption is perhaps the simplest to understand. Intestinal epithelia behave as lipid membranes that contain aqueous pores of finite size. Whereas lipophilic solutes cross the mucosa with relative ease, hydrophilic molecules are "filtered" according to size, unless a specific active mechanism of transport is present. Disaccharides have no such mechanism and are too large to undergo passive transport of any quantitative significance. Since the jejunal epithelium is freely permeable to water [a "leaky" membrane in the terminology of Diamond (1974)], there is a strong tendency for osmotic equilibrium to be established. The retention of disaccharide in the lumen provides an osmotic force for water and sodium (to which the jejunum also is freely permeable) to move into the lumen. Thus, the volume of chyme increases (Launiala 1968a, b; Christopher and Bayless 1971).

Malabsorption of lactose is an expected consequence of lactase deficiency, and quantitative or semiquantitative studies have taken several different approaches. Debongnie et al. (1979) used a test meal of milk, labeled with a nonabsorbable marker. The content of sugar was quantified as the meal passed through the distal ileum, 1 to 5 hours postprandially. A second ileal marker was used to indicate the degree to which the meal was recovered by aspiration. In healthy controls, essentially no lactose was identified in the ileum; in subjects with lactase deficiency up to 50% of lactose (10 g) in the meal escaped digestion and absorption. Bond and Levitt (1976a) showed that 0% to 8% of a 12.5 g dose of lactose was recovered in the ileum of controls; 42% to 75% was recoverable in hypolactasia.

EFFECTS OF UNABSORBED CARBOHYDRATE IN TRANSIT IN THE SMALL INTESTINE

Several different experimental approaches have been used to examine the possibility that unabsorbed lactose stimulates intestinal motor activity and hastens transit through the small bowel. Launiala (1968b, 1969) looked at transit through a perfused segment of jejunum, while Bond and Levitt (1975) used the appearance of hydrogen in the breath after a dose of lactulose as an index of mouth to cecum transit time. Debongnie et al. (1979) used the timed recovery of a meal marker to assess transit from mouth to ileum. All studies point to more rapid transit through the small bowel when lactose absorption is incomplete. Still unsettled is the location of the rapid transit; in theory, gastric emptying could be speeded, intestinal transit might be rapid, or both effects might operate. Also unanswered is the possible consequence of rapid transit through the small bowel. Does this, in turn, further impair absorption of lactose and fluid?

OSMOTIC CONSEQUENCES OF BACTERIAL FERMENTATION

Unabsorbed carbohydrate, on reaching the fecal flora, does not remain an inert, osmotic agent. Bacterial hydrolysis of sugars has a physical impact on the composition of chyme (increasing the osmolality) as well as a chemical one (biotransformation of sugar, with production of organic acids). In simple terms, 5 g monosaccharide or 10 g lactose, when dissolved in 100 ml water, yields a solution with an osmolality of approximately 280. Fermentation produces more molecules of lesser molecular weight and, since osmotic pressure is a colligative property, osmolality increases. This was shown in vivo when the osmolality of intestinal contents and stools was examined in lactase-deficient subjects (Christopher and Bayless 1971). Contents aspirated from the small bowel were isosmolar with extracellular fluid, feces were hypertonic. These studies also confirmed the decrease in pH of intestinal contents during bacterial biotransformations, due to the generation of short-chain fatty acids.

FATE OF SHORT-CHAIN (VOLATILE) FATTY ACIDS IN THE COLON

Bustos-Fernandez et al. (1971) first drew attention to the importance of organic anions (acetate, butyrate, proprionate) as major constituents of normal human stools, though it had been known before that these compounds were found in the stools of infants with diarrhea who continued to take formula (Torres-Pinedo et al. 1966). It was thus predictable that the fermentation of lactose by the fecal flora would lead to production of the same fecal anions. But questions remained. Did the colon absorb some or all of these ions? Did their presence, and the reduced pH they caused, interfere with colonic absorption, and so aggravate diarrhea?

The experiments of Bond and Levitt (1976b) showed clearly the ability of the human colon to absorb the gaseous byproducts of lactose fermentation. Another group (Ruppin et al. 1980), using colonic perfusion, reached the same conclusion for organic anions. Moreover, they showed that concentrations of organic anions in the range found in stools (up to 90 mM) do not impair absorption of sodium chloride and water by the human colon. In fact, sodium and water absorption was increased. In earlier studies, the same group had demonstrated effective absorption of organic anions in the human ileum (Schmitt et al. 1977).

Thus, following the bacterial fermentation of lactose, some end products are absorbed, some are excreted in the stools, but colonic absorption of sodium, chloride, and water was unimpaired. As to whether loose stools develop or not in susceptible subjects after a lactose load, a balance might have to be struck. On each occasion, the reabsorptive properties of the colon will minimize symptoms; however, important but poorly documented additional factors in any individual will include the nature of the fecal flora and transit time of material through the colon.

LACTOSE MALABSORPTION AND THE ABSORPTION
OF OTHER NUTRIENTS

Studies to evaluate the bioavailability of the nutrients in lactase-deficient sub- jects have relied primarily on measurement of fecal excretion of fat and nitrogen. When adults with lactase deficiency are given a diet containing lactose, fecal fat excretion generally remains normal (Ringrose et al. 1972, Calloway and Chenoweth 1973). However, if the gastrointestinal tract is abnormal, such as in patients with previous gastric surgery or in the short bowel syndrome, fecal fat may increase significantly. Calloway and Chenoweth (1973) observed no azotorrhea when lactase-deficient adults ingested milk as the only form of dietary protein. However, similar studies in children with lactase deficiency yielded variable results (Paige and Graham 1972, Bowie 1975, Brand et al. 1977).

In addition to these balance studies, intestinal aspiration and perfusion has been used to assess directly the absorption of lactose and other nutrients. Thus, Bond and Levitt (1976a) demonstrated that only 30% to 60% of a 12.5 g load of lactose, equivalent to one glass of milk, was absorbed in the small bowel by lactase-deficient subjects, compared with 90% to 100% by healthy controls. Launiala (1969) showed that sucrase-isomaltase deficiency was associated also with decreased absorption of xylose, palmitic acid, and arginine. In a less direct approach, impaired absorption of calcium has been demonstrated in lactase- deficient subjects (Kocian et al. 1973).

Our group determined whether malabsorption of lactose, secondary to lactase deficiency, influenced absorption of other nutrients in milk, specifically, protein, fat, and minerals (Debongnie et al. 1979). An infusion-aspiration technique was used that allowed quantification of flow through the terminal ileum after a test meal of milk. Healthy and lactase-deficient volunteers were studied after the ingestion of whole milk, or a milk in which lactose had been hydrolyzed pre- viously to glucose and galactose.

In the fasting state, ileal flow of protein, carbohydrate, electrolytes, and fluid was small and not different in controls and lactase-deficient subjects. Ileal flow increased in all subjects after the test meal of milk. More fluid and nutrient were recovered from the ileum in lactase-deficient subjects after ingesting whole milk than in control subjects or in lactase-deficient subjects after ingesting lactose- hydrolyzed milk. Two deficient subjects showed marked malabsorption of lac- tose (35% and 50%); two did not. Protein, calcium, magnesium, and phosphorus also were recovered from the ileum in greater quantities in lactase-deficient subjects after ingesting whole milk.

However, over 90% of the fat and protein contained in the meal was absorbed, even by the lactase-deficient subjects after ingesting milk containing lactose and the calories remaining unabsorbed from the entire meal were 5% in healthy subjects but only 14% in lactase-deficient subjects. Thus, significant fat and protein malnutrition seems an unlikely consequence of hypolactasia. The role of disturbed mineral absorption also is unlikely to be of major nutritional significance. Osteoporosis is common in lactase deficiency (Birge et al. 1967, Newcomer et al. 1978), but reports of calcium absorption in hypolactasia are conflicting, showing a decrease (Condon et al. 1970), an increase (Pansu and Chapuy 1970), or no change (Kocian et al. 1973) when compared to controls.

SUMMARY

The maldigestion of lactose leads to an abnormal composition of chyme, which, in turn, may have a variety of effects on gastrointestinal function. Of these possible consequences, malabsorption of lactose and rapid transit of chyme through the small intestine are documented best. More speculative are effects on gastric emptying; these have not been studied extensively, but could be of importance. There are few indications that lactose malabsorption has important effects on the absorption of other nutrients. When lactose reaches the fecal flora a series of metabolic events occur. These are important in the production of symptoms, but the normal colon has the potential of limiting the consequences by absorbing volatile fatty acids, which are major fermentative end products.

REFERENCES

Bank S, Barbezat GO, Marks IN: Postgastrectomy steatorrhea due to intestinal lactase deficiency. *S Afr Med J* 40:597–99, 1966.

Birge SJ Jr, Keutmann HT, Cuatrecasas P, Whedon GD: Osteoporosis, intestinal lactase deficiency and low dietary calcium intake. *N Engl J Med* 276:445–48, 1967.

Bond JH, Levitt MD: Investigation of small bowel transit time in man utilizing pulmonary hydrogen (H_2) measurements. *J Lab Clin Med* 85:546–55, 1975.

Bond JH, Levitt MD: Quantitative measurement of lactose absorption. *Gastroenterology* 70:1058–62, 1976a.

Bond JH, Levitt MD: Fate of soluble carbohydrate in the colon of rats and man. *J Clin Invest* 57:1158–64, 1976b.

Bowie MD: Effect of lactose-induced diarrhoea on absorption of nitrogen and fat. *Arch Dis Child* 50:363–66, 1975.

Brand JC, Miller JJ, Vorbach EA, Edwards RA: A trial of lactose hydrolyzed milk in Australian aboriginal children. *Med J Aust* (spec suppl) 2:10–13, 1977.

Bustos-Fernandez R, Gonzalez E, Marzi A, dePaolo MIL: Fecal acidorrhea. *N Engl J Med* 284:295–98, 1971.

Calloway DH, Chenoweth WL: Utilization of nutrients in milk- and wheat-based diets by men with adequate and reduced abilities to absorb lactose: I. Energy and nitrogen. *Am J Clin Nutr* 26:939–51, 1973.

Christopher NL, Bayless TM: Role of the small bowel and colon in lactose-induced diarrhea. *Gastroenterology* 60:845–52, 1971.

Condon JR, Nassim JR, Millard JC, Hilbe A, Stainthorpe EM: Calcium and phosphorus metabolism in relation to lactose tolerance. *Lancet* 1:1027–29, 1970.

Debongnie JC, Newcomer AD, McGill DB, Phillips SF: Absorption of nutrients in lactase deficiency. *Dig Dis Sci* 24:225–31, 1979.

Diamond JM: Tight and leaky junctions of epithelia: A perspective on kisses in the dark. *Fed Proc* 33:2220–23, 1974.

Gudmand-Høyer E: Lactose malabsorption after gastric surgery. *Digestion* 2:289–97, 1969.

Kocian J, Skala I, Bakos K: Calcium absorption from milk and lactose-free milk in healthy subjects and patients with lactose intolerance. *Digestion* 9:317–24, 1973.

Launiala K: The mechanism of diarrhea in congenital disaccharide malabsorption. *Acta Paediatr Scand* 57:425–32, 1968a.

Launiala K: The effect of unabsorbed sucrose and mannitol on the small intestinal flow rate and mean transit time. *Scand J Gastroenterol* 3:665–71, 1968b.

Launiala K: The effect of unabsorbed sucrose or mannitol-induced accelerated transit on absorption in the human small intestine. *Scand J Gastroenterol* 4:25–32, 1969.

Newcomer AD, Hodgson SF, McGill DB, Thomas PJ: Lactase deficiency: Prevalence in osteoporosis. *Ann Intern Med* 89:218–20, 1978.

Paige DM, Graham GG: Nutritional implications of lactose malabsorption. *Pediatr Res* 6:329, 1972.

Pansu D, Chapuy MC: Calcium absorption enhanced by lactose and xylose. *Calcif Tissue Res* 4(suppl):155–56, 1970.

Pirk F, Skala I: Functional response of the digestive tract to the ingestion of milk in subjects suffering from lactose intolerance. *Digestion* 5:89–99, 1972.

Ringrose RE, Thompson JB, Welsh JD: Lactose malabsorption and steatorrhea. *Am J Dig Dis* 17:533–38, 1972.

Ruppin H, Bar-Meir S, Soergel KH, Wood CM, Schmitt MG Jr: Absorption of short chain fatty acids by the colon. *Gastroenterology* 78:1500–07, 1980.

Schmitt JG Jr, Soergel KH, Wood CM, Steff JJ: Absorption of short chain fatty acids from the human ileum. *Am J Dig Dis* 22:340–47, 1977.

Torres-Pinedo R, Lavastida M, Rivera CL, Rodriguez H, Ortiz A: Studies in infant diarrhea: I. A comparison of the effects of milk feeding and intravenous therapy on the composition and volume of the stool and urine. *J Clin Invest* 45:469–80, 1966.

Welsh JD, Hall WH: Gastric emptying of lactose and milk in subjects with lactose malabsorption. *Am J Dig Dis* 22:1060–63, 1977.

CHAPTER 5

CARBOHYDRATE DIGESTION

EFFECTS OF MONOSACCHARIDE INHIBITION

AND ENZYME DEGRADATION ON

LACTASE ACTIVITY

D. H. Alpers

The intestine has a great capacity to absorb monosaccharides. The maximum capacity for absorption of glucose and fructose, the component sugars of sucrose, has been estimated at over 10,000 g per day (Holdsworth and Dawson 1964). The capacity for absorption of glucose and galactose from lactose hydrolysis should be as great. Moreover, the majority of monosaccharide absorption follows a downhill chemical gradient, since luminal concentrations after a meal exceed 10 mM (180 mg per dl) for at least 30 minutes (Crane 1975).

The level of lactase in terms of specific activity (units per gram) is the lowest of the three major disaccharidases. It is about one-half that of sucrase and one-quarter or less that of maltase (Newcomer and McGill 1966). Within the normal enzyme range for sucrase, the rate of liberation of monosaccharide exceeds the considerable capacity of the intestine to absorb glucose. In order to see any effect on the rate of monosaccharide absorption from sucrose, the level of sucrase activity must be diminished markedly to below the lower limits of normal. Therefore the amount of sucrase activity on the brush border (and by analogy the amount of maltase activity) is not rate limiting for monosaccharide absorption.

LACTOSE DIGESTION

On the other hand, lactase activity is at least one-half that of sucrase, and the normal range of activity is quite wide for lactase. Possible reasons for the wide range among the disaccharidases will be discussed below. In the normal lactase range, the rate of hydrolysis does not exceed the capacity to absorb all of the glucose from lactose. As a result, any change in lactase activity within the normal range theoretically can affect the rate of monosaccharide absorption from lactose, and this change becomes even more critical below the normal range. Therefore, one need not be lactase deficient to suffer periodic lactose intolerance. If given enough lactose, even someone with a lactase activity that falls within the normal range may suffer from lactose intolerance.

FACTORS AFFECTING LACTASE ACTIVITY

A number of factors may affect lactose absorption by influencing the lactase enzyme. The genetic predisposition to a low level of lactase protein is discussed in chapter 2. The emphasis here is on factors that can affect lactose hydrolysis or the activity of lactase after the protein is made from the messenger RNA on the ribosomes.

Lactase is localized to the intestinal brush border. It is a glycoprotein and, arguing from the data on sucrase and maltase, the carbohydrate side chains contain about 10 or 11 sugar residues (Kelly and Alpers 1973). The protein is attached by a peptide bond to a hydrophobic region on the protein, which presumably is inserted into the membrane lipid bilayer. Although this "anchor piece" never has been demonstrated in lactase, it has been documented for other brush border proteins (Maroux and Louvard 1976). Lactase is released easily from the membrane by proteolysis; in this respect it differs from some other brush border proteins such as alkaline phosphatase, which are embedded more deeply in the lipid bilayer and require lipid solvents in order to be released.

Enzyme Inhibition. The first factor that can modify lactose hydrolysis, over and above any change in absolute lactase activity levels, is inhibition of the enzyme. The hydrolysis of lactose in a perfused system in rat intestine has been studied (Alpers and Cote 1971). Since adult rats are lactase deficient, the rate of absorption of sugar from lactose is limited by the amount of enzyme. The percentage of perfused lactose hydrolyzed is not inhibited by xylose, but it is inhibited by adding galactose, fructose, or glucose to the medium (fig. 5.1). The same results were seen when disaccharides were perfused.

Hydrolysis of other disaccharides eaten at a meal containing lactose also can inhibit lactose hydrolysis. Sucrose or maltose are hydrolyzed into their component sugars and those component sugars can inhibit further lactose hydrolysis. Thus, lactose hydrolysis is affected not only by the monosaccharides ingested

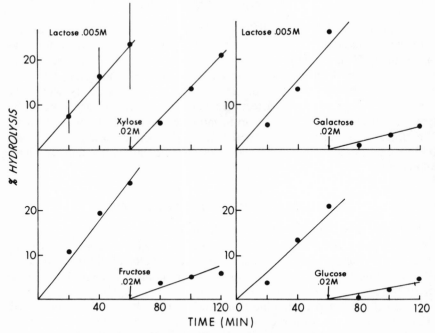

FIGURE 5.1. Inhibition of lactose hydrolysis during in vivo perfusion of monosaccharides. Experiments were done in rat using a recirculating perfusion system. Source: Alpers and Cote 1971, reprinted with permission.

and by the monosaccharides derived from lactose, but also by the monosaccharides derived from other carbohydrates (sucrose and maltose).

The monosaccharide concentration in the rat intestinal lumen after infusion of disaccharides varies between 4 mM and 11 mM, certainly a range in which the sugars can have inhibitory effects. The half maximal inhibition (K_i) occurs at about 20 mM to 25 mM (Alpers and Cote 1971). This calculation ignores the factor of the concentration in the unstirred water layer, which might be considerably higher but could not be measured during these experiments.

Monosaccharide inhibition of lactase activity is dependent on pH, with greater inhibition at pH 6 than at pH 7.4. Since pH 6 is optimal for the disaccharidases themselves, the microenvironment around the brush border is assumed to be approximately pH 6. This never has been demonstrated clearly, but seems a reasonable assumption. Not only is hydrolysis of lactose and the inhibition of the enzyme maximal at pH 6, but the transport of monosaccharides into the intestines is also maximal at pH 6, at least in experimental animals (Iida et al. 1968). Presumably the same would be true for man. Monosaccharide inhibition occurs not only at the same pH as maximal lactose hydrolysis but also at concentrations that are perfectly consistent with those of monosaccharides (20 mM to 30 mM) after a meal (table 5.1). Thus such inhibition easily could occur physiologically.

Inhibition of lactase activity may be a factor in producing some of the variable results of standard lactose tolerance tests, and in affecting tolerance of different doses of lactose. Moreover, it may play a role in the alteration of lactose intolerance noted when milk is ingested with other foods. (See chapters 10 and 11.)

Enzyme Degradation. The release of lactase from the membrane and subsequent degradation of the enzyme also influence lactose hydrolysis. The enzymes that can effect such changes are pancreatic (Alpers and Tedesco 1975) and bacterial (Jonas et al. 1978) proteases. Only the effects of pancreatic proteases will be discussed here. The experiments described below are based on the theoretical considerations developed by Arias, Doyle, and Schimke (1969) in which the turnover of membrane proteins was measured by administering the same amino acid to animals on two occasions, once labeled with ^3H, and once labeled with ^{14}C. For example, ^{14}C is given first to the animal. After a period of time, during which the labeled proteins are degraded at different rates, the other label (^3H) is given and the process of protein degradation allowed to proceed for a finite time. If the labeled proteins are degraded at different rates, the ratio of ^3H to ^{14}C is a measure of how rapidly the protein turns over. Proteins that turn over rapidly have a high ^3H to ^{14}C ratio; those that turn over slowly have a low ratio. It should be noted that this is only a relative ratio, since no absolute turnover rates are obtained in this way.

This experiment was performed in normal animals and the brush border proteins were isolated and separated. A large peak was observed, corresponding to a high ^3H to ^{14}C ratio (fig. 5.2). When the brush border is isolated and the proteins are denatured and separated on an SDS acrylamide gel, at least 20 protein bands can be seen (Alpers and Tedesco 1975). Proteins that turn over rapidly occur in the high molecular weight region of the brush border ($> 150,000$), a region

TABLE 5.1
Effect of pH on monosaccharide
inhibition of intestinal lactase

Inhibitor	pH	K_1
Glucose	6.0	0.03
	7.4	0.177
Galactose	6.0	0.022
	7.4	0.190
Fructose	6.0	0.034
	7.4	0.221

Note: Experiments were performed in an intact rat using a recirculating perfusion system as described by Alpers and Cote (1971).

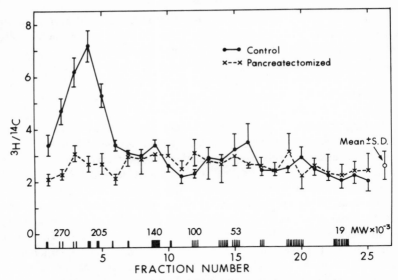

FIGURE 5.2. Effect of 95% pancreatectomy on turnover of brush border proteins. Valine was the labeled amino acid used. Brush borders from rat jejunum were isolated after double labeling and separated on SDS acrylamide gels. The mean (± SD) for a control experiment where both labels are given together is shown on the right. A high ratio means more rapid turnover. Source: Alpers and Tedesco 1975, reprinted with permission.

corresponding to that which includes all of the major disaccharidases. Sucrase has a molecular weight of 205,000, and lactase is somewhat larger. The relative turnover rate of the remaining proteins in the brush border is quite slow, since it differs not at all from control experiments in which the labels are given simultaneously.

Although 95% pancreatectomy eliminates all of the rapid turnover of the large proteins (fig. 5.2), if elastase is fed by tube to the pancreatectomized animals the normal pattern of rapid turnover is restored. Elastase restores turnover more effectively than either trypsin or chymotrypsin, but all of the proteases will reverse the findings in pancreatectomized rats. Elastase has a less specific pattern of proteolysis and exactly the same specificity (hydrolyzing next to neutral amino acids) as does papain, a plant protease that traditionally is used to solubilize disaccharidases from the brush border. Therefore, mammals appear to develop in the intestine large amounts of a protease that has the same specificity as papain and that can be partially responsible for the rapid removal and turnover of disaccharidases and other large proteins in the intestinal brush border. Since the rat makes a particularly large amount of elastase compared to trypsin and chymotrypsin, it is unclear whether elastase has an equal importance in man.

Animals with spontaneous exocrine pancreatic insufficiency, developed by Dr. Leitner at Jackson Laboratories, also have been examined (Kwong et al.

1978). The mouse with exocrine pancreatic insufficiency and normal islets has elevated levels of all three disaccharidases (table 5.2). This result is consistent with a slowing down in the rate of turnover, reaching a new steady state in which the levels of the enzymes are increased. When pancreatic enzymes are added to the feed of the animals, these levels all return towards normal.

These examples differ somewhat from the results in man with pancreatic insufficiency. Maltase and sucrase levels in man are elevated, whereas lactase levels are not. It is not clear why lactase levels rise in an experimental animal from which one can remove all or virtually all of the pancreatic enzyme activities, while in man the lactase level does not rise although the entire pancreas rarely is removed (except in a few instances where it is removed surgically). It is possible that in man whatever remaining pancreatic proteolytic activity may affect lactase activity. Before discussing that possibility, it is necessary to mention factors other than proteases that can affect the release of sucrase (and other disaccharidases) from the membrane.

The factors responsible for sucrase release probably include more than just the pancreatic enzymes, although these proteins are sufficient by themselves in vitro. Another important factor is luminal pH (fig. 5.3). The effects of the proteases on sucrase release from the brush border do not occur at the maximal 7.5 pH of the proteases themselves. The release effect occurs maximally at pH 7, and begins to rise at pH 6. These pH values may approximate the microenvironment on the surface of the brush border, since transport and digestive functions work maximally at pH 6.

In addition to pancreatic enzymes, bile acids, fatty acids, and phospholipids are important components of intestinal contents after a meal. Only studies in vitro with lysolecithin will be described, although similar enhancement of sucrase release has been obtained with bile acids. Lysolecithin, but not lecithin, will enhance the release of sucrase or lactase from brush borders by proteases. Sucrase release will increase by 27% at concentrations as low as 10 μg per ml when added to isolated rat brush borders in the presence of elastase (0.1 mg per ml). At

TABLE 5.2
Stimulation of brush border enzyme activity by exocrine
pancreatic insufficiency

Group of mice	Enzyme		
	Maltase	Lactase	Sucrase
Normal	0.16 ± 0.06	0.06 ± 0.0005	0.033 ± 0.01
Exocrine pancreatic insufficiency (Epi)	0.25 ± 0.07	0.112 ± 0.0016	0.076 ± 0.02
Epi + pancreatin	0.20 ± 0.05	0.052 ± 0.0015	0.051 ± 0.01

Note: The values reported are mean specific activities from 8 mice in each group, as described in Kwong et al. (1978).

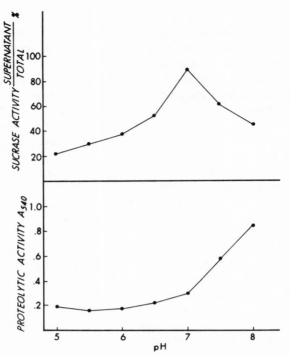

FIGURE 5.3. The effect of pH on release of sucrase activity from rat intestinal brush borders. Buffers used included acetate and phosphate. Proteolytic activity was assayed using casein as substrate.

a concentration of 50 μg per ml of lysolecithin, sucrase release increases by 46%. Thus, pancreatic enzymes in conjunction with lysolecithin and bile acids may be important in modifying the brush border surface. These substances all are present in the lumen of the intestine.

It has been suggested by Rosensweig and Herman (1969) that as the cells move up the villus, enzyme may be lost by cell extrusion from the tip (fig. 5.4). In addition, data from our laboratory suggest that as the cell moves up the villus, pancreatic proteases, along with other intraluminal factors, modify the surface proteins of the small intestine, either removing them from the membrane or destroying them either in situ or after removal from the membrane. This modification certainly could happen in the case of lactase and if so it may be an important factor in determining the amount of lactase on the brush border. In disease states such as gastroenteritis and parasitic infestations, where the surface coating of the intestine may be damaged in some way, it is conceivable that pancreatic proteases, or other intraluminal factors, may have greater access to the surface disaccharidases, and may effect a greater release and/or destruction of these enzymes.

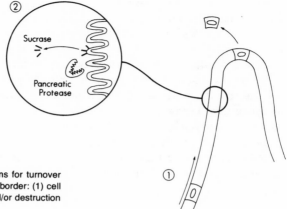

FIGURE 5.4. Proposed mechanisms for turnover of large proteins in intestinal brush border: (1) cell migration and loss, (2) removal and/or destruction by pancreatic enzymes.

Effect of Pancreatic Proteases in Man. The hypothesis that pancreatic proteases may affect lactase activity in man in vivo has been examined. Human lactase is certainly susceptible to the effects of pancreatic proteases in vitro. The effect of trypsin on lactase activity in brush borders isolated from four groups of patients, Caucasian infants and adults, and black infants and adults, has been tested (Seetharam et al. 1980). The brush borders were incubated with trypsin at a ratio of 1.3 units of trypsin per unit of lactase. The amount of lactase that remains after incubation is diminished by 25% in all groups except lactase-deficient black adults. In this case, the inhibition of activity is much greater (75%). Since there is less lactase activity (roughly one-tenth that of the other groups of patients, including the black infants), the ratio of trypsin to lactase is greater in the black adults. When the ratio of lactase to trypsin was adjusted to compare with that of the other groups, by increasing the amount of lactase (i.e., membranes) in the system, the loss of activity by trypsin was diminished and approached the inhibition found in the other groups (45%). This finding suggests that the lactase present in lactase-deficient patients has no special sensitivity to the proteases themselves, but is simply there in much smaller quantities, so that the relative ratio of protease to lactase is greater. The possibility cannot be eliminated that there is some specific sensitivity to protease involving lactase from lactase-deficient adult subjects. Whatever the reason for these results, in the case of lactase deficiency there will be more pancreatic protease in the intestinal lumen relative to the lactase than there is in normal subjects. The possibility of altering lactase activity in vivo under various physiological and pathological circumstances is greater in patients with lactase deficiency than in the normal subjects.

A group of white and black subjects who had pancreatic insufficiency was studied to determine the effect of pancreatic enzymes on lactase activity in vivo. In the absence of pancreatic enzymes (Viokase) in the white patients, results similar to those of Arvanitakis and Olsen (1974) were found, that is, the lactase levels are normal whereas sucrase and maltase levels are elevated above those of normal subjects. The lactase-deficient patients of course had low lactase activity but also had elevated sucrase and maltase compared to the controls given pancreatic extract (Viokase). With the addition of Viokase in a standard dose of five tablets with every meal, levels of all three disaccharidases fell. The absolute fall in lactase for the Caucasians was greater than that for the blacks, but the relative difference was greater in the black subjects. There was almost a 40% decrease in lactase activity in the lactase-deficient patients after the addition of pancreatic enzymes. The lactase levels were in the range (2 to 8 units per g protein) where any fall in enzyme activity could lead to an alteration in sugar absorption.

Does addition of pancreatic enzymes involve removal from the brush border membrane alone or partial proteolysis of the lactase leading to any changes in the enzyme protein itself? This question was approached by isolating lactase from

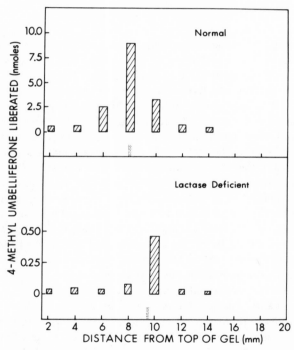

FIGURE 5.5. Lactase activity of enzyme from normal and lactase-deficient patients separated by SDS acrylamide electrophoresis. Twenty μg each of normal and low activity adult lactase previously purified on acrylamide gels were added to one pair of SDS gels. Fifty μg of protein were applied to another pair of gels. The first pair of gels was electrophoresed in SDS, and stained for protein. The protein stains are recorded graphically in the lower part of each bar graph. The other gels were electrophoresed and cut unfixed into slices using a razor blade holder with blades at 2 mm intervals. The slices were homogenized in 50mM sodium phosphate buffer pH 6.0, eluted for four hours, and the eluate dialyzed overnight against 10mM buffer. A fluorometric assay for lactase was used with unbelliferyl-β-galactoside as substrate. Incubation of 20 μl of eluate from normal enzyme gels was for two hours; eluate from gels containing enzyme from lactase-deficient patients required four hours before easily detectable hydrolysis occurred.

normal and lactase-deficient subjects. The purified enzymes from lactase-deficient and normal patients were placed on SDS acrylamide gels (fig. 5.5) where the migration towards the positive pole is dependent upon the molecular weight. Normal enzyme migrates a little more slowly than does enzyme from deficient patients, demonstrating a difference in apparent molecular weight of about 15,000. This slightly smaller size of purified enzyme from lactase-deficient patients is consistent with partial proteolysis. Whether proteolysis occurs in vivo or whether it occurs during the process of purification is unclear. The same results can be obtained in vitro whether the enzyme is dissolved by the protease papain or by detergents alone without added protease. Thus it appears that the proteolysis may occur in vivo. In addition to the change in size there is a difference in the iso-electric point of these two enzyme preparations, 5.37 for the lactase from normal subjects and 5.28 for the lactase from deficient patients. This difference again suggests limited proteolysis of the enzyme.

SUMMARY

In addition to the genetic factors that determine lactase deficiency, there appear to be other factors that can modify the activity of lactase posttranslationally in vivo. The first is inhibition by monosaccharides (mainly glucose, galactose, and fructose), whether they are eaten separately or derived from dietary disaccharides. This effect occurs maximally at pH 6, which is also the optimal pH for maximal sugar transport and lactase activity. Such monosaccharide inhibition has been demonstrated using human lactase, with a K_i of about 10 mM (Alpers and Gerber 1971). Secondly, intraluminal removal of lactase from the membrane can cause more rapid turnover of the enzyme. This is accomplished by pancreatic proteases with perhaps some help from the natural detergents, bile acids, and lysolecithin. Finally, lactase actually can be destroyed, perhaps in relation to or during removal of lactase from the membrane. This destruction of lactase also is mediated by intraluminal proteases. Data supporting each of these mechanisms have been obtained in humans as well as in experimental animals (Alpers and Tedesco 1975, Kwong et al. 1978, Seetharam et al. 1980, Arvanitakis and Olsen 1974). It is possible that these factors alter lactase activity sufficiently to account for some of the natural variation in enzyme activity and perhaps even in tolerance to lactose.

REFERENCES

Alpers DH, Cote MN: Inhibition of lactose hydrolysis by dietary sugars. *Am J Physiol* 221:865-68, 1971.

Alpers DH, Gerber J: Monosaccharide inhibition of human intestinal lactase. *J Lab Clin Med* 78:265-74, 1971.

Alpers DH, Tedesco FJ: The possible role of pancreatic proteases in the turnover of intestinal brush border proteins. *Biochim Biophys Acta* 401:28-40, 1975.

Arias IM, Doyle D, Schimke RT: Studies on the synthesis and degradation of protein of the endoplasmic reticulum of rat liver. *J Biol Chem* 244:3303–15, 1969.

Arvanitakis C, Olsen WA: Intestinal mucosa disaccharidases in chronic pancreatitis. *Am J Dig Dis* 19:417–21, 1974.

Crane RK: The physiology of the intestinal absorption of sugars. In *Physiological Effects of Food Carbohydrates,* A Jeanes, J Hodge (eds). Washington, D.C.: American Chemical Society, Symposium ser. no. 15, 1975, pp 1–19.

Holdsworth CF, Dawson AM: The absorption of monosaccharides in man. *Clin Sci* 27:371–79, 1964.

Iida H, Moore EW, Broitman SA, Zamcheck N: Effect of pH on active transport of d-glucose in the small intestine of hamsters. *Proc Soc Exp Biol Med* 127:730–32, 1968.

Jonas A, Krishnan C, Forstner G: Pathogenesis of mucosal injury in the blind loop syndrome. *Gastroenterology* 75:791–95, 1978.

Kelly JJ, Alpers DH: Blood group antigenicity of purified human disaccharidases. *J Biol Chem* 248:8216–21, 1973.

Kwong WKL, Seetharam B, Alpers DH: Effect of exocrine pancreatic insufficiency on small intestine in the mouse. *Gastroenterology* 74:1277–82, 1978.

Maroux S, Louvard D: On the hydrophobic part of amino peptidase and maltases which bind the enzyme to the intestinal brush border membrane. *Biochim Biophys Acta* 419:189–95, 1976.

Newcomer AD, McGill DB: Distribution of disaccharidase activity in the small bowel of normal and lactase-deficient subjects. *Gastroenterology* 51:481–88, 1966.

Rosensweig NS, Herman RH: Timed response of jejunal sucrase and maltase activity to a high sucrose diet in normal man. *Gastroenterology* 56:500–506, 1969.

Seetharam B, Perrillo R, Alpers DH: The effect of pancreatic proteases on intestinal lactase activity in man. *Gastroenterology* 79:827–32, 1980.

CHAPTER 6

CAUSES OF ISOLATED LOW LACTASE LEVELS
AND LACTOSE INTOLERANCE

Jack D. Welsh

An isolated low lactase level signifies a total intestinal lactase activity that is insufficient to hydrolyze usual amounts of dietary lactose or amounts of lactose used in acute testing. The other disaccharidases and the mucosal histology are normal. The deficiency develops in the first few years of life, and is inherited. A secondary deficiency results either from a decrease in the concentration of all disaccharidases or from the removal of enough intestine that the total lactase activity is insufficient. Lactose malabsorption signifies unhydrolyzed lactose reaching the colon. Lactose intolerance is the production of gastrointestinal symptoms, except constipation, associated with lactose ingestion. The intolerance is related to the dose of lactose ingested, associated medical or surgical conditions, and as yet unidentified factors.

ISOLATED LOW LACTASE

The term *isolated low lactase* is one of many that have been used in an attempt to describe the deficiency succinctly and to explain its causes. Other terms include primary lactase deficiency, acquired low lactase levels, and isolated lactase deficiency. On the basis of absolute number of adult individuals around the world with an isolated low lactase, such a deficiency should be considered the norm for adults.

Isolated low lactase encompasses a condition in which a low lactase activity is associated with lactose maldigestion/malabsorption following ingestion of "usual" amounts of dietary lactose and/or following acute testing using oral lactose. The mucosal histology is normal. There is no decrease of other disaccharidase activities, except for cellobiase; and the sucrase/lactase ratio is over 4.2 to 5.0.

It is important to emphasize that this deficiency represents a level of mucosal lactase activity, obtained from a specified area of the small intestine, that has been correlated with evidence of lactose maldigestion/malabsorption by history and/or acute testing with oral lactose. The exact lower limits of adequate lactase activity vary somewhat between laboratories, as do results of the acute testing using oral lactose.

Congenital Isolated Lactase Deficiency (Alactasia).   Alactasia is a rare enzyme defect that is present at birth and probably is inherited (Holzel et al. 1959). Unfortunately, reports describing the histology of the intestinal mucosa and results of mucosal enzyme assays are few, while long-term follow-up studies are nonexistent. This deficiency should not be confused with infantile familial lactose intolerance, which is characterized by a critically ill infant who presents with vomiting, failure to thrive, disacchariduria, and amino aciduria (Berg et al. 1979). In the latter cases intestinal lactase levels are normal. Oral lactose produces normal blood glucose responses but marked lactosuria, while intraduodenally administered lactose also yields normal blood glucose responses but without increased lactosuria.

Isolated Low Lactase (Acquired).   Evidence supports the concept that individuals with acquired isolated low lactase have adequate lactase activity during infancy but that the levels decrease during early childhood. The lactase decline is inherited, and the racial incidence varies from 5% to 95%. Many reports have suggested that this decline in lactase activity takes place between 1 and 5 years of age, depending on the subject's race. Unfortunately, most of these studies have been based on oral lactose tolerance tests or breath hydrogen tests and have not been correlated with examinations of intestinal mucosal histology and enzyme assays. Therefore, it is not possible to determine whether any of the reported individuals have a secondary disaccharidase deficiency. Two studies do provide comprehensive information on white persons from the United States. The first reported on intestinal disaccharidase activities of 172 white individuals from New England, aged 6 weeks to 50 years (Lebenthal et al. 1975). All had normal intestinal histology by light microscopy. One hundred seven of the subjects were 5 years of age or less. These investigators documented that all those below 5 years of age had high lactase levels, while a group with low activity emerged after 5 years of age. In the second report, intestinal disaccharidase activity levels were presented on 339 white subjects with normal intestinal mucosal histology who ranged from 2 months to 93 years of age (Welsh et al. 1978). All of the 117 children between 2 months and 5 years of age had lactase activities of 22 units per g protein or more (fig. 6.1). Those over 5 years of age could be divided into three groups: 142 (64%) had high lactase activity levels (22 units per g protein or more); 63 (28%) had low lactase levels (less than 13 units per g protein); and 17 (8%) had intermediate levels of activity. The high and intermediate levels of lactase activity were associated with normal blood glucose rises with oral lactose tolerance tests, while those with low activity levels had flat blood glucose responses. Those with intermediate activity levels illustrated an interesting group that had decreased lactase levels, but did not have lactose malabsorption or intolerance. Similar findings have been demonstrated in a more limited group of 53 blacks (Welsh et al. 1978). See fig. 6.2. Regrettably, few black subjects were studied in the 3- to 12-year age group.

Even these studies are limited, because the interpretations are based on individual lactase determinations from a single location in the intestine. No repeat studies are included on the same individual, nor are there data on possible changes in enzyme distribution along the intestine over time. Such investigations

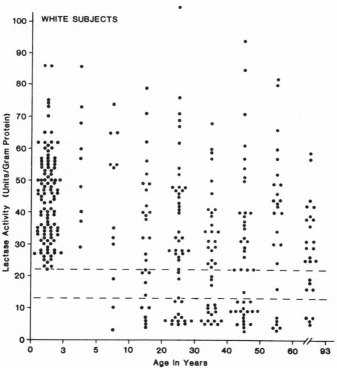

FIGURE 6.1. Lactase activity in normal small intestinal mucosa from 339 white subjects between the ages of 2 months and 93 years. The results are arranged by decades to 60 years of age, and those older are grouped together. Source: Welsh et al. 1978, fig. 1, reprinted with permission.

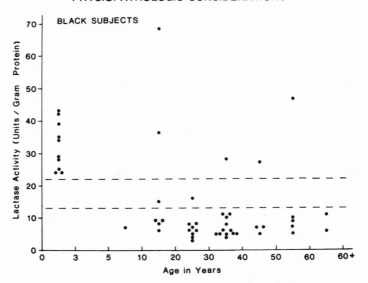

FIGURE 6.2. Lactase activity in normal small intestinal mucosa from 53 black subjects between the ages of 4 weeks and 68 years. Source: Welsh et al. 1978, fig. 2, reprinted with permission.

probably will not be possible in humans, but can be undertaken in animals. Changes with age in intestinal disaccharidase activity in the baboon (*Papio papio*) are of interest in this regard (Welsh et al. 1974). Eight healthy male baboons 1, 2, 3, 4, 8, 9, 12, and 36 months of age were sacrificed. The small intestines were removed, measured, and divided into 10 equal segments. Concentration and distribution of disaccharidases (sucrase, maltase, palatinase, and trehalase) were essentially similar in all ages. With increasing age, however, there was a decrease in lactase activity and a change in its topographical distribution. In comparison with the 1- to 4-month-old animals, lactase activities were less in the duodenum and ileum in the 8- to 12-month-old animals, and levels were the lowest along the intestine of the 36-month-old animal (fig. 6.3). A similar age-related change in the lactase concentration and distribution, as seen in the baboon, probably occurs in humans who develop low lactase levels during childhood. Examination of the activities along the intestine in patients with low lactase activity (Newcomer and McGill 1966) shows a similar distribution (fig. 6.4).

For completeness, a few comments on the role of mucosal damage should be made, since many consider it a factor in the etiology of this enzyme defect. One of the reasons for this interpretation is the concept that lactase is more susceptible to damage than the other disaccharidases. Evidence has suggested that in the human this may be more apparent than real, and related in part to the initial low lactase levels. Studies on children under 5 years of age with abnormal mucosal

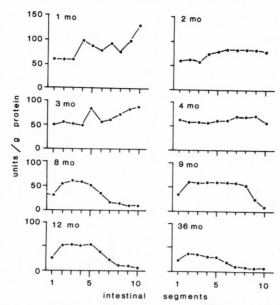

FIGURE 6.3. Relationship of intestinal lactase activity
and age in the baboon.

histology did not support damage as an important cause of an isolated low lactase
deficiency (Welsh et al. 1978). One American Indian child has been studied who
demonstrated an interesting relationship between mucosal damage and the development of an isolated low lactase (Welsh 1978). Each mucosal biopsy specimen was divided so that the histologic interpretations and enzyme assays were
performed on portions of the same specimen (fig. 6.5). At 4 months of age there
were severe mucosal changes, reduced disaccharidase activities, and a normal
sucrase/lactase ratio. Repeat mucosal biopsies at ages 10, 21, and 47 months
revealed gradual improvement in histology, until the last specimen was histolog-
ically normal. Sucrase and maltase activities also improved, but lactase activity
gradually decreased, while the sucrase/lactase ratios increased. The histologi-
cally normal mucosal specimen, obtained at age 47 months, met the criteria for
an isolated low lactase. In this case, lactase activity was the highest when there
was the most damage, and, despite improving mucosal histology, the lactase
decreased to low levels at a time when it would have been expected to increase.
Thus, age and race, more than mucosal damage, appear to be the determining
factors.

Secondary Low Lactase Activity. Secondary low total lactase activity may
result from two conditions. In the first, low concentrations of lactase produce
insufficient total lactase activity. There is an associated decrease of other disac-

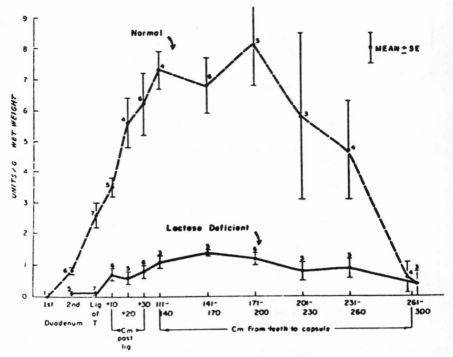

FIGURE 6.4. Lactase activity in the small bowel of seven normal and seven lactase-deficient subjects. Source: Newcomer and McGill 1966, fig. 2, reprinted with permission.

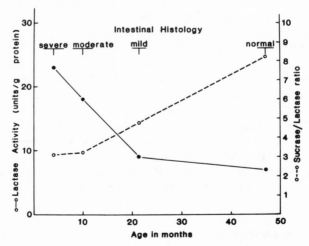

FIGURE 6.5. Secondary disaccharidase deficiency in an American Indian child.

charidases and it is reversible. This secondary deficiency may be caused by an intestinal bacterial or viral infection, giardiasis, gluten-sensitive enteropathy, tropical sprue, protein-sensitive enteropathy, some drugs, alcohol, or starvation. The histology may be normal by light microscopy, such as in cases of long-term starvation, or there may be severe mucosal changes, as seen in gluten-sensitive enteropathy (Welsh et al. 1969). Refeeding the starved patient, or eliminating gluten or the offending protein from the diet, will improve the mucosal lesion, and return all enzymes to normal (Poley et al. 1978). The second circumstance is manifest by high lactase concentrations, but low total lactase activity. Lactase and other disaccharidases have high concentrations, but since enough of the bowel has been removed ("short bowel"), inadequate total lactase activity results. In these patients the total available lactase is not adequate to hydrolyze dietary amounts of lactose or the amount given with acute testing.

LACTOSE INTOLERANCE

Lactose malabsorption occurs when orally ingested lactose reaches the colon. Lactose intolerance is manifest by gastrointestinal symptoms (except constipation) following ingestion of lactose or lactose-containing products. The presence and severity of the symptoms are influenced by a number of factors which will be discussed.

Factors in the Onset of Intolerance.   Unidentified factors seem to delay the onset of intolerance. One hundred individuals were studied who had biopsy-proven isolated low lactase activities (Welsh 1970). Historically, 22 of these individuals were not lactose intolerant. A few did not drink milk or took only small amounts, but the majority were healthy 18- or 19-year-old males who were drinking fairly large quantities of milk each day. This lack of recognized lactose intolerance in some subjects with an isolated low lactase activity also has been noted by others (Bayless et al. 1975). The reason or reasons for the lack of symptoms are not clear; however, there appears to be a progressive decrease in lactose tolerance as the lactase-deficient individual grows older (Newcomer et al. 1977).

There is poor correlation between the onset of an acquired isolated low lactase activity and the onset of lactose intolerance. It is sometimes difficult to identify the time when an individual develops recognizable lactose intolerance, because of differences in milk drinking habits and lack of recognition by patients and physicians alike that milk is the offending agent. Of the subjects studied who have had symptomatic milk intolerance, the age of recognized onset varied from early childhood to the sixties (fig. 6.6).

The onset of lactose intolerance in the individual with isolated low lactase activity may occur without any recognizable associated event or onset may be associated with other intestinal disease or following antibiotics, diet changes, or

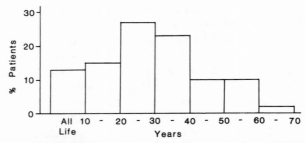

FIGURE 6.6 Age of recognized onset of lactose intolerance in 60 adults with isolated lactase deficiency.

gastrointestinal surgery. The reason for the onset occurring with some of these events is not known. The onset is easier to understand when it occurs following intestinal surgery or in association with intestinal disease, where there is altered function.

Social and Economic Factors. In North American society there is an emphasis on drinking milk and ingesting dairy products. This poses no problem for those with adequate lactase activity, but it can lead to problems in those with low lactase levels. In other parts of the world and in nonmilking societies, milk is less available and there is little social pressure to drink it.

As shown in fig. 6.7 there are wide variations in the amounts of oral lactose that produce symptoms (Bedine and Bayless 1973). Some individuals experience symptoms of lactose intolerance with as little as 3 g lactose, while the rare patient may ingest as much as 90 g at one time before experiencing symptoms.

There are few hard data on intolerance in relation to the frequency of lactose consumption since most information is anecdotal and obtained from patients.

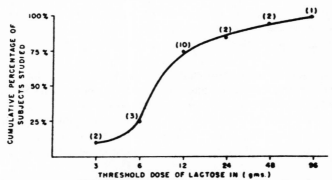

FIGURE 6.7. Threshold doses of lactose in 20 subjects with low intestinal lactase levels. Source: Bedine and Bayless 1973, fig. 1, reprinted with permission.

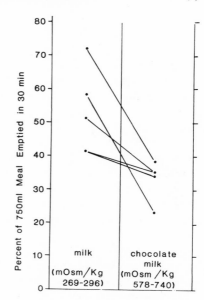

FIGURE 6.8. Gastric emptying of chocolate milk compared to regular milk in lactose malabsorbers.

Some individuals can drink half a glass of milk three or four times a day with minimal difficulty, but will have severe symptoms if a similar amount is drunk at one sitting. This is not too surprising given the wide variations in the amounts of lactose that produce symptoms (Bedine and Bayless 1973).

Supposedly, the lactose in fermented dairy products is tolerated better than regular milk by some individuals with lactose malabsorption; however, the reasons for this are not clear. The lactose content in buttermilk, for example, is similar to that in regular milk (Welsh 1978). When the lactose content of the milk has been at least 90% hydrolyzed, it is well tolerated by many patients with lactose malabsorption (Payne-Bose et al. 1977).

Lactose intolerance is less obvious in lactose malabsorbers when they drink chocolate milk, although the lactose content in regular milk and chocolate milk may be the same (Welsh and Hall 1977). The osmolarity of the chocolate milk studied ranged from 578 mOsm per kg to 740 mOsm per kg, mainly because of its sucrose content. This was from two to three times greater than that of regular milk. As a consequence the chocolate milk emptied much slower, so the lactose entered the duodenum in smaller amounts per time period (fig. 6.8). An additional factor, not examined in these studies, is the possible role of the simultaneous hydrolysis and absorption of the sucrose.

LACTOSE INTOLERANCE IN POSTGASTRECTOMY PATIENTS

For many years it has been recognized that the onset of milk intolerance occurs in some patients following gastric surgery. Only some of these patients have isolated low lactase activity, and the proportion depends on the racial composition of the surgical population. Present evidence has shown that these patients had isolated low lactase activity prior to the surgery, although frequently they were not intolerant (Bergoz and DePeyer 1979). However, with the postsurgical alteration in gastric emptying, they became intolerant. Most of the patients with postgastrectomy milk intolerance have normal lactase activity. Some postgastrectomy patients malabsorb glucose after surgery (Bond and Levitt 1972). It is not surprising that the same patients also malabsorb lactose. Figure 6.9 compares the results of simultaneous oral lactose tolerance tests and breath hydrogen tests in three postgastrectomy patients. The first patient had no milk intolerance and a normal sucrase/lactase ratio of 1.9. The blood glucose response following oral lactose was high and there was no increase in breath hydrogen. In contrast, the second patient, a black male who had a history of milk intolerance, had a sucrase/lactase ratio of 19.0, supporting the diagnosis of an isolated low lactase activity. There was a flat blood glucose response to oral lactose and an increase in breath hydrogen. The last patient illustrated the typical findings in patients with milk intolerance and normal lactase activity. This patient developed milk intolerance right after his gastric surgery; the sucrase/lactase ratio was normal; and the blood glucose response with oral lactose was normal. However, there was a marked increase in the breath hydrogen, signifying lactose malabsorption. This supports the idea that milk intolerance in these individuals is due to altered gastrointestinal function leading to lactose malabsorption.

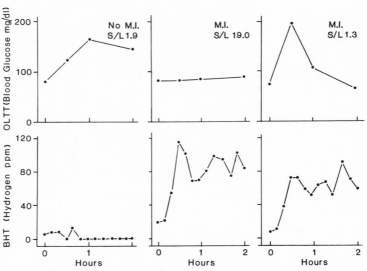

FIGURE 6.9. Oral lactose tolerance test and breath hydrogen test results in three postgastrectomy patients; two had milk intolerance (M.I.).

REFERENCES

Bayless TM, Rothfeld B, Massa C, Wise L, Paige DM, Bedine MS: Lactose and milk intolerance: Clinical implications. *N Engl J Med* 292:1156–59, 1975.

Bedine MS, Bayless TM: Intolerance of small amounts of lactose by individuals with low lactase levels. *Gastroenterology* 65:735–43, 1973.

Berg NO, Dahlqvist A, Lindberg T: A boy with severe infantile gastrogen lactose intolerance and acquired lactase deficiency. *Acta Paediatr Scand* 68:751–58, 1979.

Bergoz R, DePeyer R: Lactase intestinale et consommation de lait avant et apres gastrectomie. *Schweiz Med Wochenschr* 109:605–06, 1979.

Bond JH Jr, Levitt MD: Use of pulmonary hydrogen (H_2) measurements to quantitate carbohydrate absorption: Study of partially gastrectomized patients. *J Clin Invest* 51:1219–25, 1972.

Holzel A, Schwarz V, Sutcliffe KW: Defective lactose absorption causing malnutrition in infancy. *Lancet* 1:1126–28, 1959.

Lebenthal E, Antonowicz I, Shwachman H: Correlation of lactase activity, lactose tolerance and milk consumption in different age groups. *Am J Clin Nutr* 28:595–600, 1975.

Newcomer AD, McGill DB: Distribution of disaccharidase activity in the small bowel of normal and lactase-deficient subjects. *Gastroenterology* 51:481–88, 1966.

Newcomer AD, Thomas PJ, McGill DB, Hofmann AF: Lactase deficiency: A common genetic trait of the American Indian. *Gastroenterology* 72:234–37, 1977.

Payne-Bose D, Welsh JD, Gearhart HL, Morrison RD: Milk and lactose-hydrolyzed milk. *Am J Clin Nutr* 30:695–97, 1977.

Poley JR, Bhatia M, Welsh JD: Disaccharidase deficiency in infants with cow's milk protein intolerance. *Digestion* 17:97–107, 1978.

Welsh JD: Isolated lactase deficiency in humans: Report on 100 patients. *Medicine* (Baltimore) 49:257–77, 1970.

Welsh JD: Diet therapy in adult lactose malabsorption: Present practices. *Am J Clin Nutr* 31:592–96, 1978.

Welsh JD, Hall WH: Gastric emptying of lactose and milk in subjects with lactose malabsorption. *Am J Dig Dis* 22:1060–63, 1977.

Welsh JD, Poley JR, Bhatia M, Stevenson DE: Intestinal disaccharidase activities in relation to age, race, and mucosal damage. *Gastroenterology* 75:847–55, 1978.

Welsh JD, Russell LC, Walker AW Jr: Changes in intestinal lactase and alkaline phosphatase activity levels with age in the baboon (*Papio papio*). *Gastroenterology* 66:993–97, 1974.

Welsh JD, Zschiesche OM, Anderson J, Walker A: Intestinal disaccharidase activity in celiac sprue (gluten-sensitive enteropathy). *Arch Intern Med* 123:33–38, 1969.

CHAPTER 7

࿇

QUANTITATIVE MEASUREMENT
OF LACTOSE ABSORPTION AND COLONIC SALVAGE
OF NONABSORBED LACTOSE
DIRECT AND INDIRECT METHODS

Michael D. Levitt and John H. Bond

There are two mechanisms whereby lactose, or its constituent carbons, can move from the gut into the blood. The first is via the absorption of the component monosaccharides, glucose and galactose, from the small bowel. The lactose that escapes such absorption in the small bowel passes into the colon. A second mechanism then comes into play when the colonic flora metabolize lactose to products that may be absorbed from the colonic lumen. Ordinarily, absorption refers to the net removal of a substance from the lumen without particular reference to the form in which the substance is removed. Thus, in the most general sense, absorption of lactose from the gastrointestinal tract probably should include both of the above mechanisms. In this chapter, lactose absorption refers only to the absorption of the component monosaccharides, glucose and galactose, from the small bowel, while the absorptive process that occurs in the colon is referred to as colonic salvage of nonabsorbed lactose.

Presumably the symptoms induced by lactose malabsorption should be related to the quantity of lactose that escapes absorption in the small bowel and passes into the colon and/or to what happens to that lactose in the colon. Thus, it was somewhat surprising several years ago to find that, despite the many papers written on lactose malabsorption, there was not a single quantitative measure of the amount of a lactose load that was absorbed by control subjects or patients with lactase deficiency.

DIRECT MEASUREMENT OF LACTOSE ABSORPTION

To assess how much lactose passed the terminal ileum subjects were intubated with a narrow calibre, polyvinyl tube weighted with a mercury-filled bag that was allowed to pass to the very terminal ileum (Bond and Levitt 1976a). The subject then ingested 12.5 g 1-^{14}C-lactose and 4 g polyethylene glycol (PEG), a nonabsorbable marker. By comparing the ratio of ^{14}C to PEG in fluid aspirated from the ileum to that of the ingested material, one can estimate the percentage of lactose absorbed in the small bowel. For example, if the ratio of ^{14}C to PEG ingested was 1:1 and the ratio of ^{14}C to PEG in the material passing the terminal ileum is 0.5:1, roughly one-half the lactose must have been absorbed.

There are several problems with this technique. A question that seldom is considered, despite the widespread use of intestinal tubes for absorption studies, is the problem of whether the intestine functions normally with a tube running from the mouth to the terminal ileum. Certainly the subject does not feel ''normal'' when the intestine is so intubated. Anorexia, abnormal cramps, diarrhea, headache, and depression are among the complaints of intubated subjects. Nevertheless, it is assumed, without evidence, that the intubated bowel functions normally. Since there is no other way to obtain material from the terminal ileum, intubation appears to be a necessary evil if one wishes to distinguish the functions of the small bowel from those of the large bowel in the removal of carbohydrate from the gut.

The second problem with the technique described above is that the ^{14}C to PEG ratio in the material passing the terminal ileum is not absolutely constant. If it were constant, the ^{14}C to PEG ratio in one small aliquot of ileal contents would indicate accurately the percentage of lactose absorbed. However, the ratio tends to vary, usually reaching its lowest value (highest lactose absorption) as the tail of the ingested load passes the terminal ileum. Since the volume passing the terminal ileum at any moment is not known, it is not possible to weight each ileal collection accurately for volume—a correction necessary to calculate exactly the overall percentage of absorption. Therefore, it was assumed that the rate of passage of ileal contents was constant—an assumption that seemed to minimize the possible error to roughly ± 15% of the true value. The only other way to obtain data on the movement of lactose past the terminal ileum is by means of a constant, slow perfusion of the terminal ileum, a technique that has its own problems, but that might yield somewhat more accurate results.

Figure 7.1 shows the results of the studies of lactose absorption in four control subjects with normal lactose tolerance tests and in six lactase-deficient subjects, as demonstrated by a flat tolerance test (Bond and Levitt 1976a). Normal subjects absorbed from 92% to 100% of the 12.5 g lactose load, indicating that absorption

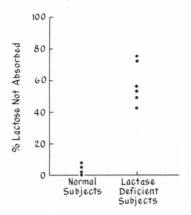

FIGURE 7.1. Quantity of lactose not absorbed by the small bowel as determined by ileal aspiration in normal and lactase-deficient subjects after ingestion of 12.5 g 1-^{14}C-lactose.

of lactose is quite good in lactose-tolerant subjects. Conversely, the data may be interpreted as showing that control subjects do not absorb lactose completely. Thus, in certain conditions such as ulcerative colitis, where the goal is to limit the amount of carbohydrate reaching the colon to an absolute minimum, lactose restriction might be in order even in subjects with normal lactose tolerance tests. In the six subjects with lactase deficiency, 40% to 78% of the 12.5 g lactose load was not absorbed in the small bowel.

COMPARISION WITH INDIRECT MEASURES

The measurements of small bowel lactose absorption shown in figure 7.1 were compared with the results of several indirect measurements of lactose absorption in an effort to provide a simple substitute for the complex and uncomfortable tube measurement. The indirect methods were: (1) breath $^{14}CO_2$ excretion; (2) fecal ^{14}C excreted for four days after the lactose ingestion, corrected for incomplete recovery by the recovery of PEG; and (3) the amount of hydrogen gas excreted by the lungs following lactose ingestion, measured by having the subjects rebreathe into a closed system.

The results of each of the three indirect tests are shown in fig. 7.2 (Bond and Levitt 1976a). Much less ^{14}C was excreted in the stool of the normal subjects than was excreted by the six lactose malabsorbers using this test, which can distinguish lactose absorbers from malabsorbers. However, the greatest amount of ^{14}C ever recovered in the stool, corrected for incomplete stool collections by PEG recovery, was only about 13% of the ingested ^{14}C—appreciably less than the quantity of lactose that appeared to be malabsorbed, based on the tube measurements.

Figure 7.3 shows the excretion curves of breath $^{14}CO_2$ after 1-^{14}C-lactose ingestion. The curves for the two groups of subjects are roughly the same shape, although the curve of the lactose-intolerant subjects is shifted to the right (Bond

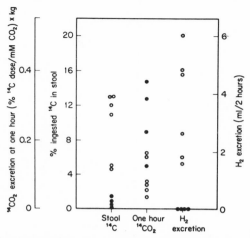

FIGURE 7.2. Comparison of stool excretion of ^{14}C, breath $^{14}CO_2$ at 1 hour, and pulmonary excretion of H_2 for 2 hours after ingestion of 12.5 g 1-^{14}C-lactose by normal (closed circle) and lactase-deficient (open circle) subjects.

and Levitt 1976). As is shown in fig. 7.3, at one hour there are highly significant differences between lactose absorbers and nonabsorbers. However, the total amount of $^{14}CO_2$ excreted over 24 hours is the same for the control subjects as for those with lactase deficiency (see fig. 7.3). The most likely explanation for this finding is that a large fraction of $^{14}CO_2$ excreted by the lactose malabsorbers was derived from malabsorption of ^{14}C-lactose reaching the colon. The shift to the right of the curve for lactase-deficient subjects (fig. 7.3) and the fact that its shape is similar to that for normal subjects suggest that transit through the small bowel delays the generation of this $^{14}CO_2$ from malabsorbed lactose but that once it reaches the colon, $^{14}CO_2$ is liberated at the same rate as that for lactose absorbed from the small bowel.

Breath hydrogen measurements also distinguish absorbers from nonabsorbers qualitatively (see fig. 7.2). Thus, qualitatively each of these simple indirect tests does a reasonable job of distinguishing normal from abnormal absorption of lactose.

To determine if any of the indirect tests could estimate the amount of lactose not absorbed, a correlation coefficient was developed using the results of the indirect test and the quantity of lactose calculated not to be absorbed based on analysis of ileal contents. Studies with lactulose, a nonabsorbable disaccharide, indicated that some people excrete more H_2 than others from a given malabsorbed dose of carbohydrate. Thus, to ascertain carbohydrate malabsorption from H_2 excretion, the H_2 excretion of an individual following lactose ingestion was compared with H_2 excretion following ingestion of a known quantity of lactulose. Thus, the lactulose calculations were used as a standard of the amount of

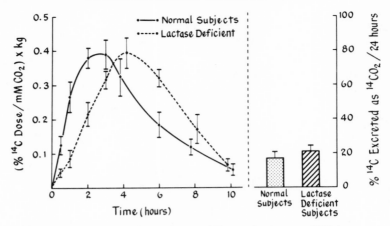

FIGURE 7.3. *Left panel,* pulmonary $^{14}CO_2$ excretion (mean ± SEM) by normal and lactase-deficient subjects for 10 hours after ingestion of 12.5 g 1-^{14}C-lactose. *Right panel,* percentage of ^{14}C excreted as $^{14}CO_2$ during 24 hours after ingestion of 12.5 g 1-^{14}C-lactose by normal and lactase-deficient subjects (mean ± SEM).

hydrogen produced by an individual when a known amount of carbohydrate reached the colon.

As shown in table 7.1, there was not a significant correlation at the 0.05 level for any of the three indirect measurements, although breath hydrogen excretion approached significance.

Figure 7.4 shows the quantity of ^{14}C entering and exiting from the colon of six lactose-intolerant subjects. An average of about 55% of the ingested ^{14}C passed the terminal ileum but only about 10% of the ^{14}C was passed in feces. Thus, appreciable conservation of the carbons of lactose occurred during colonic transit.

TABLE 7.1
Correlation between lactose absorption determined by the three indirect methods and that determined from terminal ileal aspiration

	Correlation coefficients (r values)	
Indirect measure	Normal plus lactase-deficient subjects	Lactase-deficient subjects
Pulmonary H_2 excretion	0.94 (P < 0.05)	0.68 (N.S.)*
Pulmonary $^{14}CO_2$ excretion at one hour	−0.77 (P < 0.05)	−0.3 (N.S.)*
Stool ^{14}C excretion	0.76 (P < 0.05)	0.25 (N.S.)*

*Not significant, P > 0.05.

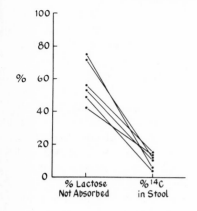

FIGURE 7.4. Comparison of the quantity of lactose not absorbed as determined by ileal aspiration with that derived from measurement of stool ^{14}C after ingestion of 12.5 g 1-^{14}C-lactose by six lactase-deficient subjects.

COLONIC SALVAGE OF NONABSORBED LACTOSE

The mechanism whereby the colon salvages nonabsorbed carbohydrate was studied in conventional and germ-free rats. A cannula was implanted permanently in the cecum of rats and, via a subcutaneous tunnel, brought out through the back of the neck. Several weeks following surgery, carbohydrates were instilled directly through this tube into the cecum of conscious rats, thus simulating carbohydrate malabsorption. Figure 7.5 shows that $^{14}CO_2$ excretion curves were virtually identical for the intracecal versus the intragastric route of administering 200 mg [U-^{14}C] glucose (Bond and Levitt 1976b). Thus, glucose instilled into the cecum is converted to $^{14}CO_2$ as rapidly as is glucose placed in the stomach. This result compares with that observed in known lactose absorbers versus nonabsorbers in which the curves of $^{14}CO_2$ were similar, although $^{14}CO_2$ excretion was delayed in the lactose malabsorbers, apparently due to small bowel transit.

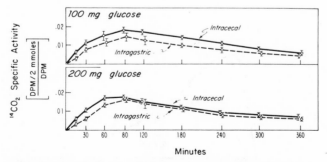

FIGURE 7.5. Comparison of the specific activity of $^{14}CO_2$ excreted by rats after intracecal or intragastric administration of 100 mg or 200 mg [U-^{14}C] glucose. Specific activity has been normalized for dosage instilled.

To determine if this efficient conservation of glucose in the rat colon was dependent upon bacterial action, similar studies were carried out in germ-free rats. As shown in fig. 7.6, virtually no $^{14}CO_2$ was excreted when [U-^{14}C] glucose was instilled into the cecum of germ-free rats (Bond and Levitt 1976b).

There are two possible mechanisms whereby the bacteria could play a role in the metabolism of intracecally administered glucose to CO_2. The bacteria could oxidize the glucose to CO_2, which would be absorbed rapidly and excreted. In this situation, the bacteria would derive most of the energy from the nonabsorbed carbohydrate. In contrast, the bacteria could merely ferment glucose to organic acids and other anaerobic metabolites, which then could be absorbed and oxidized to CO_2 by the host. In this case the host, rather than the bacteria, would receive the bulk of the caloric value of the carbohydrate.

In an attempt to determine which of these two processes was predominant, the rate was calculated at which O_2 would have to diffuse into the colonic lumen to support the observed rate of oxidation of colonically instilled carbohydrate to CO_2. An estimate then was made for the rate at which O_2 might reach the colonic lumen via transport on hemoglobin. The rate was calculated by measuring the rate of CO absorption from the colon. CO, like O_2, is transported on hemoglobin. The rate of CO absorption in rats, which averaged 28 μl per minute, tends to overestimate O_2 delivery since CO is not metabolized by mucosal tissue and the P_{CO} gradient between lumen and blood is greater than the P_{O_2} gradient. An O_2 delivery rate of 28 μl per minute to the colonic lumen would be only about 15% of that required to support the observed rate of oxidation of glucose instilled in the colon. Thus, it appears necessary to postulate that the bacteria anaerobically produce metabolic products such as organic acids, which are absorbed from the colonic lumen and then metabolized to CO_2 by the host. That these organic acids can be absorbed from the colon was confirmed by studies showing the rapid conversion of ^{14}C-acetate and ^{14}C-lactate to $^{14}CO_2$ following instillation into the cecum of germ-free rats (fig. 7.6).

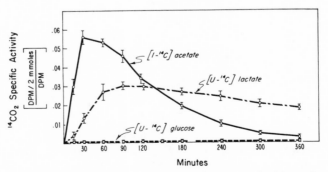

FIGURE 7.6. Specific activity of $^{14}CO_2$ of germ-free rats after intracecal administration of 200 mg [U-^{14}C] glucose, [1-^{14}C] acetate, or [U-^{14}C] lactate.

The colonic bacteria also appeared to reduce the possible osmotic load resulting from malabsorption of carbohydrate by converting more than 50% of the carbons into compounds that were not dialyzable. It is not clear if this nondialyzable form represents binding of low molecular weight compounds or actual incorporation of ^{14}C into high molecular weight compounds. In either situation the osmotic activity of the ^{14}C would be diminished.

The bacterial metabolism of nonabsorbed carbohydrates to absorbable products is crucial to the prevention of severe diarrhea following malabsorption of fairly trivial quantities of carbohydrate. Fecal water is nearly isotonic and, thus, every 100 mOsm of nonabsorbed solute necessarily carries with it about 300 ml of fecal water. The bacterial conversion of just 10 g lactose per day to organic acids and their associated cations could result in roughly 220 mOsm. If not modified, this osmotic load would result in 650 ml fecal water—very appreciable diarrhea.

The ability of many lactose malabsorbers to tolerate daily ingestion of two or more cups of milk (more than 25 g lactose) with minimal or no diarrhea presumably results from the ability of the colonic flora of these individuals to reduce the osmotic load markedly and, hence, to prevent diarrhea. Individual differences in fermentation pathways or the ability of the colon to absorb the fermentation products may be important determinants of individual differences in the susceptibility of lactose malabsorbers to symptoms following lactose ingestion.

Conserving the calories of malabsorbed carbohydrate is of little importance to lactose malabsorbers. However, this route of caloric absorption may be important in patients with massive carbohydrate malabsorption such as occurs in short bowel syndrome, where appreciable calories are removed from the fecal stream in the colon (Bond et al. 1980).

REFERENCES

Bond JH, Currier B, Buchwald H, Levitt MD: Colonic conservation of malabsorbed carbohydrate. *Gastroenterology* 78:444–47, 1980.

Bond JH, Levitt MD: Quantitative measurement of lactose absorption. *Gastroenterology* 70:1058–62, 1976a.

Bond JH, Levitt MD: Fate of soluble carbohydrate in the colon of rats and man. *J Clin Invest* 57:1158–64, 1976b.

IV

DIAGNOSIS AND SCREENING

CHAPTER 8

DIAGNOSIS AND SCREENING

TECHNIQUES FOR LACTOSE MALDIGESTION

ADVANTAGES OF THE HYDROGEN

BREATH TEST

Noel W. Solomons

A quantitative assessment of the ability of an individual to digest lactose finds its application in a variety of situations. It is important to the geneticist or the physical anthropologist interested in the enzyme lactase as a genetic marker (Flatz and Rotthauwe 1977), to the pediatrician presented with the rare infant with congenital lactase deficiency (Holzel et al. 1959), to the clinician and dietician in managing the patient with "milk intolerance," and to public health specialists and relief agencies in determining food distribution policies (Ifek-wuniqwe 1975). The extensive interest in the diagnosis of and screening for lactose maldigestion has led to a proliferation of diagnostic methodologies in the last two decades. This chapter will review and evaluate these procedures in terms of their diagnostic accuracy, clinical appropriateness, and interpretive signifi-cance.

LACTASE DEFICIENCY VERSUS LACTOSE MALDIGESTION

It is important first to define two overlapping concepts: lactase deficiency and lactose maldigestion. Lactase is the β-galactoside-specific disaccharidase in the brush border of the intestinal mucosal cell. A marked reduction of the activity of this enzyme in assay in vitro is the hallmark of congenital lactase deficiency (Durand 1958, Holzel 1959, Lebenthal 1978), of the primary lactase deficiency in various populations (Flatz and Rotthauwe 1977), and of the secondary (acquired) lactase deficiency resulting from nutritional (Jones and Latham 1974) or infectious (Lebenthal 1975) insults. Since lactase is distributed over the length of the small intestine (Newcomer and McGill 1966), even when mucosal lactase is diminished, there is often sufficient activity to hydrolyze relatively small amounts of dietary lactose. Conversely, changes in intestinal transit time or massive doses of oral lactose can result in incomplete digestion of lactose despite a normal intestinal complement of lactase. Glucose-galactose malabsorption (Gray 1967), a rare congenital disease characterized by a specific transport defect in monosaccharide absorption, functionally results in lactose malabsorption. Lactase levels and lactose hydrolysis are intact, but, as the monosaccharide constituents are not absorbed actively, net carbohydrate absorption after lactose ingestion is impaired severely. Thus, lactase deficiency and lactose maldigestion are not strictly equivalent terms. As the following review will illustrate, the use of the terms *lactase deficiency* or *lactose maldigestion* must be qualified in terms of the clinical setting and the conditions of the diagnostic procedures.

DIAGNOSTIC PROCEDURES

The procedures available for clinical or investigational assessment of lactase deficiency or lactose malabsorption are outlined in table 8.1. They fall into five classes: intubation studies, radiographic studies, blood tests, breath tests, and fecal analyses.

Intubation Studies. *Lactase Assay:* Intubation procedures probably allow the most precise quantitative data. Burgess and Dalhqvist are largely responsible for the development and standardization of the lactase assay (Burgess et al. 1964, Dalhquist 1964), which is performed on fresh intestinal biopsy tissue. A rate of in vitro hydrolysis of the lactose substrate of less than 2 μmoles per minute per gram of wet tissue at 37°C (Protein Advisory Group 1972) or of less than 5 μmoles per minute per gram of protein at 37°C (Kern and Struthers 1966) is considered to represent deficiency.* Thus, the assay provides explicitly quantitative data on the specific activity of the intestinal enzyme (Newcomer and McGill 1967). Often, the activities of the intestinal hydrolases for maltose and sucrose are assayed simultaneously for reference (Keusch et al. 1969, Flatz and Rotthauwe 1977, Sheehy and Anderson 1965). The lactase assay requires a biochemistry laboratory and is invasive to the subject insofar as it requires intestinal intubation and biopsy. An additional disadvantage is the radiation exposure to the

---

*Hydrolysis of 1 μmole of carbohydrate per minute at 37°C = 1 unit of disaccharidase activity.

TABLE 8.1
Clinical procedures for diagnosis and screening for lactose absorption and lactase status

Class	Test	Lactose dosage	Analytical procedures	Criteria for abnormality
Intubation studies	Lactase assay	—	in vitro hydrolysis of lactose in the presence of mucosal homogenates at 37°C	<2 units/ g wet tissue <5 units/ g protein
	Intestinal perfusion	variable (12.5 g; 30 g)	change in lactose concentration in the perfusate	<95% absorption
Radiographic studies	Barium-lactose meal	variable (50 g; 25 g)	abdominal radiographs	"dilution" of barium; progression of the head of the barium column
Blood tests	Plasma glucose test	1.75 g or 2 g/ kg up to 50 g in children; 50 g, 100 g, or 50 g per m² in subjects over 25 kg	determination of plasma glucose at intervals (variable) during a 2-hour period	<20 mg/ dl increment or <25 mg/ dl increment
	Plasma galactose test	variable (20 g/ m², 50 g) plus ethanol p.o.	determination of plasma galactose at intervals, or once at 45 min.	<5 mg/ dl increment
Breath tests	Hydrogen breath test	variable (12.5 g to 50 g)	determination of breath H_2 concentration by gas chromatography	>20 ppm increment in $[H_2]$ >0.31 ml of H_2/min. excretion rate
	$^{14}CO_2$ breath test	5 μCi of 1-^{14}C-lactose in a variable (12.5 g, 25 g, or 50 g) carrier dose of lactose	breath $^{14}CO_2$ excretion determined by liquid scintillation	less than the range of "normals" at a given time interval after the lactose dose
	$^{13}CO_2$ breath test	1-^{13}C-lactose, variable amount in a variable dose of unlabeled lactose	breath $^{13}CO_2$ excretion determined by mass spectrometry	less than the range of "normals" at a given time interval
Fecal analysis	Fecal pH	customary dietary milk intake	indicator litmus pH paper	pH < 6
	Fecal reducing substances	customary dietary milk intake	stool reducing substances in vitro	+ to ++++
	Fecal ^{14}C	5 μCi 1-^{14}C-lactose in carrier lactose	stool ^{14}C by liquid scintillation	not established

subject and operator when fluoroscopic control of the biopsy tube or capsule is included.

Intestinal Perfusion: Intestinal perfusion has been used in both adults (Bond and Levitt 1976, Kern and Struthers 1966) and children (Rodriguez-de-Curet et al. 1970, Torres-Pinedo et al. 1971). The test involves the insertion of a multilumen tube into the small bowel. Lactose is infused into the intestinal lumen through the proximal port (or administered by mouth), and intestinal fluid is aspirated through a distal port. The rate and dose of infusion, and the length and location of the intestinal segment perfused can be adjusted by the experimenter.

Ordinary natural lactose or ^{14}C-labeled substrate can be used as a tracer. A nonabsorbable reference marker such as polyethylene glycol is perfused simultaneously to correct for intestinal water movement. Thus, precise rates of lactose absorption over a given segment of intestine can be calculated with perfusion techniques.

As with the lactase assay, the invasive aspects of intubation and fluoroscopic radiography are inherent. The use of radio-labeled lactose implies additional radiation exposure. Although the conditions are somewhat artificial and nonphysiologic, they do permit adjustment of transit rates and total lactose doses that reasonably reflect the dietary situation.

Radiographic Studies. Laws and associates introduced a procedure for diagnosing lactose malabsorption based on intestinal radiography (Laws and Neale 1966, Laws et al. 1967). In their method, 25 g lactose were ingested along with 4 fluid ounces of a fine barium sulfate suspension. Abdominal films were taken at intervals, and the dilution of the barium and progression of the head of the barium column were assessed radiographically. These were correlated with lactase assay results; an excellent correlation of abnormal x-ray criteria with deficient lactase levels was . reported. Other investigators have used various modifications of this procedure (Reddy and Pershad 1972, Lisker et al. 1975, Rosenquist 1975). The lactose dose theoretically can be varied throughout the physiological and pharmacological ranges, and even skim milk has been used as a source of lactose (Reddy and Pershad 1972).

The radiographic methodology presents a number of obvious drawbacks: (1) the conditions of this procedure are grossly nonphysiologic; (2) the barium suspension itself contributes an osmotic load; (3) evaluation of the radiographic appearance is, at best, subjective; (4) preexisting small bowel abnormalities will invalidate the interpretation; and (5) the radiation exposure is unacceptably high and inappropriate to the information being sought. The technique cannot be recommended.

Blood Tests.   *Plasma Glucose:* The oldest and most widely used indirect index of lactase status or measure of lactose absorption is the change in plasma glucose concentration following an oral challenge of lactose. The dose of lactose necessary to define a consistent separation of absorbers and nonabsorbers via plasma glucose changes is relatively large. In young children, a dosage of 1.75 g or 2 g per kg body weight up to 50 g has been used. For individuals over 25 kg in weight, aqueous lactose doses of 50 g, 100 g, and 50 g per m^2 have been used. Blood samples are taken at various intervals—even multiples of 15 or 20 minutes—over two hours. Moreover, no universal criteria for normality have been accepted. An early study (Cuatrecasas et al. 1965) used the correspondence of the area under the curve of plasma glucose change following a dose of lactose with the area under a similar curve following an equivalent equimolar dose of the monosaccharide constituents glucose and galactose. This practice required two separate tests and promptly was abandoned in favor of a single test. Increments of both ≥ 20 mg per dl and ≥ 25 mg per dl in plasma glucose at any time within the first two postdose hours have been used as criteria of normal lactose absorption.

Delayed gastric emptying can affect the plasma glucose test. Falsely abnormal test results attributed to gastric retention of the substrate have been recorded in children (Krasilnikoff et al. 1975), and even in an occasional adult subject (Kern and Struthers 1966). In such cases, intraduodenal instillation of the lactose dose resulted in a plasma glucose curve in agreement with the mucosal lactase level of the subject. The rise in plasma glucose after ingestion of 50 g lactose as milk has been used (Leichter 1973), but the inherently slower gastric emptying of a meal containing protein and fat invalidates the criteria for a normal rise in plasma glucose based on *aqueous* lactose.

The plasma glucose technique is mildly invasive, since a concentration curve implies serial blood extractions. Venipunctures and fingerpricks have been used, but McGill and Newcomer (1966) have insisted that capillary blood is more suitable than venous blood due to peripheral utilization of glucose. Glucose levels are also susceptible to a variety of hormonal influences. Despite the universal popularity of this test, it was shown early by several workers that a relatively poor correlation of the plasma glucose results with actual mucosal lactase levels (Bayless and Rosensweig 1966, Newcomer and McGill 1966).

Plasma Galactose: Attempts to develop a more sensitive and specific blood test led to the use of galactose, rather than glucose, as the indicator sugar. Fischer and Zapf (1965), exploiting the fact that ethanol inhibits intrahepatic conversion of galactose to glucose, reported a lactose absorption test involving serial determination of plasma galactose after an oral dose of lactose plus alcohol. Doses of 50 g or of 20 g per m^2 lactose were used by proponents of this technique (Kern and Heller 1968, Jussila 1969, Isokoski et al. 1972). Lactase-deficient patients generally had a plasma galactose increment of less than 5 mg per dl. The use of a single, 45-minute postdose, blood sample was possible (Kern and Heller 1968), and, in one report, the galactose modification proved to be 89% to 97% specific and 97% to 100% sensitive (Isokoski et al. 1972).

The galactose method shares some of the disadvantages of the glucose procedure. The lesser background concentration of galactose may eliminate baseline fluctuations, and the number of sampling intervals may be reduced, but the collection procedure is still blood extraction and the doses of lactose required are pharmacological. Moreover, the biochemical analysis is more complex than that for glucose, and alcohol administration may not be suitable in all patients.

Breath Tests. *Hydrogen Breath Test:* The hydrogen breath analysis test for lactose is based on the observation that certain intestinal bacteria, part of the normal human colonic flora, will ferment unabsorbed carbohydrate with the concomitant evolution of H_2 (Calloway and Murphy 1968, Levitt 1969). There is a stoichiometric relationship between H_2 evolved and the amount of carbohydrate presented to bacteria in vivo and in vitro (Levitt 1969, Bond and Levitt 1972). Between 14% and 21% of the H_2 produced in the bowel is excreted not as intestinal gas, but by way of the lungs (Levitt 1969). Thus, an increase in the rate of breath H_2 excretion after ingestion of lactose reflects bacterial fermentation of part of the substrate, i.e., malabsorption. Not only lactose, but any soluble carbohydrate, can be used with the hydrogen breath test. The method of collection is noninvasive, no radioactivity is required, and physiological doses of lactose in its usual dietary form can be employed in the challenge dose. As this technique merits special attention in the context of diagnostic and screening procedures for lactose maldigestion, the test will be discussed in expanded detail below.

$^{14}CO_2$ Breath Test: The $^{14}CO_2$ breath test for lactose absorption was introduced by Salmon et al. (1969) and Sasaki et al. (1970). It involves the administration of 50 g lactose labeled with 5 μCi of $1\text{-}^{14}C$. Expired carbon dioxide is easy to trap and can be measured readily by liquid scintillation counting. The procedure involves a simple, noninvasive collection technique. A fundamental disadvantage is the inherent radiation exposure. Another important consequence is that although hepatic metabolism will convert *absorbed* $1\text{-}^{14}C$-lactose to $^{14}CO_2$, bacterial enzymes in the colon also will oxidize *unabsorbed* radio-labeled lactose. Thus, the *rate* of excretion of $^{14}CO_2$ is crucial, and the time interval must be chosen carefully. In one study, the net 24-hour cumulative breath excretion of $^{14}CO_2$ was equivalent for both absorbers and nonabsorbers of lactose (Bond and Levitt 1976).

$^{13}CO_2$ Breath Test: Recently, investigators at Johns Hopkins and the University of Chicago have developed an analogous lactose absorption breath test using the nonradioactive, *stable* carbon isotope, carbon 13 (Klein et al. 1979). End-expiratory samples of whole breath are collected and stored in evacuated tubes. The enrichment with $^{13}CO_2$ can be measured by mass spectrometry. All of the same inherent consequences related to colonic metabolism of unabsorbed substrate that obtain for carbon 14-labeled lactose are applicable to the $^{13}CO_2$ breath test. A definite additional advantage is the absence of any radiation biohazard. Thus, the test can be used safely in infants, children, and in pregnant and lactating women. The extraordinarily high cost of the stable isotope-labeled substrate, however, is presently a limitation to its widespread utilization.

Fecal Analysis. *Stool pH and Fecal Reducing Substances:* Time-honored screening tests for assessing lactose absorption in infants and young children are the measurement of stool pH and/or fecal reducing sugars. Indicator litmus paper and Clinitest tablets (Ames) are the only reagents necessary, and the test can be performed at the bedside. Some investigators have demonstrated that fecal analyses are more consistent than blood tests in small children, and are, in fact, the only reliable indirect indices of lactose status in infants (Harrison and Walker-Smith 1977, Kerry and Anderson 1964.) Ament (1972) has suggested that the combination of pH and reducing substance determinations improves the sensitivity of screening.

The tests, however, are inherently qualitative. No standard dose of lactose is given. Changes in intestinal water secretion will influence the final fecal concentration of both hydrogen ions and fecal reducing substances. It should be remembered, moreover, that it is perfectly normal for breast-fed infants to show an acidic stool pH and to excrete small quantities of lactose (Heine et al. 1977).

Fecal ^{14}C: Bond and Levitt (1976) determined the fecal excretion of carbon 14 after administering 5 μCi of 1-^{14}C-lactose with 12.5 g of carrier lactose. As there was no overlap between the radioisotope excretion in normal individuals and in lactose malabsorbers, the test was both sensitive and specific. In quantitative terms, however, it greatly underestimated the amount of lactose malabsorbed, since only one-quarter of the isotope known to have passed out of the small bowel into the colon appeared in the feces. The remainder presumably was metabolized to $^{14}CO_2$ and excreted as fecal and pulmonary gas. Moreover, correlation between grams of lactose not absorbed and fecal isotope excreted was relatively poor. Methods now are becoming available to quantify the stable isotope, carbon 13, in a fecal matrix (Schoeller, personal communication). Thus, an analogous procedure to fecal ^{14}C monitoring has been incorporated into the use of ^{13}C-lactose in lactose absorption tests.

Analysis of Postlactose Signs and Symptoms.   *Lactose intolerance* refers to the presentation of clinical signs and symptoms with the ingestion of lactose. With any of the tests that involve challenges with discrete lactose doses, the investigator can complement any laboratory index by soliciting reports of subjective symptoms (i.e., bloating, meteorism, abdominal pain, flatulence) or observe objective signs (i.e., eructations, diarrhea). Given the nature of the testing situation, little reliance can be placed in the reporting and grading of most symptoms. Explosive diarrhea, of course, can be monitored and recorded. In the young infant, "intolerance" is assessed more reliably. Most infants will sleep peacefully following a caloric meal; distention, diarrhea, crankiness, and irritability after lactose are good evidence of incomplete digestion. The computerized assessment of bowel sounds has been introduced (Dalle et al. 1975, Polizer et al. 1976), and its application in assessing the postlactose intestinal response bears quantitative evaluation.

Because the substrate is undisguised in the conventional testing situation, psychological factors can influence the reporting and grading of subjective symptoms. Lacassie and co-workers (1978) found a correlation coefficient of 0.008 between symptoms and the rise in plasma glucose. A number of groups recently have reported correlating objective indices of symptoms with the lactose dose disguised and presented to subjects in a double-blind, randomized fashion (Newcomer et al. 1978, Lisker and Aguilar 1978, Rorick and Scrimshaw 1979, Kwon et al. 1980, Haverberg et al. 1980, Lisker, personal communication). This approach seems essential if valid symptomatic data related to lactose ingestion are to be obtained. Moreover, attention should be paid to the osmolarity of the placebo dose, since simple hydrolysis of the lactose in milk with lactase will alter the osmolarity of the beverage.

INTRAPROCEDURE COMPARISON

Attempts to correlate the lactase assay with indirect indices of lactose malabsorption and to correlate the lactose absorption tests among one another have been reported. Arvanitakis et al. (1977) compared the $^{14}CO_2$ breath test and the plasma glucose test in biopsy-proven lactase-deficient subjects, normal controls, and patients with irritable bowel syndrome (IBS); 7 of the 20 patients with IBS also had deficient lactase levels. The test dose of lactose was 50 g. The $^{14}CO_2$ breath test resulted in no falsely abnormal assessments in control or IBS groups, whereas one lactase-deficient subject falsely was diagnosed as normal. The standard glucose test provided two false positive tests among control subjects and three false positive tests among IBS patients, while it failed to diagnose one lactase-deficient individual (Arvanitakis et al. 1977).

Newcomer et al. (1975) compared the hydrogen breath test, the plasma glucose and plasma galactose tests, and the $^{14}CO_2$ breath test against the actual tissue lactase status in 25 biopsy-proven lactase-deficient adults and an equal number of proven lactose-sufficient subjects. The $^{14}CO_2$ breath test, galactose test, and glucose test provided false negative results in two, six, and one lactase-deficient subjects, respectively; in normal subjects, one false positive result was seen with the glucose method. The hydrogen breath test proved to be 100% sensitive and 100% specific (Newcomer et al. 1975). As was stated at the outset, however, divergence between biopsy results and absorption tests is not unexpected.

Bond and Levitt (1976) used the perfusion technique, the net removal of lactose along the length of the small intestine, as their standard of absorption. With a total oral lactose dose of 12.5 g (a physiologic level) labeled with 1-^{14}C-lactose tag, they compared the hydrogen breath test, the $^{14}CO_2$ breath test, and fecal ^{14}C excretion in 10 subjects. Both the hydrogen breath test and fecal ^{14}C excretion clearly separated the normal and abnormal lactose absorbers as determined by perfusion. However, with quantitative absorption data, correlations with each of the indirect indices were calculated. The correlation coefficients were 0.94, -0.77, and 0.76 for the pulmonary H_2, pulmonary $^{14}CO_2$, and fecal ^{14}C output tests, respectively. Thus, the hydrogen breath test appears to be the most sensitive and the most specific indirect index of lactase status and the best predictor of intestinal absorptive capacity for lactose.

THE HYDROGEN BREATH TEST

At least 20 studies using the hydrogen breath analysis test to study lactose absorption have been published in the decade since the test first was introduced by Calloway et al. (1969) (table 8.2). Since this technology appears to offer the most reliable indirect index of both lactase capacity and lactose absorption and has particular applicability to field screening, it deserves a more detailed examination.

Gas Collection Procedure. Many early studies have used a continuous, closed, rebreathing system to collect expired air (Bond and Levitt 1972, Newcomer et al. 1975). The rate of pulmonary H_2 excretion can be measured directly in this manner, but the approach is cumbersome and has given way to sampling at intervals after the oral administration of lactose. With interval sampling methods, the change in hydrogen concentration in expired air above the basal fasting level is used; if necessary, an estimate of total H_2 excretion can be obtained by integration under the discontinuous curve of concentration change. End-

TABLE 8.2
Published evaluations of lactose digestion using the hydrogen breath test

Citation	Population studied
Bond and Levitt 1972	2 "adult" postgastrectomy patients in Minnesota
Bond and Levitt 1976	10 "adult" subjects in Minnesota
Brown et al. 1979	331 Bangladeshi villagers: infants, children, and adults
Calloway et al. 1969	12 subjects, aged 20 to 33 yrs: 5 orientals; 5 whites; 2 blacks
Caskey et al. 1977	60 Native Americans, aged 3 to 64 yrs, in Oklahoma
Cook 1978	36 "adult" subjects of European, African, and Asian origins
Douwes et al. 1978	163 Dutch children, aged 9 mo to 14 yrs, with chronic diarrhea or pain
Fernandes et al. 1978	52 Dutch children, aged 4 to 15 yrs, with assorted gastrointestinal disease
Gearhart et al. 1976	8 Native Americans, aged 18 to 34 yrs, in Oklahoma
Levitt and Donaldson 1970	55 "young adults" including normals, hospitalized, and gastrectomy patients
Maffei et al. 1977	23 British children, aged 2 mo to 13 yrs with chronic diarrhea
Metz et al. 1975	25 persons in London
Newcomer et al. 1975	50 adults, aged 20 to 72 yrs in Minnesota: 48 whites; 2 blacks
Newcomer et al. 1977	156 Native Americans (Chippewa), 104 aged 5 to 17 yrs; 52 aged 18 to 73 yrs
Newcomer et al. 1977	104 Native Americans (Chippewa), aged 1 to 69 yrs
Payne-Bose et al. 1977	7 Native American women, aged 18 to 26 years, in Oklahoma
Rorick and Scrimshaw 1979	87 elderly subjects, aged 60 to 97 yrs, of European, Jewish, and black origins
Solomons et al. 1978	15 Guatemalan preschool children recovering from protein-energy malnutrition
Solomons et al. 1979	12 Guatemalan preschool children recovering from protein-energy malnutrition
Solomons et al. 1980	20 "adults" of Guatemalan-indigenous, Spanish-ethnic, and European origins

expiratory air essentially represents alveolar air (Solomons et al. 1977). At the
Institute of Nutrition of Central America and Panama (INCAP) air from children
is collected in gas bags (fig. 8.1) and then transferred immediately to gas-tight
containers. This technique collects air from the full respiratory cycle, including
the anatomical dead space, and thus reflects 70% of the true alveolar concentration (Solomons et al. 1977). Although hydrogen gas is the lightest and most
diffusible of all gases, a number of containers can be used to store collected
breath samples prior to analysis. Glass syringes are functionally gas tight for 12
to 24 hours. Laminated foil bags are gas-tight for seven weeks (Solomons et al.
1977) and evacuated rubber-stoppered tubes will store samples for three weeks
(Newcomer et al. 1975).

Hydrogen Analysis.   Hydrogen concentration in expired air is determined by
gas chromatography. Two systems, thermal conductivity and helium ionization
detectors, have been used. As the latter requires a tritium source, it implies a
certain environmental hazard. Instrumental modifications have permitted sensitive analysis of H_2 in whole, unconcentrated breath samples from a single exhala-

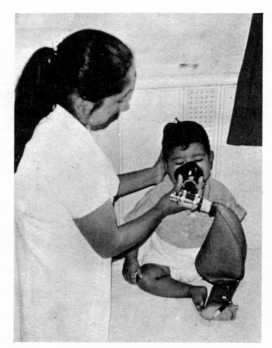

FIGURE 8.1. Procedure for collection of expired air for the
interval sampling hydrogen breath test in preschool children.
Employs mask, one-way valve, and gas bag.

tion using thermal conductivity detectors (Solomons et al. 1977, Payne-Bose et al. 1978). There has been ample demonstration of a stable level of H_2 excretion in the absence of carbohydrate malabsorption (Levitt and Donaldson 1970, Bond and Levitt 1972, Solomons et al. 1978 and 1980). A stoichiometric relationship of the H_2 response to graded doses of a nonabsorbable carbohydrate (lactulose) has been demonstrated by some groups (Bond and Levitt 1972, Solomons et al. 1978), but not by others (Cochet et al. 1978). Thus, the quantification of the amount of lactose in grams *not absorbed* by reference to a lactulose curve is only semiquantitative at best.

Application of the Hydrogen Breath Test.   The hydrogen breath test has been applied to the problem of lactose digestion in the context both of the clinical diagnosis and of screening populations. Illustrated in fig. 8.2 is a representative curve of interval sampling hydrogen breath tests performed in a 3-year-old Guatemalan with protein-energy malnutrition. Samples of expired air were collected before and at 30-minute intervals after the oral administration of a 1.75 g

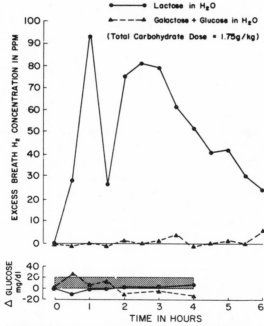

FIGURE 8.2. Change in breath H_2 concentration (upper graph) and in plasma glucose (lower graph) in a lactose-malabsorbing preschool child after oral administration of 1.75 g per kg lactose (●————●) or an equimolar mixture of galactose and glucose (▲ - - - ▲). Source: Solomons et al. 1978, reprinted with permission.

per kg dose of carbohydrate substrate. An increment in H_2 of > 20 ppm generally has been considered abnormal and indicative of fermentation of biologically significant amounts of nonabsorbed carbohydrate. Metz et al. (1975) demonstrated that a rise of > 20 ppm in breath H_2 concentration at two hours following a 50 g dose of aqueous lactose in adults corresponded to an increase in plasma glucose of < 20 mg per dl in the same subject. When the pediatric dosage of lactose was ingested by the subject, a maximum rise of 93 ppm was observed at one hour postdose. Integrating the area under the curve gave as an estimated excess pulmonary H_2 excretion rate 51.4 cc per six hours. A simultaneous plasma glucose test accompanying the H_2 breath test with lactose revealed a maximum increment of 2 mg per dl. When the same subject was given an equimolar mixture of the monosaccharide components of lactose, glucose and galactose, no significant rise in breath H_2 occurred (fig. 8.2), while plasma glucose rose to a maximum of 31 mg per dl above fasting levels.

Similar curves are seen in adult malabsorbers when challenged with 50 g lactose in water. Sampling intervals of 60 minutes are used in adult subjects. It is standard procedure at INCAP to use a six-hour observation period in all subjects. Other investigators have advocated a single two-hour postchallenge breath analysis as an index of lactose malabsorption (Metz et al. 1975, Newcomer et al. 1977a, Newcomer et al. 1977b). The INCAP experience indicates that intolerant, malabsorbing subjects often will not show the diagnostic increment in breath H_2 until some time after the two-hour interval; this is especially common in young children and in subjects receiving lactose in the form of whole milk (Solomons et al. 1980).

Lactose Challenges in Physiological Dosages and from Dietary Sources. Because the H_2 breath analysis test can demonstrate the malabsorption of as little as 2 g of carbohydrate, one can detect impaired digestion of smaller doses of lactose than are necessary for the use of blood glucose determination. Levitt and Donaldson (1970) demonstrated this in their original 1970 publication. Recently, this capability has encouraged the application of oral lactose doses in the range that one would consume in an ordinary meal, i.e., 10 g to 15 g. A 250 ml glass of milk, for instance, contains 12.5 g lactose, and Bond and Levitt (1976) used this dose in their comparison of indirect techniques. The Oklahoma group routinely uses a dosage of 0.25 g lactose per kg of body weight (Gearhart et al. 1976, Caskey et al. 1977); in a 70 kg adult, this would constitute a 17.5 g dose. Solomons et al. (1980) recently compared the sensitivity of a 12.5 g dose of lactose in detecting lactose maldigestion in individuals who had shown a positive rise in breath H_2 concentration with the conventional 50 g dose. Nine of 11 intolerant malabsorbers manifested a rise of greater than 20 ppm with both lactose loads. There was significantly less discomfort experienced with the use of the lower, more physiological dose.

The other possibility that is offered by the H_2 technology is the application of normal food sources of lactose instead of the artificial, concentrated aqueous solutions that are used with the other techniques. Calloway et al. (1969) used whole milk and cheese as sources of lactose in their pioneering report. The use of milk with the H_2 breath test recently has become increasingly popular (Gearhart et al. 1976, Caskey et al. 1977, Payne-Bose et al. 1977, Fernandes et al. 1978, Solomons et al. 1979 and 1980). In the study referred to above (Solomons et al. 1980), cow's milk providing 50 g and 12.5 g was administered to adult subjects. The higher lactose dose diagnosed 10 of 13 individuals who had an abnormal breath test with the corresponding amount of lactose in aqueous solution; 8 of 9 individuals showed abnormal tests with whole milk and aqueous forms of the 12.5 g dose. In adult subjects, no significant difference in the volume of H_2 excreted in response to either form of lactose was seen at either dose (Solomons et al. 1980). On the other hand, in preschool children a reduced rate of H_2 production has been demonstrated clearly by comparing lactose in whole milk with aqueous lactose (Solomons et al. 1979). Similar findings were demonstrated in slightly older children by Dutch investigators (Fernandes et al. 1978). Insofar as the gaseous as well as the osmotic consequences from lactose malabsorption affect the subjective symptoms, the reduced rate of H_2 production in children may explain their relatively better tolerance of milk and dietary lactose despite objective findings of impaired lactose digestion (Garza and Scrimshaw 1976). In all age groups, the combination of physiological dosages and food vehicles for lactose absorption tests provides the most realistic reflection of the dietary situation. Detection of lactose maldigestion in this context is well within the capabilities of the H_2 breath analysis technology.

Pitfalls and Caveats. A number of pitfalls to the application of hydrogen breath tests have been uncovered during the decade of experience with this technology (table 8.3). An understanding of the caveats is essential to the accurate

TABLE 8.3
Pitfalls in the application and interpretation of the hydrogen breath test for lactose absorption

Idiopathic absence of appropriate flora
  Consequence: No H_2 response to nonabsorbed carbohydrate
Use of oral antibiotics prior to the hydrogen breath test
  Consequence: Reduction in the mass of fermenting bacteria in the colon
Cigarette smoking during the hydrogen breath test
  Consequence: Abrupt increase in breath H_2 concentration not related to carbohydrate
Active diarrhea at the time of the hydrogen breath test
  Consequence: Reduced H_2 response to a given amount of nonabsorbed carbohydrate
Sleeping during the hydrogen breath test
  Consequence: Increased concentration of breath H_2
Incorporation of lactose dose into a fiber-containing meal
  Consequence: Excess of excretion of breath H_2 not related to lactose malabsorption

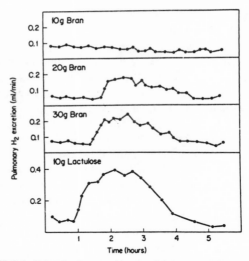

FIGURE 8.3. Rate of pulmonary H_2 excretion in a normal subject after ingestion of a standard 10 g dose of the nonabsorbable disaccharide, lactulose, and after graded doses of 10 g, 20 g, and 30 g of bran as a source of dietary fiber. Source: Bond and Levitt 1978, copyright © Am. J. Clin. Nutr. American Society for Clinical Nutrition, reprinted with permission.

implementation of the hydrogen breath test for lactose absorption. Certain rare individuals lack the appropriate colonic flora to produce H_2 (Bond and Levitt 1972). The prior use of oral antibiotics also can affect the bacterial mass (Murphy and Calloway 1972, Solomons et al. 1978). In both situations, administration of the nonabsorbable disaccharide, lactulose, can uncover the nonresponding individual. Cigarette smoking can cause an artifactual rise in breath H_2 concentration (Tadesse and Eastwood 1977). Active diarrheal disease (gastroenteritis) attenuates the H_2 response to a given dose of nonabsorbed carbohydrate (Solomons et al. 1979). Uninterrupted sleep will produce an artifactual increase in H_2 concentration in the breath (Solomons and Viteri 1976, Metz and Jenkins 1977, Solomons et al. 1978). Bond and Levitt (1978) have shown that the ingestion of bran will result in an increase in breath H_2, presumably due to bacterial digestion and fermentation of the fiber. The administration of lactose or milk in the context of fiber-rich meals will obligate H_2 evolution from the dietary fiber, thus obscuring the contribution of undigested lactose (fig. 8.3).

PRACTICAL SELECTION AND APPLICATION OF DIAGNOSTIC AND SCREENING PROCEDURES

Given the wide array of diagnostic methods available and the diverse situations in which information about lactose digestion might be sought, what are the guidelines for rational selection of procedures? In general, the strategy would be to minimize invasive procedures (intubation, blood extraction), radiation exposure (isotopes, x-rays), and cost; and to maximize simplicity, ease of administration, diagnostic sensitivity, and diagnostic specificity. Additional considerations should involve minimizing the degree of symptomatic discomfort from the challenge dose of lactose in the intolerant subject and approximating the dietary situation with regard to total carbohydrate dose and vehicle.

How can these guidelines be interpreted in terms of the various situations demanding diagnosis of or screening for lactose maldigestion? In the rare instance of a congenitally lactase-deficient infant, a definitive diagnosis demands not only demonstration of lactose malabsorption but also exclusion of other diagnoses. This justifies the use of the more aggressive diagnostic procedures, including intestinal biopsy for lactase assay and/or perfusion studies. The same justification holds for the clinical investigation of the infant suspected of having glucose-galactose malabsorption. In the child with active diarrhea, alterations in intestinal flora, small bowel transit time, and stool water make almost all procedures except intestinal perfusion unreliable. It is reasonable to assume that incomplete lactose digestion will accompany the pathophysiological changes in acute diarrhea, and elaborate attempts to confirm or quantify the malabsorption of lactose are rarely justifiable.

The correlations between abnormally low lactase levels (< 2 lactase units) and indirect tests of lactose absorption have been performed using pharmacological, i.e., 2 g per kg up to 50 g, aqueous doses of lactose. In population studies of a physical anthropological or genetic nature in which the explicit intent is to infer information about the gene frequency of the *lactase enzyme,* therefore, the larger, nonphysiologic doses are justified. It can be anticipated, however, that these tests will be associated with a higher degree of physical discomfort. Although plasma glucose determination is the traditional modality for studies of this nature, the hydrogen breath test can be substituted. This will eliminate the additional discomfort of blood sampling, reduce costs, and simplify the field operations and laboratory analysis. Moreover, breath H_2 determination probably would be more sensitive and specific than glucose measurements under these conditions (Newcomer et al. 1975, Bond and Levitt 1976).

It is in the usual clinical situation, in which the practitioner or dietician wishes to determine if milk intolerance symptoms are related to lactose maldigestion and how much lactose the patient reasonably could tolerate, that the general strategy outlined above is directly applicable. This is equally true, however, for population studies in which dietary and nutritional, rather than genetic, questions are being raised concerning the use of milk. This would include studies aimed at directing food relief efforts or for designing or evaluating subsidy programs such as the Women, Infants and Children (WIC) program of the U.S. Department of Agriculture. In both of these situations, the hydrogen breath test would be the procedure of choice. Moreover, usual rather than pharmacological doses of lactose would be appropriate to the information being sought. Torun et al. (1979) recently recommended the following lactose dosage schedule: 2 g per kg to a maximum of 12 g during the first year of life; 15 g during the second year; and 18 g thereafter. The vehicle of lactose should be whole cow's milk, assuming a 5% lactose content. In both field and office applications of the hydrogen breath test, several intervals of collection are suggested. When symptomatic as well as objective malabsorption data are required, suitably disguised, identical lactose-containing and lactose-free vehicles should be presented in a double-blind fashion and coupled to the determination of breath H_2. Occasionally, in an infant, a quick screening procedure is called for. The combination of stool pH and fecal reducing substances, although neither 100% specific nor 100% sensitive, can be worth employing at the bedside.

REFERENCES

Ament ME: Malabsorption syndrome in infancy and childhood: I. *J Pediatr* 81:685–97, 1972.

Arvanitakis C, Chen G-H, Folscroft J, Klotz AP: Lactose deficiency: A comparative study of diagnostic methods. *Am J Clin Nutr* 30:1597–1602, 1977.

Bayless TM, Rosensweig NW: A racial difference in the incidence of lactose deficiency: A survey of milk tolerance and lactase deficiency in healthy males. *JAMA* 197:968–72, 1966.

Bond JH, Levitt MD: Use of pulmonary hydrogen (H_2) measurements to quantitate carbohydrate absorption: Study of partially gastrectomized patients. *J Clin Invest* 51:1219–25, 1972.

Bond JH, Levitt MD: Quantitative measurement of lactose absorption. *Gastroenterology* 70:1058–62, 1976.

Bond JH, Levitt MD: Effect of dietary fiber on intestinal gas production and small bowel transit time in man. *Am J Clin Nutr* 31: S169–S174, 1978.

Brown KH, Parry L, Khatun M, Ahmed MG: Lactose malabsorption in Bangladeshi village children: Relation with age, history of recent diarrhea, nutritional status, and breast feeding. *Am J Clin Nutr* 32:1962–69, 1979.

Burgess EA, Levin B, Mahalanabis D, Tonge RE: Hereditary sucrose intolerance: Levels of sucrase activity in jejunal mucosa. *Arch Dis Child* 39:431–43, 1964.

Calloway DH, Murphy EL: The use of expired air to measure intestinal gas formation. *Ann NY Acad Sci* 150:82–95, 1968.

Calloway DH, Murphy EL, Bauer D: Determination of lactose intolerance by breath analysis. *Am J Dig Dis* 14:811–15, 1969.

Caskey DA, Payne-Bose D, Welsh JD, Gearhart HL, Nance MK, Morrison RD: Effects of age on lactose malabsorption in Oklahoma Native Americans as determined by breath H_2 analysis. *Am J Dig Dis* 22:113–16, 1977.

Cochet B, Beyeler S, Balant L, Loizeau E: Test de l'hydrogene expire: Sa valeur dans l'appreciation quantitative des malabsorptions glucidiques. *Schweiz Med Wochenschr* 108:1536–41, 1978.

Cook GC: Breath hydrogen concentration after oral lactose and lactulose in tropical malabsorption and adult hypolactasia. *Trans R Soc Trop Med Hyg* 72:277–81, 1978.

Cuatrecasas P, Lockwood DH, Caldwell JR: Lactase deficiency in the adult. *Lancet* 1:14–18, 1965.

Dahlquist A: Method for assay of intestinal disaccharidases. *Anal Biochem* 7:18–25, 1964.

Dalle D, Devroede G, Thibault R: Computer analysis of bowel sounds. *Comput Biol Med* 4:247–56, 1975.

Douwes AC, Fernandes J, Degenhart HJ: Improved accuracy of lactose tolerance test in children, using expired H_2 measurement. *Arch Dis Child* 53:939–42, 1978.

Durand P: Lactosuria idiopathica in una paziente con diarrea cronica et acidosi. *Minerva Pediatr* 10:706–11, 1958.

Fernandes J, Vos CE, Douwes AC, Slotema E: Respiratory hydrogen excretion as a parameter for lactose malabsorption in children. *Am J Clin Nutr* 31:597–602, 1978.

Fischer W, Zapf J: Zur erworbene lactoseintoleranz. *Klin Wochenschr* 43:1243–45, 1965.

Flatz G, Rotthauwe HW: The human lactose polymorphism: Physiology and genetics of lactose absorption and malabsorption. In *Progress in Medical Genetics, NS, II,* AG Steinberg, AG Bearn, AG Motulsky, B Childs (eds). Philadelphia: Saunders, 1977, pp 205–49.

Garza C, Scrimshaw NS: Relationship of lactose intolerance to milk intolerance in young children. *Am J Clin Nutr* 29:192–96, 1976.

Gearhart HL, Bose DP, Smith CA, Morrison RD, Welsh JD, Smalley TK: Determination of lactose by breath analysis with gas chromatography. *Anal Chem* 48:393–98, 1976.

Gray GM: Malabsorption of carbohydrate. *Fed Proc* 26:1415–19, 1967.

Harrison M, Walker-Smith JA: Reinvestigation of lactose intolerant children: Lack of correlation between lactose intolerance and small intestinal morphology, disaccharidase activity, and lactose tolerance tests. *Gut* 18:48–52, 1977.

Haverberg L, Kwon PH Jr, Scrimshaw NS: Comparative tolerance of adolescents of differing ethnic backgrounds to lactose-containing and lactose-free dairy drinks: I. Initial experience with a double-blind procedure. *Am J Clin Nutr* 33:17–21, 1980.

Heine W, Zunft HJ, Müller-Beuthow W, Grütte F-K: Lactose and protein absorption from breast milk and cow's milk preparations and its influence on the intestinal flora. *Acta Paediatr Scand* 66:699–703, 1977.

Holzel A, Schwarz V, Sutcliffe KW: Defective lactose absorption causing malnutrition in infancy. *Lancet* 1:1126–28, 1959.

Ifekwuniqwe AE: Emergency treatment of large numbers of children with severe protein-calorie malnutrition. *Am J Clin Nutr* 28:79–83, 1975.

Isokoski M, Jussila J, Sarna S: A simple screening method for lactose malabsorption. *Gastroenterology* 62:28–32, 1972.

Jones DV, Latham MC: Lactose intolerance in young children and their parents. *Am J Clin Nutr* 27:547–49, 1974.

Jussila J: Diagnosis of lactose malabsorption by the lactose tolerance test with peroral ethanol administration. *Scand J Gastroenterol* 4:361–68, 1969.

Kern F Jr, Heller M: Blood galactose after lactose and ethanol: An accurate index of lactase deficiency. *Gastroenterology* 54:1250, 1968.

Kern F Jr, Struthers JE Jr: Intestinal lactase deficiency and lactose intolerance in adults. *JAMA* 195:927–30, 1966.

Kerry KR, Anderson CM: A ward test for sugar in faeces. *Lancet* 1:981, 1964.

Keusch GT, Troncale FJ, Thavaramara B, Prinyanont P, Anderson PR, Bhamarapravathi N: Lactase deficiency in Thailand: Effect of prolonged lactose feeding. *Am J Clin Nutr* 22:638–41, 1969.

Klein PD, Schoeller DA, Niu HC: [13]C breath tests: Components, technology and comparative costs. *Gastroenterology* 76:1171, 1979.

Krasilnikoff PA, Gudmand-Hoyer E, Moltke HH: Diagnostic value of disaccharide tolerance tests in children. *Acta Paediatr Scand* 64:693–98, 1975.

Kwon PH Jr, Rorick MH, Scrimshaw NS: Comparative tolerance of adolescents of differing ethnic backgrounds to lactose-containing and lactose-free dairy drinks: II. Improvement of a double-blind test. *Am J Clin Nutr* 33:22–26, 1980.

Lacassie Y, Weinberg R, Monckeberg F: Poor predictability of lactose malabsorption from clinical symptoms for Chilean populations. *Am J Clin Nutr* 31:799–804, 1978.

Laws JW, Neale G: Radiological diagnosis of disaccharidase deficiency. *Lancet* 2:139–43, 1966.

Laws JW, Spencer J, Neale G: Radiology in the diagnosis of disaccharidase deficiency. *Br J Radiol* 40:594–603, 1967.

Lebenthal E: Small intestinal disaccharidase deficiencies. *Pediatr Clin North Am* 20:757–66, 1975.

Lebenthal E: Lactose intolerance. In *Digestive Diseases of Children,* E Lebenthal, TE Hatch, LR Romano (eds). New York: Grune and Stratton, 1978, pp 367–88.

Leichter J: Comparison of whole milk and skim milk with aqueous lactose solution in lactose tolerance testing. *Am J Clin Nutr* 26:393–96, 1973.

Levitt MD: Production and excretion of hydrogen gas in man. *N Engl J Med* 28:122–27, 1969.

Levitt MD, Donaldson RM: Use of respiratory hydrogen (H_2) excretion to detect carbohydrate malabsorption. *J Lab Clin Med* 75:937–45, 1970.

Lisker R, Aguilar L: Double blind study of milk lactose tolerance. *Gastroenterology* 74:1283–85, 1978.

Lisker R, Lopez HG, Mora MA: Correlation in the diagnosis of intestinal lactase deficiency between the radiological method and the lactose tolerance test. *Rev Invest Clin* 27:1–5, 1975.

McGill DB, Newcomer AD: Comparison of venous and capillary blood samples in lactose tolerance testing. *Gastroenterology* 53:371–74, 1967.

Maffei HVL, Metz G, Bampoe V, Shiner M, Herman S, Brook CGD: Lactose intolerance detected by the hydrogen breath test in infants and children with chronic diarrhea. *Arch Dis Child* 52:766–71, 1977.

Metz G, Jenkins DJ: Breath hydrogen during sleep. *Lancet* 1:145–46, 1977.

Metz G, Jenkins DJA, Peters JJ, Newman A, Blendis LM: Breath hydrogen as a diagnostic method for hypolactasia. *Lancet* 1:1155–57, 1975.

Murphy EL, Calloway DH: The effect of antibiotic drugs on the volume and composition of intestinal gas from beans. *Am J Dig Dis* 17:639–42, 1972.

Newcomer AD, Gordon H, Thomas PJ, McGill DB: Family studies of lactase deficiency in the American Indian. *Gastroenterology* 73:985–88, 1977a.

Newcomer AD, McGill DB: Distribution of disaccharidase activity in the small bowel of normal and lactase-deficient subjects. *Gastroenterology* 51:481–88, 1966.

Newcomer AD, McGill DB: Disaccharidase activity in the small intestine: Prevalence of lactase deficiency in 100 healthy subjects. *Gastroenterology* 53:881–89, 1967.

Newcomer AD, McGill DB, Thomas PJ, Hofmann AF: Prospective comparison of indirect methods for detecting lactase deficiency. *N Engl J Med* 293:1232–35, 1975.

Newcomer AD, McGill DB, Thomas PJ, Hofmann AF: Tolerance to lactose among lactase-deficient American Indians. *Gastroenterology* 74:44–46, 1978.

Newcomer AD, Thomas PJ, McGill DB, Hofmann AF: Lactase deficiency: A common genetic trait of the American Indian. *Gastroenterology* 72:234–37, 1977b.

Payne-Bose D, Tsegaye A, Morrison RD, Waller GR: An improved method for determining breath H_2 as an indicator of carbohydrate malabsorption. *Anal Biochem* 88:659–67, 1978.

Payne-Bose D, Welsh JD, Gearhart HL, Morrison RD: Milk and lactose-hydrolyzed milk. *Am J Clin Nutr* 30:695–97, 1977.

Polizer JP, Devroede G, Vasseur C, Gerard J, Thibault R: The genesis of bowel sounds: Influence of viscus and gastrointestinal content. *Gastroenterology* 71:282–85, 1976.

Protein Advisory Group of the United Nations: PAG statement 17 on low lactase activity and milk intake. *PAG Bull* 2(2):9–11, 1972.

Reddy V, Pershad J: Lactase deficiency in Indians. *Am J Clin Nutr* 25:114–19, 1972.

Rodriguez-de-Curet H, Lugo-de-Rivera C, Torres-Pinedo R: Studies on infant diarrhea: IV. Sugar transit and absorption in small intestine after a feeding. *Gastroenterology* 59:396–403, 1970.

Rorick M, Scrimshaw NS: Comparative tolerance of elderly from differing ethnic backgrounds to lactose-containing and lactose-free dairy drinks: A double-blind study. *J Gerontol* 34: 191–96, 1979.

Rosenquist CJ: Lactose-barium study as a screening test for lactase deficiency. *West J Med* 122:319, 1975.

Salmon PR, Read AE, McCarthy CF: An isotope technique for measuring lactose absorption. *Gut* 10:685–89, 1969.

Sasaki Y, Iio M, Kameda H, Veda H, Aoyagi T, Christopher NL, Bayless TM, Wagner HN: Measurement of ^{14}C-lactose absorption in the diagnosis of lactase deficiency. *J Lab Clin Med* 76: 824–35, 1970.

Sheehy TW, Anderson PR: Disaccharidase activity in normal and diseased small bowel. *Lancet* 2:1–4, 1965.

Solomons NW, Garcia R, Schneider R, Viteri FE, von Kaenel VA: H_2 breath tests during diarrhea. *Acta Paediatr Scand* 68:171–72, 1979.

Solomons NW, Garcia-Ibanez R, Viteri FE: Reduced rate of breath hydrogen (H_2) excretion with lactose tolerance tests in young children using whole milk. *Am J Clin Nutr* 32:783–86, 1979.

Solomons NW, Garcia-Ibanez R, Viteri FE: Hydrogen (H_2) breath test of lactose absorption in adults: The application of physiological doses and whole cow's milk sources. *Am J Clin Nutr* 33:545–54, 1980.

Solomons NW, Viteri FE: Breath hydrogen during sleep. *Lancet* 2:636, 1976.

Solomons NW, Viteri FE, Hamilton LH: Application of a simple gas chromatographic technique for measuring breath hydrogen. *J Lab Clin Med* 90:856–62, 1977.

Solomons NW, Viteri FE, Rosenberg IH: Development of an interval sampling hydrogen (H_2) breath test for carbohydrate malabsorption in children: Evidence for a circadian pattern of breath H_2 concentration. *Pediatr Res* 12:816–23, 1978.

Tadesse K, Eastwood M: Breath-hydrogen test and smoking. *Lancet* 2:91, 1977.

Torres-Pinedo R, Lugo-de-Rivera C, Rodriguez-de-Curet H: Intestinal absorptive defects associated with enteric infections in infants. *Ann NY Acad Sci* 176:284–98, 1971.

Torun B, Solomons NW, Viteri FE: Lactose malabsorption and lactose intolerance: Implication for general milk consumption. A position paper. *Arch Latinoam Nutr* 29:445–94, 1979.

CHAPTER 9

LIMITATIONS OF THE HYDROGEN

BREAST TEST AND OTHER TECHNIQUES

FOR PREDICTING INCOMPLETE

LACTOSE ABSORPTION

Ronald G. Barr

Analysis of the techniques available for diagnosis and screening of "lactose maldigestion" confirms that the lactose hydrogen breath test has a number of distinct advantages over other available methods. Indeed, it was partly these important advantages that led to the consideration of the potential application of the hydrogen breath test to some common clinical problems of childhood (Barr et al. 1979 and 1978, Perman et al. 1978). Consequently, this chapter is illustrated with examples from the lactose hydrogen breath test literature, although the principles would be equally applicable with but slight modification to the other diagnostic and screening methods.

Asking the question, "Diagnosis and screening *for what?*" leads to three observations. The first two are important in any discussion, not just of the techniques themselves, but of their actual *use* in diagnosis and screening. The first observation is a semantic one, namely that "incomplete lactose absorption" rather than "lactose maldigestion" is a more appropriate description of what is being diagnosed and screened for. Second, when discussing diagnostic use and screening, the more relevant measure of a test's efficiency is positive and negative predictive accuracy rather than the more common indices of sensitivity and specificity. The third observation is that the "normal" rise in breath H_2 excretion should be defined in terms of the technique's variability and the time of the H_2

rise. Calling a rise of < 20 ppm H_2 normal, regardless of the time of occurrence, may deprive investigators of much useful information. These three points are illustrated briefly below.

INCOMPLETE LACTOSE ABSORPTION VERSUS LACTOSE MALDIGESTION

There have been other semantic arguments in the literature on lactose intolerance, notably around what to call the lactase levels found in the majority of the world's adult population. The argument that the phrase *lactose maldigestion* should be replaced by *incomplete lactose absorption* may seem like a semantic quibble, but in fact there are important real life consequences when the tests described are applied in the clinical context. There is no very good evidence that lactose arriving in the large intestine is abnormal, wrong, or indicative of malfunction or disease. Indeed, probably the opposite is true. Consider the following:

(1) Utilizing an ileal intubation method, Bond and Levitt (1976a) demonstrated that up to 8% of a physiologic 12.5 g lactose load could reach the colon in lactose-tolerant individuals.
(2) Based on tests using breath H_2 methods, both Engel and Levitt (1970) and Chiles et al. (1979) have reported that all normal newborn infants absorb lactose incompletely in the first week of life. Can it be claimed reasonably that something *all* infants do is in any way unusual or abnormal?
(3) Bond and Levitt (1976b) also demonstrated that carbohydrate reaching the colon probably is not lost to the energy pool of the body, but rather is transformed, by the bacteria that produce the H_2 rise, into potentially useful short-chain fatty acids, which then are absorbed from the colon and oxidized by the host.

The case for the term *incomplete lactose absorption* is that, at best, that is what is being measured, more or less directly, by the techniques described in chapter 8. Indeed, besides its other advantages of noninvasiveness and safety, the hydrogen breath test is the most direct assessment clinically available of incomplete lactose absorption, or, for that matter, of the functional lactase activity of the complete small intestine. The so-called direct assessment provided by enzyme determinations on small intestinal biopsy tells only about one small part of the intestine, and nothing about lactose maldigestion. In sum, the use of the term *lactose maldigestion* imports to the data observed a level of interpretation that is neither inherent in the phenomenon or justified by the evidence. Thus, in describing the hydrogen breath test, one could paraphrase Dr. Solomons as follows: an increase in the rate of breath H_2 excretion after ingestion of lactose reflects bacterial fermentation of part of the substrate, i.e., *incomplete lactose absorption*. Whether that incomplete absorption was actually malabsorption would depend on whether it was due to a disease process, which, in a majority of cases, it is not.

SENSITIVITY AND SPECIFICITY VERSUS PREDICTIVE ACCURACY

The second observation concerns the efficiency of the tests. Sensitivity and specificity, the indices of efficiency (sometimes ambiguously labeled "accuracy") that are used in papers describing these tests, are not what are most important to practicing physicians (Feinstein 1977). Sensitivity and specificity usually are derived from trying the prospective test after the patient's condition is known. Thus, in their important study, Newcomer et al. (1975) compared hydrogen breath test results in 25 patients known to have isolated lactase insufficiency with 25 known not to have it. In contrast, what the clinician wants to know is the *predictive accuracy* of the test in a patient not yet diagnosed as having isolated lactase insufficiency. In other words, one wants to know (1) if the test is positive, what is the chance that the patient will have the condition; and (2) if the test is negative, what is the chance that the patient will not have that condition.

To illustrate the practical importance of this difference, consider the application of the hydrogen breath test to two populations, one black American and one Caucasian American in a "best of all possible worlds" situation. Taking account of observations concerning colonic bacteria by Bond and Levitt (1977), assume that the only source of error will be the 2% of individuals who do not have the appropriate bacteria to produce the H_2 signal. In this situation, the sensitivity of the test is 98% and the specificity is 100%. Assume, secondly, that the prevalence of incomplete lactose absorption is 10% in a Caucasian population, and 90% in a black population.

Despite the test's excellent sensitivity and specificity ratings, its predictive accuracy differs in black and Caucasian populations: the positive predictive accuracy will be 100% in both groups, but the negative predictive accuracy will be 100% in Caucasians, but only 84% in blacks. The calculations are based on the assumption that these subjects did not present with a complaint, or have any condition, that might compromise the use of the test.

The predictive accuracy of the hydrogen breath test would be reduced further under certain less ideal conditions: (1) in children not cooperative with the collection procedure, who could hyperventilate to produce a false negative result; (2) in a patient who "forgot" about the medicine prescribed by another doctor, medicine that suppressed the bowel flora; or (3) in the teenager who says he does not smoke, but out of sight of the technician may take a puff between samples.

Similarly, problems might arise when the test is applied to *clinical* populations, rather than epidemiologically in otherwise well populations. Solomons et al. (1979) noted that the breath hydrogen response is attenuated in children with acute diarrhea. Fernandes et al. (1975) reported a "false positive" case of Crohn's disease where the hydrogen breath test was positive, but the decreased lactase activity was (presumably) limited to the distal small bowel. In addition, Barr et al.

(1979a) reported that only 70% of children presenting with chronic nonspecific diarrhea show concordance between breath hydrogen and enzyme data. With a small bowel overgrowth, a "false positive" hydrogen breath test is possible, as pointed out by Levitt (1969) and others.

Finally, problems may arise if the test is used for a different reason than that for which it was used in the original study defining sensitivity and specificity. For example, if the hydrogen breath test were used to screen for celiac disease in 2-year-olds, would it be equally sensitive in demonstrating "mild" changes on biopsy as in demonstrating "severe" changes? In summary, there are many factors not included in earlier descriptions of the efficiency of the test, factors that must be taken into account when it is applied in the clinical situation.

The important principle is that the efficiency of any test, even a test with a very high sensitivity and specificity, is highly dependent on the conditions of the testing, such as the type of population being screened and the condition for which the population is being screened. If, for example, all of these factors together result in the test still having a sensitivity of 95% and a specificity of 95%, the predictive accuracy then changes. In Caucasians or some clinical population in which the condition is unlikely to be present, the positive predictive accuracy becomes 68%, while the negative predictive accuracy is about 100%; whereas in blacks or some population in which the condition is likely to be present, the positive predictive accuracy remains about 100%, while the negative predictive accuracy falls to 68%.

THE "NORMAL" RISE

The third and final observation concerns the definition of a "normal" value for a breath H_2 rise after a lactose load. Using the techniques reported by Perman et al. (1978), a rise of 10 ppm over baseline is greater than can be accounted for by variability in the technique. Therefore, the author, along with Douwes (1979), recommends a rise of 10 ppm over baseline as indicative of incompletely absorbed lactose. The recommendation that a rise of 20 ppm be taken as an "abnormal" finding appears to have been based on a comparison with concurrent lactose tolerance test results. In view of the inaccuracy of the latter test, one is hesitant to accept that criterion as meaningful. Similarly, it is not clear why "an increment in H_2 of > 20 ppm generally has been considered . . . indicative of fermentation of *biologically significant* amounts of nonabsorbed carbohydrate" (chapter 8). Using as a criterion a 20 ppm rise above baseline will make the test less sensitive for reasons related not to the test itself, but rather to the insensitivity of the lactose tolerance test. This will be even more important if one wants to explore the possibility of lactose hydrogen breath test screening using a smaller test dose that does not provoke symptoms, but will identify populations with isolated lactase insufficiency. However, data in a normal school population (Barr, unpublished observations) support the suggestion (chapter 8) that some sensitivity will be lost with smaller doses.

Secondly, it is recommended that the *time* of the rise as well as the height (or area under the curve) of rise be considered. In children with biopsy-proven isolated lactase insufficiency, the H_2 rise occurred uniformly by 120 minutes (Barr et al. 1979b). Late rises occurred only in patients with partial pandissacharidase deficiency and in patients whose lactose tolerance tests reached normal values by 30 minutes postingestion. Therefore, ''late rises'' may constitute incomplete absorption in the face of normal functional lactase activity, at least when aqueous lactose solutions are used as the test dose. The early blood glucose rises also make gastric delay an unlikely explanation.

In conclusion, despite its increasing popularity, experience with the lactose hydrogen breath test is still limited. Rapid dissemination of this promising technology no doubt will increase awareness of its limitations. Careful consideration of the clinical questions these techniques are being required to answer will permit their rational and appropriate use.

REFERENCES

Barr RG, Levine MD, Watkins JD: Recurrent abdominal pain of childhood due to lactose intolerance: A prospective study. *N Engl J Med* 300:1449–52, 1979.

Barr RG, Perman JA, Schoeller DA, Watkins JB: Breath tests in pediatric gastrointestinal disorders: New diagnostic opportunities. *Pediatrics* 62:393–401, 1978.

Barr RG, Watkins JB, Perman JA, Boehme C: Prediction of assayed lactase activity by interval breath hydrogen sampling in children. *Pediatr Res* 13:395, 1979a.

Barr, RG, Watkins JB, Perman JA, Boehme C: Mucosal function and breath hydrogen (H_2) excretion: Criteria for a normal response. *Pediatr Res* 13:394, 1979b.

Bond JH, Levitt MD: Quantitative measurement of lactose absorption. *Gastroenterology* 70:1058–62, 1976a.

Bond JH, Levitt MD: Fate of soluble carbohydrate in the colon of rats and man. *J Clin Invest* 57:1158–64, 1976b.

Bond JH, Levitt MD: Use of breath hydrogen (H_2) in the study of carbohydrate absorption. *Digestive Diseases* 22:379–82, 1977.

Chiles C, Watkins JB, Barr RG: Lactose utilization in the newborn: Role of colonic flora. *Pediatr Res* 13:365, 1979.

Douwes AC: Respiratory hydrogen excretion as a parameter for sugar malabsorption in children. Ph.D. dissertation in Medicine, University of Groningen. 's-Gravenhage: J. H. Passmans, 1979.

Engel RR, Levitt MD: Intestinal trace gas formation in newborns. In *American Pediatric Society and Society for Pediatric Research Combined Program and Abstracts*, 1970, p 226.

Feinstein AR: On the sensitivity, specificity, and discrimination of diagnostic tests. In *Clinical Biostatistics*, AR Feinstein (ed). St. Louis: C. V. Mosby, 1977, ch 15.

Fernandes J, Vos CE, Douwes AC, Slotema E: Respiratory hydrogen excretion as a parameter for lactose malabsorption in children. *Am J Clin Nutr* 31:597–602, 1978.

Levitt MD: Production and excretion of hydrogen gas in man. *N Engl J Med* 281:122–27, 1969.

Newcomer AD, McGill DB, Thomas PJ, Hofmann AF: Prospective comparison of indirect methods for detecting lactase deficiency. *N Engl J Med* 293:1232–35, 1975.

Perman JA, Barr RG, Watkins JB: Sucrose malabsorption in children: Noninvasive diagnosis by interval breath hydrogen determination. *J Pediatr* 93:17–22, 1978.

Solomons NW, Garcia R, Schneider R, Viteri FE, von Kaenel VA: H_2 breath tests during diarrhea. *Acta Paediatr Scand* 68:171–72, 1979.

V

CLINICAL CONSEQUENCES
IN ADULTS

CHAPTER 10

LACTOSE MALABSORPTION,
MILK INTOLERANCE, AND SYMPTOM
AWARENESS IN ADULTS

Theodore M. Bayless

Lactose intolerance indicates that a subject has both definite intestinal symptoms and a blood sugar rise of less than 26 mg per dl with a lactose tolerance test of 50 g per square meter of body surface, 2 g per kg body weight, or 50 g total dose. If there is a low blood sugar rise without symptoms, the term *lactose malabsorber* is applied. No precise quantitative definition is used for the term *milk intolerance*. An individual who has noted that ingestion of one or two glasses of milk will cause gastrointestinal symptoms, excluding nausea or constipation, is considered to have a history of an "awareness of milk intolerance."

RESULTS OF TRADITIONAL LACTOSE TOLERANCE TESTS

Most subjects with low lactase levels will be unable to digest a lactose load of 50 g per square meter of body surface. Almost all will have a peak blood sugar rise of less than 20 mg or 25 mg per dl and most will be symptomatic (fig. 10.1). A few "controls" with normal jejunal lactase levels also will be symptomatic (Bayless and Rosensweig 1966). With a total lactose dose of 50 g, equivalent to one quart of milk, a lesser number, perhaps 90% to 95%, will have a flat blood sugar curve and 85% to 90% will have symptoms. At this dosage some people who have low lactase levels will not be symptomatic (Bedine and Bayless 1973). In terms of breath hydrogen rise with 50 g lactose, the results have been excellent

117

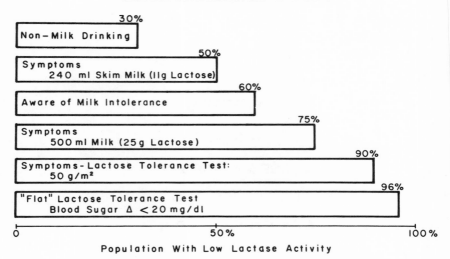

FIGURE 10.1. The consequences of low intestinal lactase activity in adults, given as the frequency of responses to varying amounts of milk and lactose. The data derived from Bayless and Rosensweig 1966, Bayless et al. 1975, Bedine and Bayless 1973, Payne-Bose and Welsh 1973, Cheng et al. 1979, Gudmand-Høyer and Simony 1977, Jones et al. 1976, Lisker et al. 1978, and Welsh 1970.

but the data have varied somewhat. Utilizing a rise of over 20 ppm as evidence that undigested lactose has reached the colon, 100% of persons with lactose intolerance are said to have a positive test (Metz et al. 1975). When a lactose tolerance test and a breath hydrogen test are done simultaneously, there is generally a good correlation between a breath hydrogen rise over 20 ppm and blood sugar rise under 20 mg per dl. In studies at Johns Hopkins some subjects have had a low blood sugar rise and symptoms during the tolerance test but have not experienced a breath hydrogen rise over 20 ppm. These individuals, perhaps 5% of those tested, have falsely negative breath hydrogen tests as a measure of lactose tolerance. Another factor that could create false negative test results is the use of only a 120-minute value, as suggested by Newcomer et al. (1975) and by Metz et al. (1975). Some patients show a peak rise in breath hydrogen at another time, and the 120-minute value is below 20 ppm.

TESTS WITH REDUCED LACTOSE LOAD

There are also data on the ability of lactose-intolerant individuals to digest smaller amounts of lactose. In a recent double-blind study (Cheng et al. 1979), over 90% of the lactose-intolerant subjects who received 25 g lactose as skim milk were symptomatic, as contrasted to only 16% of the control subjects. When the lactose-intolerant subjects received lactose-hydrolyzed milk on a double-blind basis, only 13% were symptomatic. In a Cornell study (Jones et al. 1976) 88% of lactose-intolerant adult subjects were symptomatic with 30 g lactose as skim milk. In this same study, a more selected population of lactose-intolerant adults was examined and 76% were symptomatic with 25 g lactose. Workers in Copenhagen reported that 92% of lactose-intolerant adults were symptomatic with 25 g lactose in milk given on a double-blind basis (Gudmand-Høyer and Simony 1977). Thus, data from a number of groups in different countries indicate that 25 g lactose given as skim milk or whole milk to fasting subjects will produce symptoms in over three-fourths of adults with lactose intolerance and presumed low lactase levels.

CLINICAL CONSEQUENCES OF DIETARY LACTOSE TESTS

Studies using a 12 g lactose dose are most relevant to clinical situations, since a glass of whole milk (240 ml) contains 12 g lactose while a glass of skim milk contains 11 g. When 12 g lactose, as an electrolyte solution equivalent to the electrolyte concentrations in milk, were given to 20 adult subjects with biopsy-confirmed low lactase levels, 75% were symptomatic (Bedine and Bayless 1973). It should be noted, however, that this population was selected in part because the subjects were aware of milk intolerance. In separate studies in 44 randomly selected lactose-intolerant male adults, 68% had symptoms with 12 g lactose in a water-electrolyte solution, while only 1 (2%) had symptoms with an equivalent solution of glucose and galactose, the monosaccharide components of lactose. Utilizing skim milk that contained 12 g lactose, 59% of the lactose-intolerant men were symptomatic, while none of the 27 lactose-tolerant controls reported symptoms (Bayless et al. 1975). Although these studies were not conducted on a double-blind basis, the results are almost identical to those obtained by Gudmand-Høyer and Simony (1977). They gave 10 g lactose in milk powder to 13 lactose-intolerant adults on a double-blind basis and 75% were symptomatic. In a study by Latham and colleagues, sponsored in part by the National Dairy Council (Jones et al. 1976), 69% of lactose-intolerant adult subjects were symptomatic with 15 g lactose in skim milk. In all these studies the main symptoms that the lactose-intolerant subjects noted after drinking 240 ml milk or 12 g lactose solution were flatulence, distention, or cramps. Diarrhea was not a prominent symptom in this dosage range. Some of the subjects were symptomatic with as little as 3 g or 6 g lactose (Bedine and Bayless 1973) (please see fig. 6.7 in chapter 6).

Measurement of breath hydrogen excretion after ingestion of lactose provides a somewhat more objective measure of inadequate lactose digestion than recording symptoms (Solomons et al. 1977). In our studies utilizing 240 ml skim milk containing 11 g lactose, 40% of lactose-intolerant adults had a peak breath hydrogen rise of over 20 ppm. If one considers a rise of over 10 ppm as an indication that unabsorbed lactose has reached the colon, then 58% of the subjects tested positive with 240 ml skim milk. Dr. Solomons (Solomons et al. 1980) also has reported that over one-half the lactose-intolerant subjects tested had a rise in breath hydrogen with a glass of milk. Earlier work by Levitt and Donaldson (1970) also had suggested that approximately one-half the lactose-intolerant people tested had a rise in breath hydrogen after 240 ml milk. Thus, there is objective evidence of inadequate lactose digestion of dietary quantities of milk by one-half the adults who are lactose intolerant. The reason why half the lactose-intolerant adults are unable to digest and absorb the lactose in 240 ml skim milk adequately while the other half can do so, will be considered below.

In terms of abnormal levels of breath hydrogen, our data agree with those of Barr et al. (1979), that with a small dosage of lactose, a rise over 10 ppm indicates that undigested lactose has reached the colon. With a larger dose of lactose, such as 50 g, a rise of over 20 ppm seems to be a reasonable cut-off level.

AWARENESS OF MILK INTOLERANCE

When one carefully questions a population of lactose-intolerant adults living in an environment where milk is available and milk consumption is encouraged, as in the United States, one finds that the majority give a history of being aware that milk will cause intestinal symptoms. In chapter 6, Welsh described his study of 100 adults with low lactase levels, of whom 55% gave a clear history of milk intolerance (Welsh 1970). Usually, this milk intolerance was recognized in the late teenage years or in the subject's early twenties. In another study, Bose and Welsh (1973) reported that 65% of the lactose-intolerant American Indian adults studied were aware of milk intolerance. The results were similar in 89 hospitalized male veterans with lactose intolerance who were being fed milk every day. Some 72% were aware, prior to testing, that they were milk intolerant. This history is not specific for lactose intolerance because one-third of the lactose-tolerant adults also gave a history of milk intolerance (Bayless et al. 1975). These cumulative results on an awareness of milk intolerance fit well with the estimate that at least one-half the lactose-intolerant adults would be symptomatic with a glass of skim milk taken when fasting.

VARIATIONS IN MILK TOLERANCE AMONG LACTOSE-INTOLERANT INDIVIDUALS

The fact that one-half a lactose-intolerant population is unable to digest completely 240 ml skim milk taken when fasting while the other half of the subjects can digest this amount, indicates that the adult population with low lactase levels is not homogeneous in terms of the consequences of their lactose intolerance. In chapter 4 on the pathophysiology of lactose intolerance, Phillips mentions variables such as size of the lactose load; rate of gastric emptying; actual lactase levels throughout the small intestine; and the rate of small bowel transit, all of which would affect substrate enzyme interactions. In addition, one must consider the role of the colonic flora in the fermentation of unabsorbed lactose; the fate of the short-chain fatty acids that result from the breakdown of lactose in the colon; colonic motility; and the absorptive response to this increased load. In work with Dr. Marshall Bedine (Bedine and Bayless 1973), the threshold dose of lactose needed to produce symptoms (3 g, 6 g, 12 g, or 25 g) did not correlate with the jejunal lactase levels as measured by assays of biopsy material. Those who were symptomatic with the smaller amounts of lactose did not necessarily have the lowest lactase levels at the ligament of Trietz. It is possible that the lactase levels lower in the jejunum or in the ileum were different, but the multiple biopsy studies required to obtain that type of information were not performed. Based on the available data, the jejunal lactase levels did not explain the different symptoms with varying amounts of lactose.

DIFFERENCES IN BREATH HYDROGEN EXCRETION AFTER LACTOSE INGESTION

In lactose-intolerant subjects a relatively high peak rise in breath hydrogen (over 70 ppm) during a 50 g lactose tolerance test tended to be associated with a greater likelihood of a breath hydrogen rise (over 10 ppm) with 240 ml skim milk than did only a modest rise in breath hydrogen (less than 70 ppm) on the 50 g tolerance test. For example, 77% of the people whose breath hydrogen on the tolerance test was over 70 ppm had a rise in breath hydrogen of over 10 ppm with 240 ml skim milk containing 11 g lactose versus only 17% of those who were also lactose intolerant but had lower breath hydrogen increases with the 50 g lactose load (Bayless and Paige 1979). The reason for these differences in breath hydrogen production has not been delineated. It is possible that those with the high levels absorbed less of the lactose or alternatively that their colonic flora reacted differently. In addition to a greater percentage of these subjects having a rise in breath hydrogen with 240 ml skim milk, a greater percentage of the subjects who were aware of milk intolerance showed a breath hydrogen rise over 70 ppm on the lactose tolerance test. The majority of this group already was aware of milk intolerance, that is, that a glass of milk or two would cause gas, cramps, or laxative effect. In contrast, only one-fourth of the other lactose-intolerant subjects were aware of milk intolerance.

These differences in milk intolerance might become important if the clinical consequences of lactose intolerance were studied in a medically knowledgeable volunteer population such as medical students, hospital laboratory technicians, or nutritionists (Stephenson and Latham 1974). These types of health care personnel probably would be aware of the concepts of lactose and milk intolerance. It is possible that the lactose-intolerant individuals in the population who already were aware that they were milk intolerant might not "volunteer" to be studied if the protocol included a lactose tolerance test equivalent to four or more glasses of milk. In fact, at Johns Hopkins some potential study subjects do not volunteer because they realize that they probably will become extremely symptomatic. Thus, if one is using a medically knowledgeable population as a source of lactose-intolerant volunteers, the study population has the potential for being unduly weighted with those least likely to respond to dietary quantities of milk.

FORMAT OF MILK ADMINISTRATION

The type of milk used also influences the responses in terms of breath hydrogen rise and possibly in terms of symptoms. Fasting subjects are more symptomatic with skim milk than with whole milk (Leichter 1973), chocolate milk, or milk taken with a meal (Bedine and Bayless 1972). The breath hydrogen response also decreases, in approximately the same order, with the various types of milk (Bayless unpublished data).

Since symptoms and breath hydrogen rise are reduced if lactose or skim milk is taken after a meal, studies done with fasting subjects should not be compared with those in which the test sugar is given with food or other materials that may delay gastric emptying (Newcomer et al. 1978).

MILK CONSUMPTION

Data suggest that lactose or milk intolerance is one of several variables that may influence an individual's milk drinking habits. In a study of hospitalized male veterans, one-third of the lactose-intolerant subjects drank less than one-quarter of the 240 ml glass of milk on their trays in contrast to only 11% of lactose-tolerant controls (Bayless et al. 1975). Similar results were reported from Mexico (Lisker et al. 1978). They found that 46% of their lactose-intolerant subjects drank less than one glass of milk per day in contrast to only 24% of the lactose-tolerant test subjects.

SUMMARY

Thus, it may be estimated that approximately one-half of a group of lactose-intolerant adults would be symptomatic if they took 240 ml skim milk fasting (fig. 10.1). One-half of the original group, and mostly the same subjects, also would have evidence of a breath hydrogen rise with that same amount of milk. Data from Johns Hopkins indicate variations in lactose absorption and/or fermentation in the population defined by standard lactose tolerance testing as lactose intolerant. These variations in groups of lactose-intolerant adults may be major factors in the conflicting answers obtained when similar questions are asked by different groups with slightly different protocols.

REFERENCES

Barr RG, Levine MD, Watkins JB: Recurrent abdominal pain of childhood due to lactose intolerance: A prospective study. *N Engl J Med* 300:1449–52, 1979.

Bayless TM, Paige DM: Consequences of lactose malabsorption: Breath hydrogen excretion after milk ingestion. *Gastroenterology* 76:1097, 1979.

Bayless TM, Rosensweig NS: A racial difference in the incidence of lactase deficiency: A survey of milk tolerance and lactase deficiency in healthy males. *JAMA* 197:968–72, 1966.

Bayless TM, Rothfeld B, Massa C, Wise L, Paige DM, Bedine MS: Lactose and milk intolerance: Clinical implications. *N Engl J Med* 292:1156–59, 1975.

Bedine MS, Bayless TM: Modification of lactose tolerance by glucose or a meal. *Clin Res* 20:448, 1972.

Bedine MS, Bayless TM: Intolerance of small amounts of lactose by individuals with low lactase levels. *Gastroenterology* 65:735–43, 1973.

Bose DP, Welsh JD: Lactose malabsorption in Oklahoma Indians. *Am J Clin Nutr* 26:1320–22, 1973.

Chen AHR, Brunsor O, Espinoza J, Fones HL, Monckeberg F, Chichester CO, Rand AG, Hourigan JA: Long-term acceptance of low-lactose milk. *Am J Clin Nutr* 32:1989–93, 1979.

Gudmand-Høyer E, Simony K: Individual sensitivity to lactose in lactose malabsorption. *Am J Dig Dis* 22:177–81, 1977.

Jones DV, Latham MC, Kosikowski FV, Woodward G: Symptom response to lactose-reduced milk in lactose-intolerant adults. *Am J Clin Nutr* 29:633–38, 1976.

Leichter J: Comparison of whole milk and skim milk with aqueous lactose solution in lactose tolerance testing. *Am J Clin Nutr* 26:393–96, 1973.

Levitt MD, Donaldson RM: Use of respiratory hydrogen (H_2) excretion to detect carbohydrate malabsorption. *J Lab Clin Med* 75:937–45, 1970.

Lisker R, Aguilar L, Zavala C: Intestinal lactase deficiency and milk drinking capacity in the adult. *Am J Clin Nutr* 31:1499–1503, 1978.

Metz G, Jenkins DJA, Peters TJ, Newman A, Blendis LM: Breath hydrogen as a diagnostic method for hypolactasia. *Lancet* 1:1155–57, 1975.

Newcomer AD, McGill DG, Thomas PJ, Hofmann AF: Prospective comparison of indirect methods for detecting lactase deficiency. *N Engl J Med* 293:1232–35, 1975.

Newcomer AD, McGill DB, Thomas PJ, Hofmann AF: Tolerance to lactose among lactase-deficient American Indians. *Gastroenterology* 74:44–46, 1978.

Solomons NW, Garcia-Ibanez R, Viteri FE: Hydrogen (H_2) breath test of lactose absorption in adults: The application of physiological doses and whole cow's milk sources. *Am J Clin Nutr* 33:545–54, 1980.

Solomons NW, Viteri FE, Hamilton LH: Application of a simple gas chromatographic technique for measuring breath hydrogen. *J Lab Clin Med* 90:856–62, 1977.

Stephenson LS, Latham MC: Lactose intolerance and milk consumption: The relation of tolerance to symptoms. *Am J Clin Nutr* 27:296–303, 1974.

Welsh JD: Isolated lactase deficiency in humans: Report on 100 patients. *Medicine* (Baltimore) 49:257–77, 1970.

CHAPTER 11

IMMEDIATE SYMPTOMATIC
AND LONG-TERM NUTRITIONAL CONSEQUENCES
OF HYPOLACTASIA

Albert D. Newcomer

In this chapter, the terms *lactase deficiency* and *hypolactasia* will be used in reference to a decline in lactase activity that occurs in most population groups, generally in early childhood but occasionally as late as the teenage years. This decline is controlled by an autosomal recessive gene. Since the pattern is seen in all land mammals and in about 70% of humans, it is the "normal" pattern. Thus, lactase deficiency and hypolactasia do not imply an abnormal state. In fact, the persistence of lactase activity throughout adulthood would have to be considered the "abnormal" state. The advantage in using these two terms is that they are more specific in describing the basic mechanism than are commonly used terms such as *lactose nondigestion, lactose malabsorption,* and *lactose intolerance.* In my opinion, the term *lactose intolerance* should be used only in reference to a symptomatic response to a defined load of lactose. For example, a lactase-deficient subject may be tolerant to one glass of milk and yet intolerant to two glasses. Thus, it becomes confusing when *lactose intolerance* is used synonymously with lactase deficiency or hypolactasia.

The clinical consequences of hypolactasia can be divided into immediate and long-term. This chapter will consider these consequences primarily in adults. The immediate consequences have been described clearly and refer to the intestinal symptoms that develop when a lactase-deficient subject ingests a *sufficient amount* of lactose. However, there is little agreement as to the actual clinical significance of this when a "physiologic" amount of lactose, such as that in one glass of milk, is ingested. In an attempt to focus more clearly on this controversy, the following two specific questions will be addressed: (1) How frequently can lactase-deficient subjects drink nutritionally helpful amounts of milk, such as one glass, without experiencing symptoms? (2) How often is occult lactase deficiency the cause of irritable bowel-type symptoms? The effect of malabsorbed lactose on the absorption of other nutrients in milk is reviewed in chapters 4, 13, and 14.

In contrast to these immediate effects of hypolactasia, relatively little attention has been given to the possibility of long-term consequences, such as osteoporosis. The relationship of lactase deficiency and osteoporosis will be reviewed in terms of the possible long-term nutritional consequences of lactase deficiency.

CONSUMPTION OF NUTRITIONALLY HELPFUL AMOUNTS OF MILK

To determine the amount of lactose that could be tolerated in a meal, a Mayo Clinic group conducted a study among a group of lactase-deficient American Indians living on Leech Lake Indian Reservation in northern Minnesota (Newcomer et al. 1978b).

Selection of Subjects. Bias in selection of the subjects during recruitment was avoided by initially asking volunteers to participate in a "nutrition study"; no mention was made of milk intake or milk intolerance. However, immediately before the study, the specific details of the project were explained to each volunteer, and at that point no one refused to participate. In an initial screening study, a total of 103 lactase-deficient Indian subjects were identified and 59 were available for participation in this tolerance study (Newcomer et al. 1977). The degree of intolerance was equivalent among those who did and those who did not participate in the tolerance study. For example, among those who participated, 88% experienced symptoms when challenged with a 50 g lactose load and 19% had a history of milk intolerance. Corresponding figures for the group not studied were 71% and 27%. The ages of the participants ranged from 5 to 62 years, but most were either teenagers or adults.

The diagnosis of lactase deficiency rested on measurement of hydrogen excretion in the breath after a lactose load of 2 g per kg body weight (maximum of 50 g; all but three received 50 g) (Newcomer et al. 1975). The 59 subjects excreted 0.26 ml to 1.56 ml hydrogen per minute above the fasting level (mean, 0.79 ml per min).

Conduct of Tolerance Study. On six consecutive mornings between 8 a.m. and 9 a.m., each subject ingested a breakfast that consisted of a lactose-free sweet roll and 8 ounces of Ensure, a commercial preparation that contains no lactose. To the Ensure was added a packet of sugar that contained 0 g, 3 g, 6 g, 9 g, 12 g, or 18 g lactose along with a reciprocal quantity of glucose and galactose in equal amounts to make a total of 18 g sugar in each packet.

Each sugar packet was coded so that neither the investigator nor the volunteer knew the amount of lactose it contained. The flavor of Ensure masks the taste of the sugar, so that the subject could not distinguish the packet containing 18 g lactose from the one containing 18 g glucose and galactose. The order of the six breakfasts was randomized, and each subject ingested the entire packet. After breakfast, the subjects were instructed to eat according to their usual habit but to avoid dairy products until the evening meal. Between 4 p.m. and 5 p.m. each day, each subject was interviewed by an observer—who was ignorant of the quantity of lactose ingested—regarding any gastrointestinal symptoms that had occurred between breakfast and the time of the interview. A subject was considered to have a positive symptomatic response if he or she had one or more loose stools or had a grade of +2 or higher in at least one of the following symptoms: cramps or abdominal pain, bloating or gas, borborygmi or flatus.

The subjects graded the severity of their symptoms from 0 to +4 according to the following criteria: 0—no trouble; +1—slight or questionable symptoms; +2—mild symptoms, yet not sufficient to bother the subject enough to avoid this breakfast in the future; +3—moderate symptoms such that the subject normally would avoid a breakfast causing these symptoms; and +4—severe symptoms such that the subject was unable to carry on usual activities and had to sit or lie down.

The same criteria were used in judging symptomatic response to the lactose load used in the hydrogen breath test.

Results. Seventeen subjects (29%) experienced positive symptomatic responses some time during the day after eating 31 (9%) of the aggregate 354 breakfasts (table 11.1). Four subjects noted diarrhea, usually consisting of one loose stool. Eleven additional subjects experienced only +1 symptoms and were

TABLE 11.1
Number of subjects with symptoms after indicated lactose dose at each grade level of symptoms

Symptom grade	Lactose (g)					
	0	3	6	9	12	18
+1	6	7	5	3	3	4
+2	2	1	5	5	2	1
+3	1	0	0	1	0	1
+4	0	1	1	1	1	1
Diarrhea	0	1	2	2	1	1

Source: Newcomer et al. 1978b, table 2, reprinted with permission.

not considered to have a positive response. There was no correlation between the amount of lactose ingested and symptoms (table 11.1, fig. 11.1); about the same number of subjects had symptoms after 0 g as after 18 g lactose, whereas after the large dose of 2 g per kg (maximum 50 g), a significantly higher percentage (88%) had symptoms (fig. 11.1).

Discussion. This study shows that lactase-deficient American Indians may, under conditions of the study, tolerate an amount of lactose equivalent to one or one and one-half glasses of milk taken with a meal, without intestinal symptoms that can be attributed to lactose. Although some subjects did experience symptoms after 9% of the breakfasts were consumed, these were not related to the lactose content of the breakfasts. It is not unexpected that volunteer subjects occasionally should experience mild or even moderate gastrointestinal symptoms when given an unknown test meal in an unfamiliar setting. These findings are consistent with the observation that the average daily intake of lactose in the 59 lactase-deficient subjects was 20.6 g per day, and only 19% of the group had a history of intolerance to milk. Clearly, the dose at which half of lactase-deficient American Indian subjects become symptomatic, the "LD_{50}," is between 18 g and 50 g and can be defined by further studies.

In studies of food tolerance, it is absolutely essential to give the test item under blinded conditions. Lactose often is given in water for tolerance testing, and thus it can be distinguished readily from glucose and galactose. Also, it is difficult to be certain of the level of tolerance to lactose by giving different volumes of milk.

Variations in Estimates of Milk Intolerance. The literature offers controversial opinions about tolerance to physiologic loads of lactose. Among the various published studies, the prevalence of intolerance to one glass of milk or the equivalent amount of lactose (12 g) ranges from 0% to 75% (table 11.2), with an overall mean of 19%. Certain regional differences are apparent; for example, the mean for Baltimore blacks in 4 studies was 48%, whereas the average for the remaining 10 studies was 13%. Another factor that may result in discrepancies is related to the nonblinded nature of the majority of the studies in which lactose is given either in the form of milk or as lactose in a water solution that has a

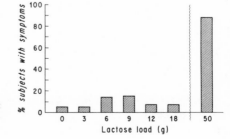

FIGURE 11.1. Tolerance to various doses of lactose in 59 subjects with lactase deficiency. Source: Newcomer et al. 1978b, p. 45, reprinted with permission.

TABLE 11.2
Prevalence of milk intolerance in various ethnic groups with hypolactasia

			% Intolerant	
Study	Ethnic group	Lactase-deficient subjects, no.*	0 g†	12 g‡
Double-blind				
Lisker and				
Aguilar 1978	Mexican	97 A, T	0	37
Paige et al. 1975	Black, USA	22 T	14	14
Rorick and				
Scrimshaw 1979	Mixed	23 A	30	22
Newcomer et al.				
1978b	American Indian	59 A, C, T	5	7
Garza and				
Scrimshaw 1976	Black, USA	12 C	ND§	8
Not blinded				
Lisker et al. 1978	Mexican	121 A, T		15
Desai et al. 1970	India	64 A		5
Reddy and				
Pershad 1972	India	20 C		0
Stephenson and				
Latham 1974	Mixed	15 A		20
Bell et al. 1973	Eskimo	20 A		5
Pieters and				
Rens 1973	Black, Kenya	53 C		0
Bayless et al. 1975	Black (primarily), USA	44 A		59
Bedine and				
Bayless 1973	Black (primarily), USA	20 A		75
Mitchell et al. 1975	Black, USA	13 T		54
				Mean 19%‖

*A = adults; T = teenagers; C = children.
†0 g to 1 g.
‡10 g to 15 g.
§ND = Not done; assume 0% for calculation of means.
‖In calculating the mean among double-blind studies, the percentage intolerant to 0 g is subtracted from the percentage intolerant to 12 g.

distinctive taste; in the blinded studies lactose is given in the form that makes both its presence and its amount indistinguishable from the placebo. If all the studies had been double-blind, the percentage of subjects truly intolerant to 12 g lactose probably would have been lower than 19%, perhaps in the 10% to 15% range.

A double-blind study by Gudmand-Høyer and Simony (1977) showed that 75% of 20 subjects with lactase deficiency were intolerant to 10 g lactose. This study is not included in the table because all of their patients presented with diarrhea and other irritable bowel-type symptoms. This group of 20 subjects obviously was selected from one end of the tolerance spectrum.

A number of other factors also may play a role in the broad range of intolerance that has been reported. For example, the form in which lactose is given will have an important influence on gastric emptying. Several studies have shown that delayed gastric emptying improves tolerance to lactose. For example, whole milk (containing fat) is tolerated better than skim milk, which, in turn, is tolerated better than lactose in water (Leichter 1973, Bayless et al. 1975). Milk taken with a meal is tolerated better than milk taken by itself. Chocolate milk, which has an osmolality around 600 mOsm per kg, is tolerated better than regular milk, which has an osmolality of 300 mOsm per kg (Welsh and Hall 1977).

Yet another factor that influences the degree of intolerance is age. Children and teenagers with lactase deficiency are more tolerant to lactose than are adults (Flatz et al. 1969, Newcomer et al. 1977). Although a progressive decline in lactase activity over several years during early childhood may play some role in this age difference, other factors appear to be important. In a study done among American Indians, 10% of the children and teenagers with lactase deficiency had noted milk intolerance, in contrast to 53% of adults (P < 0.005) (Newcomer et al. 1977). The average daily lactose intake in these subjects was 19 g, which is equivalent to one and one-half glasses of milk. Following a lactose load of 2 g per kg (maximum 50 g), 76% of children and teenagers had symptoms, compared with 93% of adults (P = 0.05). In another study among adults with lactase deficiency, the average age when milk intolerance first was noted was 33 years, although loss of lactase activity presumably occurred in early childhood (Welsh 1970). Perhaps there is a difference in bacterial flora of the gut, a difference that allows children to absorb a larger percentage of short-chain fatty acids formed in the colon as compared with adults. Or possibly children may have a higher threshold for intestinal discomfort. Whatever the mechanism, children with lactase deficiency are more tolerant of lactose than are adults.

Prolonged ingestion of milk has been shown to improve tolerance to milk among lactase-deficient subjects. Individuals who do not tolerate physiologic amounts of milk initially may tolerate the same amount without symptoms after continuous ingestion for several weeks. The mechanism by which this occurs is not clear.

Finally, it has been suggested that tolerance to lactose may vary among ethnic groups, although this is not supported in table 11.2.

Several studies have reported intolerance to milligram amounts of lactose, but these subjects have not been challenged in double-blind fashion. It would be difficult to explain this extreme degree of intolerance on the basis of the usual pathophysiologic explanation of retained intraluminal lactose causing osmotic-induced symptoms.

Effects of Lactase Deficiency on Milk-Drinking Habits.   The effect of lactase deficiency on milk-drinking habits has been analyzed in a number of studies. In the Mayo Clinic study of American Indians, lactase-sufficient subjects were ingesting 25 g lactose per day (equivalent to two glasses of milk), which was slightly more than the 19 g taken by the lactase-deficient subjects (P < 0.05) (Newcomer et al. 1977). Some studies have shown this same trend, yet others have found no relationship between milk intake and lactase activity (Bolin et al.

1970; Paige et al. 1971, 1972; Sahi et al. 1972; Stephenson and Latham 1974; Bayless et al. 1975; Lebenthal et al. 1975; Paige et al. 1977; Stephenson et al. 1977).

Lactose Intolerance in Lactase-Sufficient Individuals.   Intolerance to lactose is not limited to lactase-deficient subjects. In subjects with lactase sufficiency, a large load of lactose may overwhelm small-intestinal lactase activity. For example, when 150 g to 225 g (equivalent to three to four quarts of milk) of lactose is given to lactase-sufficient subjects through a nasogastric tube over a period of 24 hours, intestinal symptoms, including diarrhea, may result (Walike and Walike 1977).

OCCULT LACTASE DEFICIENCY AND IRRITABLE BOWEL-TYPE SYMPTOMS

Many people with hypolactasia who have symptoms after physiologic amounts of milk already have recognized the relationship between milk intake and intestinal symptoms and have decreased milk intake to the tolerance level. From the clinical standpoint, a more important group would be those subjects who have unrecognized lactase deficiency and secondary intestinal symptoms that mimic irritable bowel syndrome. A much-debated question is how commonly occult lactase deficiency accounts for chronic nonspecific abdominal complaints. Review of the literature does not provide a clear answer to this important question. Some studies conclude that from 20% to 95% of subjects with irritable bowel-type symptoms have underlying lactase deficiency, and many of these patients are reported to improve with lactose restriction (McMichael et al. 1965, Weser et al. 1965, Jussila et al. 1969, Fung and Kho 1971, Gudmand-Høyer et al. 1973, Arvanitakis et al. 1977, Gudmand-Høyer and Simony 1977). In contrast, other studies report that only 5% to 6% of patients with symptoms of an irritable bowel have underlying lactase deficiency as the cause (Peña and Truelove 1972, Fairman et al. 1975). The early studies did not include information on ethnic background, and most of the studies contain no data on control groups. Another problem is that almost all of the studies include subjects who already are aware of intolerance to milk. Finally, the diet studies that showed improvement with lactose restriction were not double-blind. The well-known placebo effect could well have played a role in this improvement.

Currently, a study is being conducted at the Mayo Clinic to provide further insight into the relationship of irritable bowel syndrome and lactase deficiency. This study is incomplete, and preliminary results are presented here as a progress report. The two objectives of this study are (1) to determine the prevalence of hypolactasia in adults with nonspecific abdominal symptoms (irritable bowel syndrome) and (2) to determine whether lactose restriction is helpful in patients with irritable bowel-type symptoms and hypolactasia. Seventy-four adults with irritable bowel syndrome and no history of milk intolerance were screened for hypolactasia. The subjects ranged in age from 20 to 82 years, were of white European and non-Jewish descent, and gave no history of milk intolerance. On the basis of hydrogen breath testing, 4 of the 74 (5%) had hypolactasia compared with 6% of 100 control subjects who were of comparable ethnic background. Elimination of milk in the diets of the 4 subjects with lactase deficiency did not alleviate the gastrointestinal symptoms. Hypolactasia does not appear to be a common cause of irritable bowel syndrome in adults of white European and non-Jewish descent who are not aware of milk intolerance. The unexpected finding of hypolactasia in patients with irritable bowel syndrome is frequently incidental, and subsequent elimination of milk does not improve the intestinal symptoms. It is important to point out that the subjects were studied during 1979, and the negative results may relate in part to the increasing awareness of hypolactasia among both physicians and patients.

LONG-TERM NUTRITIONAL CONSEQUENCES OF LACTASE DEFICIENCY

Although the immediate side effects of lactase deficiency are well recognized, potential long-term complications have received little attention. One such long-term effect was described by Birge and colleagues (1967), who reported that 9 of 19 osteoporotic subjects had lactase deficiency, whereas all 13 of the control subjects had "normal" lactase. At the time of this study, it was not fully appreciated that the prevalence of lactase deficiency ranges widely among various ethnic groups; thus, the authors made no mention of ethnic background.

Later, a similar study was conducted at the Mayo Clinic but with control of ethnic background (Newcomer et al. 1978a). The prevalence of lactase deficiency was determined by analysis of breath hydrogen in 30 women with idiopathic postmenopausal osteoporosis and in 31 female control subjects who had no evidence of metabolic bone disease. Eight subjects with osteoporosis and only one control subject were found to be lactase deficient ($P < 0.05$). Although none of the lactase-deficient subjects were aware of milk intolerance, their intake of both lactose and calcium was significantly lower than that of the "lactase-normal" group.

Additional support for a relationship between lactase deficiency and osteoporosis comes from Kocián and colleagues (1973), who reported that the cortical thickness of the clavicle in subjects after gastric resection was significantly thinned in subjects with lactase deficiency compared with those with sufficient lactase.

None of these studies proves a cause-and-effect relationship between lactase deficiency and osteoporosis. However, hypolactasia could conceivably predispose a person to osteoporosis through either reduced intake of milk secondary to intolerance or impaired calcium absorption. Investigations into the effect of lactose on the absorption of calcium have produced conflicting results both in animals and in man. Debongnie et al. (1979) reported that four subjects with lactase deficiency did not absorb calcium contained in regular milk as well as calcium in lactose-free milk. This question of absorption needs to be clarified with more sophisticated techniques.

The observation that blacks, who are frequently lactase deficient, have a low prevalence of osteoporosis, argues against a simple cause-and-effect relationship between hypolactasia and osteoporosis. However, greater bone density in blacks (thicker cortices) at maturity would offer relative protection from osteoporosis later in life despite the presence of lactase deficiency (Trotter et al. 1960). Obviously, further studies will be necessary to resolve these questions.

REFERENCES

Arvanitakis C, Chen G-H, Folscroft J, Klotz AP: Lactase deficiency: A comparative study of diagnostic methods. *Am J Clin Nutr* 30:1597–1602, 1977.

Bayless TM, Rothfeld B, Massa C, Wise L, Paige DM, Bedine MS: Lactose and milk intolerance: Clinical implications. *N Engl J Med* 292:1156–59, 1975.

Bedine MS, Bayless TM: Intolerance of small amounts of lactose by individuals with low lactase levels. *Gastroenterology* 65:735–43, 1973.

Bell RR, Draper HH, Bergan JG: Sucrose, lactose, and glucose tolerance in northern Alaskan Eskimos. *Am J Clin Nutr* 26:1185–90, 1973.

Birge SJ Jr, Keutmann HT, Cuatrecasas P, Whedon GD: Osteoporosis, intestinal lactase deficiency and low dietary calcium intake. *N Engl J Med* 276:445–48, 1967.

Bolin TD, Morrison RM, Steel JE, Davis AE: Lactose intolerance in Australia. *Med J Aust* 1:1289–92, 1970.

Debongnie JC, Newcomer AD, McGill DB, Phillips SF: Absorption of nutrients in lactase deficiency. *Dig Dis Sci* 24:225–31, 1979.

Desai HG, Gupte UV, Pradhan AG, Thakker KD, Antia FP: Incidence of lactase deficiency in control subjects from India: Role of hereditary factors. *Indian J Med Sci* 24:729–36, 1970.

Fairman M, Scott B, Losowsky M: Lactase activities in the irritable colon syndrome (letter to the editor). *Br Med J* 26:227, 1975.

Flatz G, Saengudom CH, Sanguanbhokhai T: Lactose intolerance in Thailand. *Nature* 221:758–59, 1969.

Fung W-P, Kho KM: The importance of milk intolerance in patients presenting with chronic (nervous) diarrhoea. *Aust NZ J Med* 4:374–76, 1971.

Garza C, Scrimshaw NS: Relationship of lactose intolerance to milk intolerance in young children. *Am J Clin Nutr* 29:192–96, 1976.

Gudmand-Höyer E, Riis P, Wulff HR: The significance of lactose malabsorption in the irritable colon syndrome. *Scand J Gastroenterol* 8:273–78, 1973.

Gudmand-Høyer E, Simony K: Individual sensitivity to lactose in lactose malabsorption. *Am J Dig Dis* 22:177–81, 1977.

Jussila J, Launiala K, Gorbatow O: Lactase deficiency and a lactose-free diet in patients with "unspecific abdominal complaints." *Acta Med Scand* 186:217–22, 1969.

Kocián J, Vulterinová M, Bejblová O, Skála I: Influence of lactose intolerance on the bones of patients after partial gastrectomy. *Digestion* 8:324–35, 1973.

Lebenthal E, Antonowicz I, Shwachman H: Correlation of lactase activity, lactose tolerance and milk consumption in different age groups. *Am J Clin Nutr* 28:595–600, 1975.

Leichter J: Comparison of whole milk and skim milk with aqueous lactose solution in lactose tolerance testing. *Am J Clin Nutr* 26:393–96, 1973.

Lisker R, Aguilar L: Double blind study of milk lactose intolerance. *Gastroenterology* 74:1283–85, 1978.

Lisker R, Aguilar L, Zavala C: Intestinal lactase deficiency and milk drinking capacity in the adult. *Am J Clin Nutr* 31:1499–1503, 1978.

McMichael HB, Webb J, Dawson AM: Lactase deficiency in adults: A cause of "functional" diarrhoea. *Lancet* 1:717–20, 1965.

Mitchell KJ, Bayless TM, Paige DM, Goodgame RW, Huang SS: Intolerance of eight ounces of milk in healthy lactose-intolerant teen-agers. *Pediatrics* 56:718–21, 1975.

Newcomer AD, Hodgson SF, McGill DB, Thomas PJ: Lactase deficiency: Prevalence in osteoporosis. *Ann Intern Med* 89:218–20, 1978a.

Newcomer AD, McGill DB, Thomas PJ, Hofmann AF: Prospective comparison of indirect methods for detecting lactase deficiency. *N Engl J Med* 293:1232–36, 1975.

Newcomer AD, McGill DB, Thomas PJ, Hofmann AF: Tolerance to lactose among lactase-deficient American Indians. *Gastroenterology* 74:44–46, 1978b.

Newcomer AD, Thomas PJ, McGill DB, Hofmann AF: Lactase deficiency: A common genetic trait of the American Indian. *Gastroenterology* 72:234–37, 1977.

Paige DM, Bayless TM, Ferry GD, Graham GG: Lactose malabsorption and milk rejection in Negro children. *Johns Hopkins Med J* 129:163–69, 1971.

Paige DM, Bayless TM, Huang SS, Wexler R: Lactose hydrolyzed milk. *Am J Clin Nutr* 28:818–22, 1975.

Paige DM, Bayless TM, Mellits ED, Davis L: Lactose malabsorption in preschool black children. *Am J Clin Nutr* 30:1018–22, 1977.

Paige DM, Leonardo E, Cordano A, Nakashima J, Adrianzen B, Graham GG: Lactose intolerance in Peruvian children: Effect of age and early nutrition. *Am J Clin Nutr* 25:297–301, 1972.

Peña AS, Truelove SC: Hypolactasia and the irritable colon syndrome. *Scand J Gastroenterol* 7:433–38, 1972.

Pieters JJL, Van Rens R: Lactose malabsorption and milk tolerance in Kenyan school-age children. *Trop Geogr Med* 25:365–71, 1973.

Reddy V, Pershad J: Lactase deficiency in Indians. *Am J Clin Nutr* 25:114–19, 1972.

Rorick MH, Scrimshaw NS: Comparative tolerance of elderly from differing ethnic backgrounds to lactose-containing and lactose-free dairy drinks: A double-blind study. *J Gerontol* 34:191–96, 1979.

Sahi T, Isokoski M, Jussila J, Launiala K: Lactose malabsorption in Finnish children of school age. *Acta Paediatr Scand* 61:11–16, 1972.

Stephenson LS, Latham MC: Lactose intolerance and milk consumption: The relation of tolerance to symptoms. *Am J Clin Nutr* 27:296–303, 1974.

Stephenson LS, Latham MC, Jones DV: Milk consumption by black and by white pupils in two primary schools. *J Am Diet Assoc* 71:258–62, 1977.

Trotter M, Broman GE, Peterson RR: Densities of bones of white and Negro skeletons. *J Bone Joint Surg [Am]* 42:50–58, 1960.

Walike BC, Walike JW: Relative lactose intolerance: A clinical study of tube-fed patients. *JAMA* 238:948–51, 1977.

Welsh JD: Isolated lactase deficiency in humans: Report on 100 patients. *Medicine* (Baltimore) 49:257–77, 1970.

Welsh JD, Hall WH: Gastric emptying of lactose and milk in subjects with lactose malabsorption. *Am J Dig Dis* 22:1060–63, 1977.

Weser E, Rubin W, Ross L, Sleisenger MH: Lactase deficiency in patients with the "irritable-colon syndrome." *N Engl J Med* 273:1070–75, 1965.

CHAPTER 12

USE OF SYMPTOM RESPONSES TO CLASSIFY ADULT LACTOSE ABSORBERS AND NONABSORBERS

L. S. Stephenson

Relatively low levels of intestinal lactase activity are extremely common in adult non-Caucasians world-wide, while the majority of adult Caucasians maintain the high levels of intestinal lactase that are common to infants of all races. Lactase levels can decrease in two ways: (1) naturally with age, as in primary lactose malabsorption; or (2) as a result of pathogenic organisms, as in gastroenteritis, malabsorption syndromes, and other gastrointestinal diseases. This chapter is concerned with primary malabsorption, that is, the natural, nonpathological decrease in lactase activity that occurs gradually with age in those destined to be lactose malabsorbers in adult life.

There was great concern in the late 1960s and early 1970s over whether lactose malabsorbers should consume milk. This was partially because many malabsorbers developed symptoms such as diarrhea, bloating, gas, and intestinal cramps after ingesting 50 g lactose given in a standard lactose tolerance test.

Wide reporting of these symptoms during lactose tolerance testing caused concern that individuals with flat curves may not be able to drink milk without suffering abdominal symptoms. Yet 50 g lactose is the amount found in approximately one quart of milk, and few studies had been done to determine whether these people experience symptoms when drinking the smaller amounts of milk that normally are consumed with meals. Therefore, a study was undertaken to determine the symptomatic responses of healthy adult lactose absorbers and nonabsorbers to varying quantities of lactose (Stephenson and Latham, 1974, 1975b).

The term *lactose malabsorption* generally indicates a rise of less than 20 mg per dl with a lactose tolerance test; and the term *lactose intolerance* is used for a lactose malabsorber who has symptoms with the tolerance test. Since the term *malabsorption* implies a pathological state when none may exist, the term *lactose nonabsorption* is used here to refer to persons with a mean rise in blood glucose of less than 20 mg per dl during the lactose tolerance test.

STUDY OBJECTIVES

The major objectives of the lactose ingestion study were: (1) to test the possibility of using symptoms resulting from a 50 g dose of lactose as criteria for classifying lactose absorption; and (2) to determine the amounts of lactose in water and lactose as milk that lactose absorbers and nonabsorbers could ingest without notable symptoms occurring.

The subjects participating in the study were 35 healthy adult volunteers ranging in age from 19 to 44 years, with a median age of 25 years. Twenty-five were Caucasian, and 10 were non-Caucasians of varying ethnicities, including Africans and Orientals.

In order to determine the largest amount of lactose that could be ingested comfortably by each subject, subjects were given different doses of lactose in water and lactose as milk on eight occasions and a placebo on two occasions (Stephenson and Latham 1974, 1975a).

METHODOLOGY

Subjects reported to the laboratory, fasting, one morning a week for 10 weeks. For the first 6 weeks subjects received varying doses of lactose in water on 4 days and a randomly distributed placebo on 2 days. For the last 4 weeks they received varying amounts of milk. Subjects were allowed to eat 3 hours after ingestion of the test dose.

On each study day, subjects were given a form on which to record incidence, times of occurrence, and severity of diarrhea, bloating, gas, cramps, and also normal bowel movements. They recorded symptoms for 8 hours after the test dose, and were unaware of the amounts of lactose they received.

On day one of the study, all subjects received 50 g lactose in water and were divided into two groups; those reporting notable symptoms and those reporting few or no symptoms. Subjects reporting notable symptoms on day one then received 15 g, 30 g, and/or 50 g lactose in water and then as milk until the highest amounts that caused zero, one, or two mild symptoms were ascertained. Subjects reporting only zero, one, or two mild symptoms on day one received 100 g, 150 g, and/or 200 g lactose, both in water and as milk. The concentration was 1 g lactose to 4 ml water. Lactose given as milk consisted of reconstituted nonfat dry milk. Two placebos were randomized for each subject.

Absorption and nonabsorption were determined by a lactose tolerance test using 50 g lactose. Venipunctures were taken at 0, 20, 45, and 75 minutes, and blood glucose determinations were carried out on the autoanalyzer with the Hoffman ferricyanide method. Nonabsorption was defined as a maximum rise in blood glucose over fasting level of less than 20 mg per dl.

LACTOSE TOLERANCE TEST RESULTS

With the lactose tolerance tests, 16 of the 35 subjects were nonabsorbers and 19 were absorbers. As expected, non-Caucasian ancestry was significantly associated with prevalence of nonabsorption at the 0.05 level, using a chi-square test. Eight of the 10 non-Caucasians (80%) were nonabsorbers, while 8 of the 25 Caucasians (32%) were nonabsorbers. Symptoms after the 50 g lactose dose were compared for day one to test the possibility of using symptoms as criteria for classifying nonabsorption. Prevalence of each symptom, the number of symptoms per subject, and the severity of symptoms were studied. As shown in table 12.1, nonabsorbers reported each symptom much more often than did absorbers, and nonabsorption was significantly associated with prevalence of each of the four symptoms at the 0.01 level. Diarrhea and bloating were much more common in nonabsorbers, the prevalence differing by factors of 10 and 6, respectively. Gas and cramps were also more common, but only by factors of 2 and 3.

When number of symptoms reported per subject was compared for nonabsorbers and absorbers, it was found that 80% of nonabsorbers reported two to four symptoms each, while almost 80% of absorbers reported either zero or one

TABLE 12.1
Symptoms resulting from 50 g lactose in absorbers and nonabsorbers

Subject group	Percentage reporting each symptom			
	Diarrhea*	Gas†	Bloating*	Cramps†
Nonabsorbers‡				
N = 15	53	87	60	67
Absorbers				
N = 19	5	42	10	21
All subjects				
N = 34	26	62	32	41

Source: Stephenson and Latham 1974, table 3, reprinted with permission.
*P <0.005.
†P <0.01.
‡One subject is omitted due to failure to follow instructions.

symptom each. Nonabsorption was significantly associated with higher numbers of symptoms (two to four) per subject at the 0.01 level.

The subjects themselves rated their symptoms mild, moderate, or severe, and nonabsorbers reported moderate or severe symptoms much more frequently. Ninety percent of the absorbers reported either no symptoms or mild symptoms, but 60% of nonabsorbers reported at least one moderate or severe symptom.

To compare number and severity of symptoms in the two groups a lactose score was devised. A subject received one point for each symptom rated mild, two points for a symptom rated moderate, and three points for a symptom rated severe. Thus, a subject with no symptoms would have a lactose score of 0. A subject with four symptoms, each rated severe, would have a lactose score of 12. The mean lactose score in the nonabsorbers was highly significantly different from that in the absorbers (4.4 versus 0.9). However, the ranges of the two distributions did overlap considerably, since some absorbers reported more symptoms than did some nonabsorbers. So it appears that on an individual basis, symptom response to 50 g lactose will not necessarily differentiate between those who have flat lactose tolerance test curves and those who do not.

THRESHOLD FOR LACTOSE-INDUCED SYMPTOMS

The most important objective of the study was to determine the largest amounts of lactose in water and lactose as milk that each subject could ingest without experiencing moderate to severe symptoms. In the nonabsorbers, it was found that all subjects could ingest at least 15 g lactose in water with no or negligible symptoms (see table 12.2). This amount is equal to the lactose in 300 ml milk. Ninety-three percent of nonabsorbers consumed 30 g or more of lactose in water with no or negligible symptoms. Negligible symptoms were defined as symptoms rated mild by the subject. No symptoms or mild gas occurred in three-quarters of the individuals. All of the subjects reported that the degree of discomfort, if any, caused by these doses of lactose would not prevent them from drinking milk regularly.

When these subjects were given milk, it was found that all could consume at least 15 g and 66% could consume at least 30 g lactose as milk with no or negligible symptoms. All subjects reported here had either no symptoms or one to two mild symptoms.

Profound differences in symptom response were found between lactose absorbers and nonabsorbers. Twenty-six percent of the absorbers ingested 200 g lactose in water, equal to one gallon of milk, with no or negligible symptoms resulting (table 12.3).

This was a relatively small sample of subjects, but it does seem to show that quite a few healthy adults with flat curves can consume 240 ml or more of milk on an empty stomach without experiencing symptoms that would prevent them

TABLE 12.2
Largest amounts of lactose causing zero, one, or two mild symptoms in
lactose nonabsorbers

Lactose (g)	Lactose in water N = 14* (%)	Lactose as milk N = 15† (%)
15	7	20
30	58	66
50	14	7
100	14	7
150	7	0
200	0	0
Total	100	100

Source: Stephenson and Latham 1974, table 2, reprinted with permission.
*Due to failure to follow instructions or illness previous to a study day, 2
of 16 subjects did not fit the criterion of two or fewer mild symptoms with
any doses of lactose in water: 1 reported moderate gas and bloating with
15 g lactose but said he would not stop drinking milk with such symptoms;
the second subject reported mild gas, bloating, and cramps with 15 g and
30 g lactose in water. Both subjects reported no symptoms with 15 g
lactose as milk.
†One subject reported moderate gas with 30 g lactose as milk and was not
given 15 g lactose as milk. However, the subject stated that she would not
discontinue drinking milk regularly with moderate gas.

from drinking milk regularly. From a public health point of view this is an
important finding.

CLINICAL CONSIDERATIONS

From a clinical point of view there are other considerations because one then
has to consider individuals, rather than groups of people. When should a clinician advise a patient to decrease his or her intake of milk? How can a clinician be
certain that a patient who complains of symptoms with milk ingestion is really
milk intolerant? This is a problem because gastrointestinal symptoms, especially
stomach pains and gas, obviously can be caused by a number of factors not
related to lactase levels. Some of these factors are physiologic, others are
psychological in nature. The fact that an individual has symptoms with the
lactose tolerance test is not conclusive proof because the lactose load (50 g) is so
high. The fact that a patient reports symptoms with a single glass of milk also is
not conclusive proof. Both the absorbers and the nonabsorbers in this study were
given two placebos, consisting of water flavored with saccharin and lemon juice.
One placebo was equal in volume to the solution of 15 g lactose in water (65 ml).
The other placebo was equal in volume to the highest dose of lactose in water
taken by each subject. One-quarter of the subjects in each of the two groups
(absorbers and nonabsorbers) reported that a symptom resulted after drinking the

TABLE 12.3
Largest amounts of lactose causing zero, one, or two mild symptoms in
lactose absorbers

Lactose (g)	Lactose in water N = 19 (%)	Lactose as milk N = 16* (%)
15	0	0
30	5	13
50	16	6
100	21	31
150	32	31
200	26	19
Total	100	100

Source: Stephenson and Latham 1974, table 2, reprinted with permission.
*Three of 19 subjects did not receive a dose of lactose as milk low enough to produce only two or fewer mild symptoms. Two received 150 g lactose as milk; one reported moderate gas and the other reported mild diarrhea with moderate gas. One subject received 50 g lactose as milk and reported mild gas with moderate cramps.

lower volume placebo. There were no differences between the groups in number of symptoms reported, but 25% of each group reported that the placebo caused symptoms. This placebo response clearly can lead to confusion when one asks a patient, ''Does drinking milk ever give you stomach problems?'' It also can give false positive results if one asks the patient to drink a glass of milk and record symptom response.

There was a definite pattern to the placebo responses in this study, and it may be helpful in clinical situations. Three-fourths of the symptom responses to placebos were reports of intestinal gas. No subjects reported diarrhea, only 6% (2 subjects) reported bloating, and 6% reported cramps. Thus, it may be wise to doubt that the patient is genuinely intolerant to normally consumed quantities of milk if the only symptom reported is occasional gas.

NUTRITIONAL CONSIDERATIONS

Another issue of importance in the area of lactose research is whether nonabsorbers in general voluntarily lower their milk intakes, and if they do voluntarily drink less milk than absorbers how does this affect their nutrient intakes? This is important in the United States because milk and other dairy products are important sources of calcium, riboflavin, and vitamins A and D for many Americans. Milk is also an excellent source of balanced protein even though there is no shortage of protein in most adult diets in this country. The nonabsorbers in this study were not drinking less milk as adults than were the absorbers. A 24-hour dietary recall survey also was done on each subject as an index of nutrient intake (Stephenson and Latham 1974).

TABLE 12.4
Nutrient intakes of absorbers and nonabsorbers (based on 24-hr diet recall)

Nutrient	Absorbers N = 19	Nonabsorbers N = 16
Calories		
mean	2,194	2,094
SD	1,092	846
Protein, g		
mean	97.7	83.4
SD	50.0	24.4
Calcium, mg		
mean	1,021	727
SD	932	279
Riboflavin, μg*		
mean	2,222	1,542
SD	1,345	622
Vitamin A, IU		
mean	8,373	5,495
SD	5,850	4,220
Vitamin D, IU		
mean	165	128
SD	249	141

*Difference between subject groups statistically significant ($P < 0.05$).

The quantities of calories, protein, calcium, riboflavin, vitamin A, and vitamin D were calculated. As table 12.4 indicates, there were no significant differences in nutrient intakes between groups, except for riboflavin (2,222 μg in absorbers, 1,542 μg in nonabsorbers). Even so, 1,500 μg is very close to the RDAs for the reference man and woman (1,700 μg and 1,300 μg, Food and Nutrition Board 1980), and 24-hour recalls tend to underestimate nutrient intakes. Therefore, one need not be concerned that healthy adult lactose nonabsorbers consuming a variety of foods will have less adequate diets than those of lactose absorbers. There may be problems in the rare person who is, for example, a lactovegetarian, depends heavily on dairy products as sources of calcium and riboflavin, and is also genuinely milk intolerant. But this would be a rare situation and would be easily dealt with by dietary manipulation.

LACTOSE TOLERANCE IN EAST AFRICAN MASAI AND BANTU

Most of the people in East Africa (Kenya and Tanzania) are Bantu people and are lactose nonabsorbers as adults. They regularly consume small amounts of milk, daily if it is available and affordable, but usually in tea. The Masai, the nomadic people who are famous for drinking cow's blood mixed with milk as their staple food, have a different genetic origin from the Bantu tribes. Recently, Jackson and Latham (1978, 1979) completed a study of lactose tolerance in a sample of the Masai population. One might expect, since they regularly consume large quantities of milk, that they are mostly lactose absorbers. It appears that they are not.

Lactose tolerance tests were done in Tanzania on Bantu and Masai children over 5 years of age. As expected, 92% of the Bantus were nonabsorbers. Contrary to what one might expect for the Masai, 62% were also nonabsorbers, even though they are unquestionably a milk-drinking people. However, the mean rise in blood glucose during the lactose tolerance test was twice as high in the Masai (16 mg per dl) as in the Bantu (7 mg per dl). Although this work needs expansion to include a larger number of subjects, it does provide additional evidence that milk can and does make an important nutritional contribution to the diets of people with relatively low levels of intestinal lactase.

CONCLUSIONS

The decade of the 1970s has been an exciting and fruitful one in the area of lactose research. From the public health perspective, one of the most important discoveries is that many healthy persons with flat lactose tolerance test curves (the majority of the world's adults) can consume useful quantities of milk if they wish to do so. This does not mean that all people should drink milk any more than that they all should consume any other single food. The best nutritional advice is for people to choose a varied diet. This research indicates that milk and other dairy products can continue to have their place in the diets of lactose absorbers and nonabsorbers alike.

REFERENCES

Food and Nutrition Board: *Recommended Dietary Allowances*. Washington, D.C.: National Research Council, National Academy of Sciences, 1980.

Jackson RT, Latham MC: Lactose and milk intolerance in Tanzania. *East Afr Med J* 55:298–302, 1978.

Jackson RT, Latham MC: Lactose malabsorption among Masai children of East Africa. *Am J Clin Nutr* 32:779–82, 1979.

Stephenson LS, Latham MC: Lactose intolerance and milk consumption: The relation of tolerance to symptoms. *Am J Clin Nutr* 27:296–303, 1974.

Stephenson LS, Latham MC: Lactose tolerance tests as a predictor of milk tolerance. *Am J Clin Nutr* 28:86–88, 1975a.

Stephenson LS, Latham MC: Rapid and portable methods of lactose tolerance test administration. *Am J Clin Nutr* 28:888–93, 1975b.

CHAPTER 13

EFFECTS OF LACTOSE ON
THE ABSORPTION OF OTHER NUTRIENTS
IMPLICATIONS IN LACTOSE-INTOLERANT
ADULTS

Joseph Leichter

The prevalence and etiology of adult lactose intolerance in different population groups has been studied quite extensively over the last 15 years. Relatively few researchers have studied the tolerance of a normal serving of milk as part of a meal and the possible effect of lactose malabsorption on the absorption of other nutrients under such conditions.

SIGNIFICANCE OF LACTOSE INTOLERANCE TESTS

Lactose intolerance is commonly identified by a lactose tolerance test utilizing an aqueous lactose solution. The criteria used for the diagnosis of lactose malabsorption usually consist of a maximum rise in blood glucose of no greater than 20 mg per 100 ml above fasting level, coupled with gastrointestinal symptoms after an oral administration of 50 g lactose dissolved in about 400 ml water.

The maximum rise of blood glucose levels and the intensity of symptoms among lactose-intolerant adults vary following a lactose tolerance test. This indicates that the actual amount of lactose critical for symptoms varies among lactose malabsorbers. A review of the literature indicates that most lactose-intolerant adults can consume moderate amounts of milk without experiencing symptoms (Stephenson and Latham 1974, Reddy and Pershad 1972, Garza and Scrimshaw 1976, Leichter 1973, Lisker et al. 1978, Bayless and Paige 1972).

From our own experience with lactose-intolerant adults it seems that normal consumption of dairy products rarely causes symptoms. This can be explained by the fact that most adults have about one glass of milk at a time, i.e., a quantity of lactose that corresponds to no more than about 25% of the lactose load given in the lactose tolerance test. In addition, there is evidence that lactose in milk, and particularly with a meal, is tolerated better than an equivalent amount of lactose in water after an overnight fast (Reddy and Pershad 1972, Leichter 1973, Bayless and Paige 1972). The reason for this is probably twofold: the delay in gastric emptying due to the presence of food in the stomach and the consequent dilution effect. Thus, lactose intolerance (as defined by the lactose tolerance test or by lactase activity of intestinal biopsies) and milk intolerance are not the same (Reddy and Preshad 1972, Garza and Scrimshaw 1976, Lisker et al. 1978). In fact most lactose-intolerant adults can tolerate more than a glass of milk per day provided it is not ingested all at once but rather in small quantities with breakfast, lunch, and dinner. Therefore, from a practical and nutritional point of view, one should not try to limit this type of milk consumption among healthy lactose-intolerant adults as it is not a significant factor in the production of symptoms.

NUTRITIONAL IMPLICATIONS OF LACTOSE INTOLERANCE

Relatively little is known about the possible effect of unabsorbed lactose on the absorption of other nutrients in the diet. There have been a limited number of studies on the influence of lactose on the absorption of protein, fat, calcium, and other minerals (Calloway and Chenoweth 1973, Kocián et al. 1973, Debongnie et al. 1979, Paige and Graham 1972, Bowie 1975). Some investigators have reported decreased absorption of fat and protein (Paige and Graham 1972), while others have shown that dietary lactose had no effect on the absorption of these nutrients (Kocián et al. 1973, Calloway and Chenoweth 1973, Bowie 1975). The variability in the design of the experiments may have had an effect on the results obtained. In order to determine the effect of unabsorbed lactose on the absorption of other nutrients, the losses of nutrients in fecal matter frequently are measured (Calloway and Chenoweth 1973, Kocián et al. 1973, Paige and Graham 1972, Bowie 1975, Tolensky 1974, Leichter and Tolensky 1975). Recently Debongnie et al. (1979) employed an ileal perfusion technique to study the absorption of protein, calcium, magnesium, and phosphorus from whole milk.

EFFECT OF LACTOSE ON PROTEIN ABSORPTION

In our laboratory we attempted to measure the effect of lactose on the absorption of protein in lactose-tolerant and intolerant adults by determining the maximum rise of plasma urea levels as an index of protein absorption. It has been well established that blood urea level increases in proportion to the amount of protein in a meal (Eggum 1970).

A test drink consisting of 50 g lactose and 55 g gelatin dissolved in 400 ml water was given to seven lactose-tolerant and five lactose-intolerant subjects after an overnight fast. Venous blood samples were drawn while the subjects were still fasting and at 60, 120, 180, and 240 minutes after ingestion of the test drink. One week later the procedure was repeated with the same subjects except that 50 g sucrose replaced the lactose in the test drink. The mean rise in plasma urea above the fasting plasma urea level following the ingestion of the test drinks were compared (table 13.1). There were no statistically significant differences in the peak plasma urea levels in either the lactose-tolerant or intolerant groups, whether lactose or sucrose was consumed with the protein. There were also no significant differences in peak plasma urea levels between the lactose-tolerant and intolerant groups. It should be pointed out that none of the subjects experienced symptoms when the lactose was consumed with the gelatin.

EFFECT OF LACTOSE ON VITAMIN A AND VITAMIN C ABSORPTION

We also investigated the effect of lactose on the absorption of vitamin A and ascorbic acid in lactose-tolerant and intolerant adults by measuring the peak plasma vitamin level as an index of absorption. After an overnight fast the subjects were given 50 g lactose dissolved in 400 ml water with 0.5 g ascorbic acid or a meal consisting of 45 g lactose, 15 g casein (Casilla, Glaxo-Allenburys, Toronto, Ontario), 25 g olive oil, 1 g ascorbic acid, and 200,000 IU vitamin A. Blood samples were drawn before and at 60, 120, 180, and 240 minutes after administration of the test meal. The entire experiment was repeated one week later using an equivalent amount of sucrose. There were no significant differences in the peak plasma ascorbic acid levels between the lactose-tolerant and intolerant subjects, regardless of whether ascorbic acid was ingested with lactose or sucrose. Moreover, when the subjects served as their own controls, lactose

TABLE 13.1

Mean maximum rise in plasma urea after gelatin and sugar ingestion in lactose-tolerant and intolerant subjects

| | Plasma urea (mg/100 ml) | | |
	Lactose	Sucrose	P
Lactose-tolerant subjects (N = 7)	11.7 ± 5.57	10.3 ± 2.78	>0.05
Lactose-intolerant subjects (N = 5)	9.8 ± 3.16	10.5 ± 5.03	>0.05
P	>0.05	>0.05	

Source: Tolensky (1974), reprinted with permission.
Note: Subjects were given 55 g gelatin and 25,000 IU vitamin A with either 50 g lactose or 50 g sucrose.

TABLE 13.2

Maximum rise in plasma ascorbic acid and vitamin A after sugar and liquid meal in lactose-intolerant subjects

	Lactose	Sucrose	P
Plasma ascorbic acid (mg/100 ml)	1.05 ± 0.048	1.03 ± 0.232	>0.05
Plasma vitamin A (mg/100 ml)	0.012 ± 0.009	0.031 ± 0.024	>0.05

Source: Tolensky (1974), reprinted with permission.
Note: Values refer to mean ± SD for six subjects given 1 g ascorbic acid and 200,000 IU vitamin A with a liquid meal containing 15 g protein, 25 g olive oil, and either 45 g lactose or 45 g sucrose.

seemed to have no effect on the absorption of ascorbic acid as compared to sucrose. Symptoms were reported by all the lactose-intolerant subjects when ascorbic acid was ingested with lactose in an aqueous solution.

The peak plasma ascorbic acid and vitamin A levels in four lactose-intolerant adults who ingested the vitamins with a test meal are shown in table 13.2. Again there was no significant difference in the absorption of the two vitamins, regardless of whether they were ingested with lactose or sucrose; however, the maximum rise in plasma vitamin A was slightly lower after the lactose meal. It is of interest to note that only two of the four lactose-intolerant individuals experienced symptoms when 45 g lactose was given in the test meal. On the basis of this preliminary study, one may conclude that a lactose-intolerant adult probably would not have significant losses of these nutrients while consuming products containing lactose.

ANIMAL STUDIES

The postweaning rat, which has a low level of intestinal lactase activity, also was used to study the possible effect of lactose on the absorption of vitamin A. In this experiment 72 male Sprague-Dawley rats (mean body weight 263 g) were divided randomly into two groups. Each group then was divided into nine subgroups of four animals each. After an overnight fast, the experimental group received 500 mg lactose and 2,500 IU vitamin A (Trans Retinol Palmitate Type VII Water Dispersable, Sigma Chemical Co., St. Louis, Mo.) in 2 ml water by stomach tube, while the control group was given sucrose instead of lactose. Four rats from each group were sacrificed and blood was drawn by heart puncture at the following time intervals: prior to receiving the test solution and at 1, 2, 3, 4, and 5 hours after administration of the test solution.

The mean plasma vitamin A levels reached after intragastric administration of 2,500 IU retinol palmitate with either 500 mg lactose or sucrose to postweaning rats were compared. Peak vitamin A absorption occurred for both groups at the two-hour interval. Although the plasma vitamin A level was higher in the lactose

TABLE 13.3
Fecal fat excretion of rats on diets containing lactose or sucrose

Dietary group	Fecal fat	P
10% Lactose	3.75 ± 0.94	
		<0.01
10% Sucrose	2.30 ± 0.14	
30% Lactose	4.43 ± 0.72	
		<0.05
30% Sucrose	3.51 ± 0.55	

Source: Leichter and Tolensky (1975), reprinted with permission.
Note: Values refer to mean ± SD for six rats.

group, the difference was not statistically significant. The maximum mean plasma vitamin A rise, that is, the difference between the mean fasting plasma vitamin A value and the maximum mean plasma vitamin A rise, in the experimental group also was slightly higher than the mean rise in the controls. The values for vitamin A absorption differed significantly between the controls and the experimental animals only at the five-hour interval.

Leichter and Tolensky (1975) conducted balance studies to assess the effect of dietary lactose on the absorption of protein, fat, and calcium in the postweaning rat for a period of 10 days. The experimental diets contained either 10% or 30% lactose, while in the control diets the lactose was replaced with equivalent amounts of sucrose. The fecal losses of fat and nitrogen were significantly higher in the lactose groups (tables 13.3 and 13.4). However, the fecal calcium excretion was lower in the lactose groups, the difference being significant only in the case of the 30% lactose diet (table 13.5). The urinary calcium excretion was also significantly higher in the rats fed the 30% lactose diet. This is probably a result of the increased absorption of calcium by this group of animals. These findings suggest that high levels of dietary lactose may reduce the absorption of protein and fat, but not of calcium, in subjects with lactase deficiency.

TABLE 13.4
Fecal nitrogen excretion of rats on diets containing lactose or sucrose

Dietary group	Fecal nitrogen	P
10% Lactose	5.02 ± 0.91	
		<0.05
10% Sucrose	3.71 ± 0.55	
30% Lactose	6.11 ± 0.92	
		<0.01
30% Sucrose	4.22 ± 0.48	

Source: Leichter and Tolensky (1975), reprinted with permission.
Note: Values refer to mean ± SD for six rats.

TABLE 13.5
Fecal calcium excretion of rats on diets containing lactose or sucrose

Dietary group	Fecal calcium	P
10% Lactose	45.12 ± 13.15	
		>0.05
10% Sucrose	51.42 ± 4.10	
30% Lactose	28.20 ± 6.10	
		<0.001
30% Sucrose	56.07 ± 7.03	

Source: Leichter and Tolensky (1975), reprinted with permission.
Note: Values refer to mean ± SD for six rats.

It is concluded that dietary lactose has no significant effect on the absorption of protein, ascorbic acid, and vitamin A in lactose-intolerant adults. If the unabsorbed lactose has some effect on the absorption of other nutrients it is doubtful whether this effect has significant nutritional consequences in healthy lactose-intolerant adults who consume milk and milk products in moderate amounts.

REFERENCES

Bayless T, Paige DM: Disaccharide intolerance in feeding programs. In *Proceedings of the Western Hemisphere Nutrition Congress: III*, PL White (ed.). Mount Kisco, NY: Futura, 1972, pp 183–93.

Bowie MD: Effect of lactose-induced diarrhoea on absorption of nitrogen and fat. *Arch Dis Child* 50:363–66, 1975.

Calloway DH, Chenoweth WL: Utilization of nutrients in milk- and wheat-based diets by men with adequate and reduced abilities to absorb lactose: I. Energy and nitrogen. *Am J Clin Nutr* 26:939–51, 1973.

Debongnie JC, Newcomer AD, McGill DB, Phillips SF: Absorption of nutrients in lactase deficiency. *Dig Dis Sci* 24:225–31, 1979.

Eggum BO: Blood urea measurement as technique for assaying protein quality. *Br J Nutr* 24:983–88, 1970.

Garza C, Scrimshaw NS: Relationship of lactose intolerance to milk intolerance in young children. *Am J Clin Nutr* 29:192–96, 1976.

Kocián J, Skála I, Bakos K: Calcium absorption from milk and lactose-free milk in healthy subjects and patients with lactose intolerance. *Digestion* 9:317–24, 1973.

Leichter J: Comparison of whole milk and skim milk with aqueous lactose solution in lactose tolerance testing. *Am J Clin Nutr* 26:393–96, 1973.

Leichter J, Tolensky AF: Effect of dietary lactose on the absorption of protein, fat and calcium in the postweaning rat. *Am J Clin Nutr* 28:238–41, 1975.

Lisker R, Aguilar L, Zavala C: Intestinal lactase deficiency and milk drinking capacity in the adult. *Am J Clin Nutr* 31:1499–1503, 1978.

Paige DM, Graham GG: Nutritional implications of lactose malabsorption. *Pediatr Res* 6:329, 1972.

Reddy V, Pershad J: Lactase deficiency in Indians. *Am J Clin Nutr* 25:114–19, 1972.

Stephenson LS, Latham MC: Lactose intolerance and milk consumption: The relationship of tolerance to symptoms. *Am J Clin Nutr* 27:296–303, 1974.

Tolensky AF: The nutritional implications of lactose intolerance. Master's thesis, The University of British Columbia, Vancouver, BC, Canada, 1974.

VI

CLINICAL CONSEQUENCES
IN CHILDREN

CHAPTER 14

LACTOSE MALABSORPTION IN CHILDREN

PREVALENCE, SYMPTOMS, AND NUTRITIONAL

CONSIDERATIONS

David M. Paige

A high prevalence of lactose malabsorption has been reported in various populations of children throughout the world (Huang and Bayless 1967, Keusch et al. 1969, Paige et al. 1971, Woteki et al. 1977, Ellestad-Sayed et al. 1978, Sadre and Karbasi 1979, Jackson and Latham 1979). Identification of groups at risk has relied on lactose tolerance testing. Except for very young children, the level of lactose used exceeds the level of lactose routinely consumed. This has prompted discussion within the scientific community with respect to the nutritional inferences to be drawn from prevalence data reported in the literature (Paige et al. 1971, Kretchmer 1972, Simoons et al. 1977, Committee on Nutrition 1978, National Dairy Council 1978).

Initially, many reports had treated the population studied as a single unit and had paid incomplete attention to age-specific considerations. Distinctions between secondary lactose malabsorption due to short-term intestinal injury, and primary lactose malabsorption that has a genetic basis, were not always made. This introduced additional confounding variables. Differences in an individual's capacity to hydrolyze and tolerate a lactose challenge dose compared to his or her ability to utilize lesser amounts of lactose found in usually consumed amounts of milk created additional areas of confusion (Paige et al. 1971 and 1972, *Nutrition Reviews* 1969, Protein Advisory Group 1972, Reddy and Pershad 1972, Stephenson and Latham 1974, Bayless and Paige 1978, Brown et al. 1979, 1980).

When attention is paid to the many factors associated with lactose digestion from infancy to old age, it is possible to place many of the seeming contradictions into perspective. What may have appeared to be incongruities in reported data appear to merge into a relatively predictable pattern of lactose digestion.

This pattern is influenced by age, genetics, environment, infection, size of the lactose bolus, gastric emptying time, intestinal transit time, individual sensitivities, eating habits, food ideologies, and cultural patterns. Clearly, lactose malabsorption is not a homogeneous event. Neither is it an all or none phenomenon having its origins in a single etiology. Clinical expressions of lactose malabsorption, lactose intolerance, milk intolerance, and milk rejection find their origins in one or more of the causes outlined above.

As a basis for understanding the pattern of lactose digestion in children, this chapter will report on (1) the age-specific prevalence of lactose malabsorption in black children and its relationship to socioeconomic factors; (2) the association of symptoms with incomplete lactose digestion and the pattern of reported symptoms with increasing age; (3) milk consumption practices at different ages and their nutritional implications; (4) absorption of lactose-hydrolyzed milk; and (5) comparisons and differences in reported information on lactose digestion.

AGE-SPECIFIC PREVALENCE

Age-specific prevalence data suggest a progressive decrease in lactose absorption with age in black children studied in the United States (Paige et al. 1977). This progressive decrease is seen in a study of 409 black children, 13 months to 12 years of age. The population was stratified by age to have approximately equal representation in each 12-month category. The mean age of the children studied was 6.6 years. The study subjects were drawn from four well child clinic sites and a private pediatrician's office in Baltimore, Maryland. All subjects were in good health as determined by history and a review of recent clinic visits. The children were free of any overt intestinal or allergic disorders and had no recent history of gastroenteritis.

One hundred fifty of the parents of the 409 children fell into the upper three occupational rankings of the Hollingshead Index to social position and were characterized as higher socioeconomic status families. The remaining 259 parents were judged to be of lower socioeconomic status, having been ranked in the lower three occupational positions of the Hollingshead Index.

Two hundred fifty-eight (99%) of the lower socioeconomic status families were receiving medical assistance. None of the 150 families categorized as of higher socioeconomic status were receiving such assistance. Seventy-three percent of the lower socioeconomic status mothers had less than a twelfth grade education, while all of the mothers in the high socioeconomic status category had at least a twelfth grade education. One-half of the latter category had 13 or more years of education, compared to only two mothers in the lower socioeconomic status group. The study population was equally distributed between males and females in both high and low income groups.

Lactose tolerance tests were performed in the morning after an overnight fast. Lactose, as a 20% suspension in water, was given orally at a rate of 2 g per kg body weight. Microcapillary blood samples were obtained at 0, 15, 30, and 60 minutes. A blood glucose rise of less than 26 mg per dl over fasting levels was considered a flat tolerance curve.

Clinical signs associated with the ingestion of the lactose load, such as loose stools, diarrhea, gas and symptoms of abdominal fullness, and cramping occurring during the test and for two hours following the completion of the test, were noted and recorded by trained observers.

Results of regression studies of glucose rise on age in black subjects following a lactose challenge of 2 g per kg indicate a progressive decrement in blood glucose level with increasing age (fig. 14.1). The mean glucose level over fasting values at 12 months of age was 38 mg per dl. At 5 years of age, the level was 31 mg per dl, and at 12 years of age, 20 mg per dl. The decline in blood glucose level occurs for black children of both high and low socioeconomic status, with no significant difference between the two groups at any age interval.

The prevalence of lactose malabsorption among black children studied indicates that 16 of 60 children in the 1- to 2-year age range (27%) were lactose malabsorbers. At 5 to 6 years of age, 26 of the 80 study children (33%) were malabsorbers; and at 11 to 12 years of age, 39 of 53 (74%) were malabsorbers. This progressive increase in the prevalence of malabsorption with age is noted for high and low socioeconomic status black children with no significant difference between the two groups by age or sex (fig. 14.2). In 52 low income white children, 1 to 12 years of age, only 9 (17%) were malabsorbers.

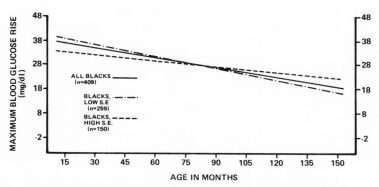

FIGURE 14.1. Maximum blood glucose rise in black children, by age and socioeconomic status.

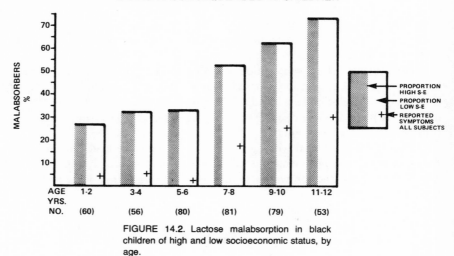

FIGURE 14.2. Lactose malabsorption in black children of high and low socioeconomic status, by age.

SYMPTOMS

The association of symptoms with lactose digestion was studied in the same population. Complete data on symptomatic response to a lactose load were recorded in 378 of the 409 subjects on whom blood glucose rise information was available. The 31 subjects on whom information was incomplete were not included in this analysis. These subjects were not identifiably different from the remainder of the children.

In children less than 4 years of age there was no difference in peak blood glucose rise in the 16 subjects with symptoms and 97 subjects without symptoms following a lactose challenge (Paige et al. 1977). Similarly, no significant differences were found in the 27 symptomatic and 125 nonsymptomatic subjects 4 to 7 years of age. At 8 years of age, however, this pattern changes. Results indicate a significantly lower peak blood glucose rise of 13.6 mg per dl in the 40 symptomatic black subjects with a lactose load, compared to a blood glucose rise of 24.6 mg per dl in the 73 black children who were asymptomatic. Data suggest that the steady decline of available lactase reaches an identifiable clinical threshold by 8 years of age. These changes result in a pattern of increasing reports of symptoms with a lactose load (table 14.1).

Despite the randomness in reported symptoms in the youngest age children, symptoms are significantly associated with a continued decline in blood glucose rise in older children. In 78 children 8 years of age and above, 35 (45%) report symptoms with a blood glucose rise < 26 mg per dl. Twenty-eight of the 35 children reporting symptoms (80%) have a peak blood glucose rise of < 15 mg per dl. This significant association suggests a relationship of decreasing lactase

TABLE 14.1
Symptoms related to level of blood glucose rise, by age groups,
in black subjects

Blood glucose rise (mg/dl)	< 4 years*		≥ 8 years†	
	No symptoms	Symptoms	No symptoms	Symptoms
<15	12	3	20	28
	(12%)	(19%)	(27%)	(70%)
15 to 25	14	3	23	7
	(14%)	(19%)	(32%)	(18%)
≥26	71	10	30	5
	(74%)	(62%)	(41%)	(12%)
Total subjects	97	16	73	40

*X^2 = 0.81, P is not significant.
†X^2 = 19.77, P < 0.001.

activity, incomplete lactose digestion, and symptoms with increasing age (table 14.2).

MILK CONSUMPTION

As a result of the associations reported above, milk-drinking patterns were reviewed to determine if there is a change in milk consumption practices with age. Levels of milk drinking in black children were obtained by history from caretakers of 102 subjects below 5 years of age and by observation during the school lunch period in 160 low income children at and above 5 years of age. A milk drinker was defined as an individual who consumed 50% or more by weight of a 240 ml glass of milk per 24 hours. This was determined by caretaker recall below 5 years of age, and by direct observation and weighing of the milk carton at the end of the school lunch period on two independent occasions in subjects 5 years of age and above.

TABLE 14.2
Percentages of black children reporting symptoms after lactose ingestion,
by age

	<4 years*	4 to 7 years†	≥8 years‡	All ages
Malabsorbers	19% (32)	24% (63)	45% (78)	32% (173)
Absorbers	12% (81)	13% (89)	14% (35)	13% (205)

Note: Figures in parentheses indicate the number of children in each group.
*X^2 = 0.34, P is not significant.
†X^2 = 2.03, P is not significant.
‡X^2 = 8.59, P < 0.001.

Results indicate that below 8 years of age, approximately 10% of black children failed to meet the above criteria and were designated non-milk drinkers. This level was similar whether information was obtained by recall or direct observation. At 8 years of age, over 20% of the observed black children are classified as non-milk drinkers (Bayless and Paige 1979).

The pattern of milk consumption in 49 low income white children in the first three grades of the study school differed. On one observation, two (4%) failed to consume more than one-half their 240 ml milk. Two additional observations were carried out with only 42 of the white children present, and during both observations one child did not consume the milk.

This overall proportion of black children rejecting milk parallels earlier reported observations of the level of milk rejection in lactose-intolerant school children. Furthermore, the number of children above 8 years of age who incompletely consume their half-pint container of milk approximates the expected number of malabsorbing children at this age with a maximum blood glucose rise below 15 mg per dl. These data, when compared to previously reported prevalence data and milk rejection patterns, do suggest an association between blood glucose rise following a lactose test and milk rejection (Lisker et al. 1978).

LACTOSE-HYDROLYZED MILK

Forty-eight of the black children 4 to 10 years of age (mean age 7.3 years) were selected at random to participate in an additional clinical study (Paige et al. 1979). This study included a lactose tolerance test and measurement of glucose absorption with 240 ml unflavored whole cow's milk and with 90% lactose-hydrolyzed milk containing 12 g and 1 g lactose, respectively. The hydrolysis of the milk was carried out as previously reported (Paige et al. 1975a).

The children were given the coded test milk in a random manner at refrigerated temperatures after an eight-hour fast. The technologist was not aware of which milk was being tested. The milk was consumed immediately following the drawing of the fasting blood sugar. Blood samples were taken at 15, 30, and 60 minutes, and testing was carried out as previously reported (Paige et al. 1975b).

The mean ($\pm$SD) glucose rise in all children following the consumption of 240 ml unflavored whole cow's milk was 11.9 mg per dl ($\pm$ 8.5). The blood glucose rise in the same children following consumption of 240 ml lactose-hydrolyzed milk was 17.5 mg per dl ($\pm$ 11.5). The difference is significant at the 0.01 level.

When the subjects are dichotomized into lactose absorber and malabsorber groups, the mean glucose rise in the 28 malabsorbers with a lactose tolerance test was 12.4 mg per dl ($\pm$ 7.8). A glucose rise of 10.9 mg per dl ($\pm$ 7.2) and 17.8 mg per dl ($\pm$ 10.8) was observed with whole cow's milk and lactose-hydrolyzed milk, respectively ($P < 0.005$). The 20 absorbers had a peak glucose rise of 37.2 mg per dl ($\pm$ 8.7) with the lactose tolerance test. There was no statistically

TABLE 14.3

Mean blood glucose rise, by age, in malabsorbers following lactose, cow's
milk, and lactose-hydrolyzed milk

	<6 years	6 to 7 years	⩾8 years	Total
Number of subjects	9	6	13	28
Mean age	5 yr 1 mo	7 yr 2 mo	9 yr	7 yr 3 mo
Lactose tolerance test	17.2	10.7	9.9	12.4
(2 g lactose/kg)	(±4.9)	(±8.7)	(±8.0)	(±7.8)
Whole cow's milk	11.7	14.0	9.0	10.9
(12.5 g lactose)	(±8.8)*	(±7.4)*	(±5.9)†	(±7.2)‡
Lactose-hydrolyzed milk	14.9	20.7	18.5	17.8
(1 g lactose)	(±14.0)*	(±9.3)*	(±9.1)†	(±10.8)‡

*N.S.
†$P < 0.001$.
‡$P < 0.005$.

significant difference between the values for whole cow's milk (13.4 mg per dl)
and lactose-hydrolyzed milk (17.1 mg per dl) in lactose absorbers.

In the malabsorbing children 8 years of age and above, the peak blood glucose
rise was significantly lower following consumption of 240 ml whole cow's milk
when compared to 90% lactose-hydrolyzed milk (table 14.3). Significant differences in the blood glucose rise between the two milks were not observed below
this age. In the 20 absorbers there was no significant difference following the
consumption of 240 ml whole cow's milk and 90% lactose-hydrolyzed milk in
any of the three age categories.

It appears that in most older lactose malabsorbing children incomplete lactose
digestion, as measured by blood glucose rise following the consumption of 240
ml whole cow's milk, can be significantly improved by substituting 240 ml of
90% lactose-hydrolyzed milk (Paige et al. 1975a, 1979).

STUDIES WITH OTHER POPULATIONS

Other investigators have presented data supporting the fact that declining
levels of lactase activity may have no clinical consequences in populations of
healthy children below 8 years of age, but that there are increasing clinical
implications above 8 years of age.

Johnson et al. (1977) report an increasing prevalence of lactose malabsorption
with age. In full-blooded Pima subjects 3 to 4 years of age, 40% were malabsorbers. This rate climbed to 71% in those aged 4 to 5 years and to 92% in those
aged 5 to 7 years. All subjects 8 years of age and older were malabsorbers.
Symptoms associated with the test rose from 58% in subjects below 12 years of
age, to 74% in those in the 12- to 18-year age range, and to 91% in those 18 years
of age or above. Malabsorbers' recognition of symptoms associated with the
consumption of milk products also increased, from 4% in subjects less than 12

years of age to 7% in the 12- to 18-year-old group and 68% in subjects 18 years of age or older.

Data presented by Garza and Scrimshaw (1976) support the inference that declining levels of lactase may have little or no clinical consequence in populations of healthy children below 8 years of age; but have increasing clinical implications above 8 years of age. The authors report: (1) an increase in the age-specific prevalence of lactose intolerance, ranging from 11% in 4- to 5-year-old blacks to 50% at 6 to 7 years of age and 72% in 8- to 9-year-olds; (2) no differences between the milk intakes of 5- to 7-year-old black and white children; (3) an increase in symptom response to graded amounts of lactose in peanut butter and whole cow's milk, with an increase in age; and (4) symptoms in 10% of blacks above 8 years of age with 12 g lactose when consumed with peanut butter.

Lisker et al. (1980) report that in rural and urban Mexican children 5 to 14 years of age no less than 15% have gastrointestinal complaints after ingesting 240 ml regular milk and that lactose-hydrolyzed milk is significantly better tolerated than other kinds of milk.

In urban children with less chronic gastrointestinal problems and better general environmental conditions, 16.8% had symptoms with regular milk and 3.9% with lactose-free milk. In rural children with a higher incidence of poor nutrition, diarrhea, and parasitosis, severe symptoms were reported almost twice as often with regular milk as with lactose-free milk (Lisker et al. 1980).

Despite general agreement on the data reported above, only limited agreement is found on the effect of lactose intolerance on milk-drinking patterns. Some investigators report that milk consumption is not influenced by lactose intolerance. The absence of symptoms with the consumption of 8 ounces of milk is cited as support for this conclusion. For example, Jones and Latham (1974) report no difference in milk consumption by race in elementary school children. The *Dairy Council Digest*'s "Perspective on Milk Intolerance" nevertheless reports, in their review of this work, "It must be reiterated that the prevalence of lactose intolerance was not distinguished in this study, lest one erroneously conclude that these results necessarily pertain to a population with a known prevalence of lactose intolerance" (National Dairy Council 1978).

Lacassie et al. (1978) also point out in their study of 436 Chilean children the low predictability of malabsorption from symptoms. The authors conclude that investigators interested in malabsorption prevalence must estimate it from blood glucose data rather than from more easily collectible data on symptoms. Such low predictability implies that many malabsorbers are asymptomatic.

Estimates of the amount of lactose needed to provoke symptoms in children remain in dispute. Symptoms are subjective and individuals' thresholds for reporting discomfort clearly may vary. Furthermore, younger individuals may make it more difficult to determine reliably the presence or absence of symptoms. This may be due in part to the fact that lactase activity is not an all or none phenomenon. What appears to be occurring is a steady decline in available lactase activity resulting in a decreasing ability to handle even usually consumed amounts of lactose. This decline may be modified further by other food consumed along with a "usual lactose load." While a smaller lactose load may not provoke threshold level symptoms in a subject, or the subject may not recognize the association, there are data suggesting that lactose is not completely hydrolyzed and that carbohydrate absorption is altered (Solomons et al. 1980).

Comparisons also are made as if the age of the subjects were the same or similar, when in fact the ages reported on are frequently quite disparate, and preclude age-specific comparisons. Another factor contributing to the difficulty and confusion in interpreting the association of symptoms and milk drinking is the practice of quantifying the reported symptoms. Many investigators have superimposed upon the patient's subjective reports their own subjective decisions regarding which symptoms, how many symptoms, and to what degree symptoms are considered sufficiently important to be included as present or absent. Attempting to quantify, grade, or score an individual's subjective feeling of discomfort by yet another set of subjective interpretations on the part of the investigator may further distort a very imprecise outcome measure. It may be better to report the individual's recognition of the presence or absence of a threshold level of discomfort following ingestion of the test product during or immediately following the test period. Attempts at quantitative or semiquantitative statements regarding symptoms associated with lactose ingestion do not appear to increase the reliability or validity of such reports.

In addition, it would be useful if a specific standard were used for test products. Since the quality and quantity of test products differ, the literature remains quite confusing and it is almost impossible to compare results from two or more studies. Comparisons are made and inferences are drawn from reports in the literature as if the tests were similar, even when different milks such as chocolate, skim, and whole milk were used in the studies compared (Guthrie 1977).

An example of this confusion is illustrated by the reports of Kwon and colleagues (1980). Inferences are drawn about levels of milk consumption and associated symptoms in teenagers. Yet, the "milk" used is a synthetic chocolate-flavored product. Bricker et al. (1949) noted that college students have experienced several side effects, such as nausea and cramps, following the consumption of one ounce of cocoa. This may help to explain Kwon's conclusions that no statistically significant differences were found in the incidence of symptoms reported by malabsorbers and absorbers after drinking 240 ml of a synthetic chocolate milk containing lactose.

SUMMARY

In summary, lactase activity declines on a continuous basis in genetically programmed populations. Its evolution can be described and monitored during three distinct clinical phases.

First, there is a decreasing ability to digest the large lactose load consumed during the screening test. It is important to recognize that this is not an all or none phenomenon but rather a slowly progressive decline in available lactase activity, and that this decline can be influenced by transit time, the vehicle in which the lactose is consumed, and/or the intake of additional foods along with lactose.

Next, with the decline of lactase activity, a point is reached when available lactase activity is no longer sufficient to hydrolyze more modest levels of lactose. Therefore, the consumption of a glass of milk or another product containing the equivalent level of lactose will result in incomplete hydrolysis of the lactose consumed. The individuals so tested frequently do not recognize signs or symptoms associated with the incomplete digestion of lactose.

Finally, with the continued decline of lactase activity with increasing age, individuals become symptomatic as a result of the undigested lactose. The decline in available lactase activity reaches a recognizable clinical threshold with increasing age.

A review of reported data on diverse populations supports the conclusion that in later childhood and adolescence an important transition in lactose digestion occurs. The older children and young adults are increasingly unable to digest even modest amounts of lactose. This results in increased symptom production, recognition of discomfort, and avoidance of lactose-containing products that provoke symptoms.

REFERENCES

Bayless TM, Paige DM: Lactose tolerance by lactose-malabsorbing Indians. *Gastroenterology* 74: 153, 1978.

Bayless TM, Paige DM: Lactose intolerance. In *Nutritional Management of Genetic Disorders,* M Winick (ed). New York: John Wiley, 1979, pp 79-90.

Bricker ML, Smith JM, Hamilton TS, Mitchell HH: The effect of cocoa upon calcium utilization and requirements, nitrogen retention and fecal composition of women. *J Nutr* 39: 445-61, 1949.

Brown KH, Khatun M, Parry L, Ahmed MG: Nutritional consequences of low dose milk supplements consumed by lactose-malabsorbing children. *Am J Clin Nutr* 33: 1054-63, 1980.

Brown KH, Parry L, Khatun M, Ahmed MG: Lactose malabsorption in Bangladeshi village children: Relation with age, history of recent diarrhea, nutritional status, and breast feeding. *Am J Clin Nutr* 32: 1962-69, 1979.

Committee on Nutrition, American Academy of Pediatrics: The practical significance of lactose intolerance in children. *Pediatrics* 62: 240-45, 1978.

Ellestad-Sayed JJ, Haworth JC, Hildes JA: Disaccharide malabsorption and dietary patterns in two Canadian Eskimo communities. *Am J Clin Nutr* 31: 1473-78, 1978.

Garza C, Scrimshaw NS: Relationship of lactose tolerance to milk intolerance in young children. *Am J Clin Nutr* 29: 192-96, 1976.

Guthrie HA: Effect of a flavored milk option in a school lunch program. *J Am Diet Assoc* 71: 35-40, 1977.

Huang SS, Bayless TM: Lactose intolerance in healthy children. *N Engl J Med* 276: 1283-87, 1967.

Jackson RT, Latham MC: Lactose malabsorption among Masai children of East Africa. *Am J Clin Nutr* 32: 779-82, 1979.

Johnson JD, Simoons FJ, Hurwitz R, Grange A, Mitchell CH, Sinatra FR, Sunshine P, Robertson WV, Bennett PH, Kretchmer N: Lactose malabsorption among the Pima Indians of Arizona. *Gastroenterology* 73: 1299-1304, 1977.

Jones DV, Latham MC: Lactose intolerance in young children and their parents. *Am J Clin Nutr* 27: 547–49, 1974.

Keusch GT, Troncale FJ, Miller LH, Promadhat V, Anderson PR: Acquired lactose malabsorption in Thai children. *Pediatrics* 43: 540–45, 1969.

Kretchmer N: Lactose and lactase. *Sci Am* 227: 70–78, 1972.

Kwon PH Jr, Rorick MH, Scrimshaw NS: Comparative tolerance of adolescents of differing ethnic backgrounds to lactose-containing and lactose-free dairy drinks: II. Improvement of a double-blind test. *Am J Clin Nutr* 33: 22–26, 1980.

Lacassie Y, Weinberg R, Monckeberg F: Poor predictability of lactose malabsorption from clinical symptoms for Chilean populations. *Am J Clin Nutr* 31: 799–804, 1978.

Lisker R, Aguilar L, Lares I, Cravioto J: Double blind study of milk lactose intolerance in a group of rural and urban children. *Am J Clin Nutr* 33: 1049–53, 1980.

Lisker R, Aguilar L, Zavala C: Intestinal lactase deficiency and milk drinking capacity in the adult. *Am J Clin Nutr* 31: 1499–1503, 1978.

National Dairy Council: Perspective on milk intolerance. *Dairy Council Dig* 49(6): 31–36, 1978.

Nutrition Reviews: Lactase deficiency in Thailand. *Nutr Rev* 27: 278–80, 1969.

Paige DM, Bayless TM, Ferry GD, Graham GG: Lactose malabsorption and milk rejection in Negro children. *Johns Hopkins Med J* 129: 163–69, 1971.

Paige DM, Bayless TM, Huang SS, Wexler R: Lactose hydrolyzed milk. *Am J Clin Nutr* 28: 818–22, 1975a.

Paige DM, Bayless TM, Huang SS, Wexler R: Lactose intolerance and lactose hydrolyzed milk. In *Physiological Effects of Food Carbohydrates*, A Jeanes, J Hodge (eds). Washington, D.C.: American Chemical Society, Symposium ser. no. 15, 1975b, pp 191–206.

Paige DM, Bayless TM, Mellits ED, Davis L: Lactose malabsorption in preschool black children. *Am J Clin Nutr* 30: 1018–22, 1977.

Paige DM, Bayless TM, Mellits ED, Davis L, Dellinger WS, Kreitner M: Effects of age and lactose tolerance on blood glucose rise with whole cow milk and lactose hydrolyzed milk. *Agric Food Chem* 27: 677–80, 1979.

Paige DM, Leonardo E, Cordano A, Nakashima J, Adrianzen TB, Graham GG: Lactose intolerance in Peruvian children: Effect of age and early nutrition. *Am J Clin Nutr* 25: 297–301, 1972.

Protein Advisory Group of the United Nations: PAG statement 17 on low lactase activity and milk intake. *PAG Bull* 2(2): 9–11, 1972.

Reddy V, Pershad J: Lactase deficiency in Indians. *Am J Clin Nutr* 25: 114–19, 1972.

Sadre M, Karbasi K: Lactose intolerance in Iran. *Am J Clin Nutr* 32: 1948–54, 1979.

Simoons FJ, Johnson JD, Kretchmer N: Perspective on milk drinking and malabsorption of lactose. *Pediatrics* 59: 98–109, 1977.

Solomons NW, Garcia-Ibanez R, Viteri FE: Hydrogen (H_2) breath test of lactose absorption in adults: The application of physiological doses and whole cow's milk sources. *Am J Clin Nutr* 33: 545–54, 1980.

Stephenson LS, Latham MC: Lactose intolerance and milk consumption: The relation of tolerance to symptoms. *Am J Clin Nutr* 27: 296–303, 1974.

Woteki CE, Weser E, Young EA: Lactose malabsorption in Mexican-American adults. *Am J Clin Nutr* 30: 470–75, 1977.

CHAPTER 15

☙

MILK VERSUS LOW-LACTOSE DIETS
FOR LACTOSE-INTOLERANT CHILDREN

Cutberto Garza

The use of cow's milk as a food supplement for young children has been endorsed as appropriate in national and international policy statements published by concerned groups (Protein Advisory Group 1972, Food and Nutrition Board 1972, Committee on Nutrition 1974, 1978). Yet, the widespread use of cow's milk in programs targeted at preschool children has been viewed by others as possibly inappropriate (Simoons et al. 1977). Three concerns emerge most often in discussions of this issue: (1) the recognition of lactose intolerance in the majority of the world's populations (Gilat 1979); (2) the uncertainty over the relative deficiencies of protein and energy in traditional diets of undernourished populations (Scrimshaw 1976, Arroyave 1972); and (3) the belief that the use of cow's milk as a supplement promotes it and leads to an undesirable decrease in the use of human milk (Jelliffe and Jelliffe 1978). This discussion will focus on the practical significance of lactose intolerance in children. This limitation should not be misinterpreted to reflect a lack of appreciation for the other concerns listed. Each is important and must be considered within appropriate contexts.

ACCEPTABILITY OF COW'S MILK

Cow's milk has been utilized in food supplement programs because it apparently meets three of the criteria applied in choosing food supplements. The first is

This work is a publication of the USDA/SEA, Children's Nutrition Research Center, Department of Pediatrics, Baylor College of Medicine and Texas Children's Hospital.

that cow's milk is acceptable and is an accessible food that can be made to meet storage and transportation requirements. The question of acceptability has been linked to cultural factors and to symptomatic responses associated with lactose intolerance. Consideration of acceptability requires that a clear distinction be made between primary and secondary lactose intolerance. It is important to keep in mind that primary lactose intolerance occurs in the presence of a normal gastrointestinal tract and that secondary lactose intolerance is a result of a decrease in intestinal lactase activity observed during, and transiently after, stress to the gastrointestinal tract.

Table 15.1 summarizes results of studies evaluating the prevalence of primary lactose intolerance or malabsorption in black American children. Prevalence is estimated by assessing either lactose absorption or symptomatic responses to standard lactose tolerance test doses. These reports have confirmed that lactose intolerance occurs in significant proportions of the black American population by early childhood. The prevalence of lactose intolerance and lactose malabsorption is even higher in populations with rates of gastrointestinal disease that are higher than those found in this country (Gilat 1979). In these populations, lactose intolerance also seems to appear at even earlier ages than those indicated in table 15.1.

It is important to review the possibility that these higher rates of lactose intolerance are due to higher endemic levels of transient secondary lactose intolerance rather than a result of higher specific rates of "genetically programmed" and permanent primary lactose intolerance. In studies among free-living populations it is difficult to distinguish between these two conditions. However, the role of secondary lactose intolerance in explaining apparently high prevalences of primary lactose intolerance has been evaluated in studies assessing lactose tolerance status a second time in children found on initial evaluation to be either lactose intolerant or lactose malabsorbers. Brown et al. (1979) restudied 36 of 50 lactose malabsorbing children three to five months after their initial evaluation and found approximately 40% to be absorbing lactose normally at the time of the second study. Stoopler et al. (1974) performed similar studies and found 21% of

TABLE 15.1
Prevalence of primary lactose intolerance or malabsorption in selected
black American children

Study	Age (yrs)	Percentage intolerant	Percentage malabsorbers
Paige et al. 1977	1–5	18	29
Garza and Scrimshaw 1976	4–5	11	—
	6–7	50	—
	7–9	72	—
Paige et al. 1975	6–13	65	54
Haverberg et al. 1980	14–19	—	83
Kwon et al. 1980	14–19	—	81

initially lactose-malabsorbing children to be absorbing lactose normally seven months after their initial evaluation. Whether these represent true endemic rates of secondary lactose intolerance among lactose-intolerant or lactose-malabsorbing children or methodological errors is debatable. Nevertheless, the available evidence indicates that substantial numbers of children in the world have either primary or secondary lactose intolerance.

Based on information of this type, the assessment of the impact of lactose malabsorption and lactose intolerance on the acceptability of milk is appropriate. Various studies of American children have addressed this question. Paige et al. (1971) have reported that lactose intolerance adversely influences elementary school children's acceptance of the amounts of milk provided by the school lunch program. In contrast, Garza and Scrimshaw (1976) found no differences in milk consumption between lactose-tolerant and lactose-intolerant black children 6 to 9 years of age. However, 8- to 9-year-old black children consumed less milk than did a comparable group of white children, regardless of lactose tolerance status. Stephenson and co-workers (1977) reported similar results. Similarly, Paige et al. (1975) reported no differences in consumption between lactose-tolerant and lactose-intolerant black children, 1 to 5 years of age. Woteki et al. (1976) made similar observations among Mexican-Americans but found that children classified as Anglo-American drank more milk than Mexican-American children. Newcomer et al. (1978) studied American Indians and found lactose malabsorbers had mean lactose intake of 19 g in contrast to daily intakes of 25 g by lactose absorbers. Lebenthal et al. (1975) reported greater milk consumption by individuals and their families with high intestinal lactase levels than by patients and families with low lactase levels. In a recent study in Iran by Sadre and Karbasi (1979), a high rate of milk rejection by lactose-intolerant school children was noted. These authors report that initial rates of milk rejection fell as the supplementary milk program was continued. However, they did not identify whether this decreased rejection rate resulted from a decrease in symptomatic responses to milk, and/or an increased familiarity with a food not previously included in the diet on a regular basis.

The question of the acceptance of milk would be answered easily if symptomatic responses to normally consumed amounts of milk were as dramatic as responses to test doses of lactose. In my experience, this is seldom the case. In fact, in our studies of 4- to 9-year-old black children, symptomatic responses to 250 ml milk were not observed. In contrast, Mitchell et al. (1975) found that 21% of 11- to 18-year-old lactose-intolerant blacks had symptoms after 240 ml milk. This is in contrast to studies by Haverberg et al. (1980) and Kwon et al. (1980) who reported double-blind studies of adolescents in which comparable percentages of lactose absorbers and lactose malabsorbers had similarly mild symptomatic responses to 240 ml of lactose-containing and lactose-free dairy drinks. Newcomer and co-workers (1978) found that American Indians, 5 to 62 years of age, tolerated 240 ml to 300 ml milk, taken with a meal, without developing intestinal symptoms attributable to lactose. However, Peruvian children studied by Paige et al. (1972) were tolerant to lactose only at levels lower than the lactose content in 240 ml milk.

The most striking aspect of these studies is the mild symptomatic responses reported by most investigators evaluating the incidence of "milk tolerance" among young lactose-intolerant and lactose-malabsorbing children. However, there is a group of children who may have more marked symptomatic responses after the consumption of normal amounts of foods containing lactose. Two reports published recently have evaluated prospectively the rate of lactose intolerance in children with recurrent abdominal pain. Both studies concluded that lactose intolerance played a significant role in this condition. Barr et al. (1979) studied 80 children, 4 to 15 years of age, and found 40% to be lactose malabsorbers. Twenty-eight of 32 lactose malabsorbers underwent a six-week low-lactose diet trial. Seventy-one percent of those participating reported greater pain frequency with diets containing lactose. Twenty-nine percent had unchanged pain frequency on the test diet. In the study by Liebman (1979), 10 of 11 lactose malabsorbers with recurrent abdominal pain reported significant relief when placed on a low-lactose diet, in contrast to 0 of 6 lactose absorbers with similar initial complaints. Children with this type of complaint obviously often improved on low-lactose diets.

While these studies did not demonstrate conclusively that lactose was responsible for aggravating or causing these complaints, they do suggest that a responsible agent is to be found in foods containing lactose. Until more controlled studies are possible, lactose remains a good "marker" for foods to be avoided on a trial basis. Based on available evidence, lactose remains the more probable "culprit."

Taken collectively, these studies indicate that there is a wide spectrum of responses to milk that may influence its acceptability. From studies thus far published, children with significant symptomatic responses to normally consumed quantities of milk appear to be in the minority. At most 2% to 4% of children 3 to 14 years of age may be affected if one assumes that recurrent abdominal pain occurs in 9% to 15% of the pediatric population and that the elimination of lactose will help approximately 25% of those with this complaint.

NUTRIENT BIOAVAILABILITY

A second criterion used in selecting supplemental food is an acceptable bioavailability level of key nutrients. In the absence of overt lactose intolerance, this concern focuses on the assessment of the absorption of nutrients in the presence of amounts of lactose that surpass the lactose hydrolyzing capacity of the gastrointestinal tract, but do not produce symptoms. The best controlled data have been obtained in adults by Calloway and Chenoweth (1973). In these metabolic balance studies, milk provided all dietary protein for both lactose-tolerant and lactose-intolerant adults. After adjustments were made for metabolizable energy, no effect on nitrogen balance was demonstrable. Furthermore, calcium, phosphorus, and magnesium absorption was unaffected by the presence of lactose. Bowie (1975) obtained results consistent with those reported by Calloway and Chenoweth (1973). Definitive studies evaluating specific nutrient bioavailabilities in children with primary lactose intolerance have not been done. Studies that come closest to meeting this objective are those of Paige and co-workers (1974), who measured blood glucose after milk consumption by lactose absorbers and malabsorbers. These investigators found lower maximal increases in blood glucose among lactose malabsorbers. The lower blood glucose rise observed in the lactose-malabsorbing group could be due either to slower hydrolysis of lactose or to its actual malabsorption. Measurements of breath hydrogen following the ingestion of amounts of lactose much smaller than the usual tolerance test dose (2 g per kg) indicate that lactose is malabsorbed even in the absence of overt symptoms. Assessment of possible effects of small unabsorbed quantities of carbohydrate, however, requires other experiments.

More data are available assessing nutrient bioavailability in the presence of secondary lactose intolerance. Prinsloo and co-workers (1969) placed children with kwashiorkor and diarrhea on six different formulas during the first few weeks of rehabilitation. No differences in the amount of diarrhea or the amount of weight gained during hospitalization were observed in groups fed sucrose, glucose, maltose, fructose, and 4.2 g lactose per dl. The group fed 6.8 g lactose per dl had more voluminous diarrhea and gained less weight when compared to the other groups. Sutton and Hamilton (1977) compared formulas containing 10 g lactose per dl and 10 g glucose per dl in treating Canadian children with diarrhea who were under 2 years of age. The group fed the lactose formula had more severe diarrhea, but no conclusions about weight gain could be made because of the short duration of the study. Mitchell et al. (1977) studied Australian aboriginal children 2 to 38 months of age suffering from diarrhea and malnutrition. During the first two to three weeks of treatment the children were fed either a 5.2 g lactose per dl formula or an identical formula with hydrolyzed lactose. Both groups tolerated the formula, but the group on hydrolyzed lactose formula gained 70% more weight during hospitalization than did the group on unhydrolyzed lactose. This study has been criticized because the groups were not of comparable ages; the study was of relatively short duration; and criteria for assessing tolerance to lactose were not sufficiently rigid (Anderson 1977).

In considering these studies, it seems that lactose in concentrations at or below 4 g per dl may be tolerated by children in early recovery from diarrhea and malnutrition, but that the 7.2 g per dl available in commercial formulas might exacerbate the diarrhea and be associated with less than optimal weight gain during the first two to three weeks of treatment. Lower quantities may not cause symptoms but still may influence nutrient bioavailability. This, however, is in contrast to experiences in Haiti, Uganda, Ethiopia, and Guatemala. For example, children at INCAP in Guatemala receive 0.3 g to 0.6 g lactose per kg per meal during initial recovery and 1.0 g to 1.7 g lactose per kg at full treatment. These children are reported to achieve excellent catch-up growth. However, control studies comparing lactose with other carbohydrate sources have not been published by this or other centers.

Intestinal morphology also may be expected to influence bioavailability. Few studies have attempted to relate this variable to milk tolerance as a first step in assessing nutrient bioavailability from milk (Harrison and Walker-Smith 1977). Experience in our unit with children undergoing evaluation for moderate to severe gastrointestinal disease has been reviewed (table 15.2). Lactase activities, jejunal morphology, and tolerance to milks containing lactose were compared. Tolerance was assessed on the basis of the response to milk meals containing 43 g to 63 g lactose. Intolerance was diagnosed when fecal pH dropped to 5.0 or below, when glucose greater than 10% per dl was present in feces, or when a significant increase in watery diarrhea resulted. Twenty percent of the 65 biopsies examined for lactase activity had abnormally low values; 80% had normal activity levels. However, 85% of those with low lactase levels and 41% of those with normal levels were intolerant to meals containing lactose. Results of this review support the findings of others, i.e., lactase activity measured in intestinal biopsies does not appear to be a good predictor of milk tolerance or possibly of nutrient bioavailability.

Our group, in collaboration with Alan Strickland, also has concluded a pilot study comparing growth in children fed either a commercial soy/sucrose or a casein/lactose formula at later stages of recovery from severe diarrhea. Children less than 1 year of age hospitalized for severe diarrhea and below the third percentile for weight were enrolled for study. The 21 infants admitted to the study initially were intolerant to lactose and sucrose and required treatment with either a glucose formula or total parenteral nutrition. After treatment for several weeks with a casein/glucose formula, infants studied were advanced to a soy/sucrose formula and discharged from the hospital after demonstrating weight gain. These infants were seen approximately one month after hospital discharge and were

TABLE 15.2
Relationship of lactose tolerance to lactase activity and
mucosal morphology

Morphology	Lactase deficient		Normal lactase	
	N	% intolerant	N	% intolerant
Normal	2	100	34	29
Milk injury	2	50	5	40
Moderate to severe injury	9	89	13	69
Total N and average %	13	85	52	41

given 28 ml per kg of a commercial casein/lactose formula (providing 2 g lactose per kg) at one feeding. All infants were found to be tolerant to the casein/lactose formula as determined by the absence of colic, flatus, watery stools, and stool pH below 6.5. After this tolerance test, random assignment to casein/lactose or soy/sucrose commercial formulas resulted in 9 infants in the casein/lactose group and 12 in the soy/sucrose group. The formulas are compared in table 15.3.

Monthly visits were scheduled to measure weight, length, frontal occipital circumference, arm circumference, triceps skinfold thickness, and subscapular skinfold thickness. The clinic dietician obtained a 24-hour dietary recall from the child's caretaker at each visit. One infant in the sucrose group and four in the lactose group failed to return for follow-up visits and could not be located by the clinic social worker. All infants enrolled came from a public hospital patient population. Clinic social workers determined that all patients who failed to return had moved from the address given at the time of hospitalization. Thus, the final groups consisted of 5 infants in the casein/lactose group and 11 in the soy/sucrose group. These groups are compared in table 15.4. Weight gain as well as gain in length and skinfold thickness of infants enrolled in each feeding group were compared using covariant analysis. Weight/age percentile at the time of admission to the study was found to be a significant covariant when weight gain was evaluated.

During the first month of study, weight gains for the two groups were found to differ significantly. No differences were found during the second and third months of follow-up. In the first month, the group fed the soy/sucrose formula gained 77% more weight per day than the group fed the casein/lactose formula (table 15.5). Yet it is of interest to note that the 11 infants in the sucrose group reached the 20th weight percentile in 8.0 ± 3.6 weeks; the lactose group

TABLE 15.3
Nutrient composition of soy/sucrose and casein/lactose formulas

Nutrient	Soy/sucrose	Casein/lactose
Carbohydrate conc. (g/dl)	6.8	7.2
Protein source	Soy	Bovine casein & whey
Protein conc. (g/dl)	2.0	1.5
Fat source	Soy	Soy
Fat conc. (g/dl)	3.6	3.6
Vitamin A (IU/dl)	250.0	260.0
Vitamin D (IU/dl)	40.0	42.0
Vitamin E (IU/dl)	1.5	1.0
Vitamin C (mg/dl)	5.5	5.8
Thiamine (μg/dl)	40.0	70.0
Riboflavin (μg/dl)	60.0	104.0
Niacin (μg/dl)	900.0	990.0
Pyridoxine (μg/dl)	40.0	42.0
Intestinal solute load (mOsm/l)	215.0	300.0

TABLE 15.4
Clinical characteristics of infants studied

	Sucrose (mean ± SEM)		Lactose (mean ± SEM)	
Number of infants	11		5	
Age (weeks)	23.7 ±	3.7	25.2 ±	6.6
Sex: Male	6		2	
Female	5		3	
Race: Black	4		1	
Mexican-American	4		4	
Other	3		0	
% SWFA at hospital admission*	68.0 ±	4.0	77.0 ±	5.0
% SWFA at admission to study*	78.0 ±	3.0	87.0 ±	2.0
Weight on admission to study (g)	5,555.0 ± 960.0		6,168.0 ± 1,985.0	

*% SWFA = percentage standard weight for age.

required 18.0 weeks, but the scatter was greater. Because the formulas were not identical it is not possible unequivocally to ascribe the differences in weight gain to the carbohydrate source. Also, differences in the rate of weight gain cannot be explained easily on the basis of overt milk-lactose intolerance. Both groups tolerated 2 g lactose per kg body weight when it was fed in a milk formula. Any amount of possibly unabsorbed lactose would be expected to be small enough that infants easily could compensate for losses by increasing ad libitum intakes. There is no reason to suspect mild anorexia since formula intakes were comparable in both groups.

As table 15.6 demonstrates, the group fed the casein/lactose formula had a slightly higher mean intake than the soy/sucrose group, but this difference did not reach statistical significance. The quantity of unabsorbed carbohydrate, however, may have been great enough to lower the intraluminal pH sufficiently to interfere with micronutrient absorption. In children undergoing rapid growth, decreased micronutrient absorption may prevent maximal growth when inefficient absorption is superimposed on marginal reserves. We are in the process of evaluating micronutrient absorption (when different carbohydrates are provided) using perfusion studies in these types of infants. Differences in the protein consumption of both groups also should be considered. Protein sources were different and the soy formula had a higher protein concentration to correct protein

TABLE 15.5
Weight gain (g/day) of infants on casein/lactose and soy/sucrose formulas

Group	1st month	2nd month	3rd month
Casein/lactose	16.8 ± 5.2	23.8 ± 5.3	12.5 ± 5.3
Soy/sucrose	29.8 ± 2.5	20.6 ± 4.1	14.1 ± 4.1

TABLE 15.6
Formula intake (oz/day) of infants on casein/lactose and soy/sucrose diets

Group	1st month	2nd month	3rd month
Casein/lactose	51.2 ± 5.4	46.9 ± 6.9	37.3 ± 8.2
Soy/sucrose	42.2 ± 3.3	42.7 ± 4.9	28.0 ± 4.3

quality differences between soy and casein. Any possible role this treatment difference had on the observed outcome is difficult to evaluate.

NUTRIENT DENSITY

The third criterion that has been considered in choosing cow's milk for supplementary feeding programs is its high nutrient density; the concentration of macronutrients and micronutrients per kcal is high. This advantage has a significant limitation that requires more than tacit recognition. The limitation is the relatively low energy content of cow's milk. This is important because skim milk powder often is used in food supplementation programs. Any diet that is characterized by low fat content and is limited to a few staples of high bulk foods also should be supplemented with a high calorie source. Together, a high calorie food plus milk often will provide an optimal combination.

SUMMARY

In summary, young children with primary lactose intolerance can consume usual quantities of milk with no significant adverse symptoms. Therefore this condition is often of little practical importance in considering the supplementation of preschool populations. However, in children with recurrent abdominal pain, low-lactose diets should be tried. Such children may represent 2% to 4% of the population from 4 to 15 years of age. In evaluating this estimate it is important to underscore the wide age range and to consider the observation that intolerance to products containing lactose increases within this age span.

In populations with secondary lactose intolerance, the problem is much more complex. One is dealing with a damaged gastrointestinal tract, and therefore the response to undigested carbohydrate may be very much different. It is best to consider this problem within the context of the total diet. In infants with severe gastrointestinal disease, lactose-free diets may be optimal during the convalescent period. Preliminary data suggest that a low-lactose diet should be provided at least through the second month of outpatient rehabilitation. Older children, however, are not as dependent on milk for their nutrient intake. Therefore, in older children reduction of lactose may not be as critical as in infants. Studies are needed to identify the optimal uses of milks containing lactose in the rehabilitation of children convalescing from severe gastrointestinal disease.

REFERENCES

Anderson CM: Weight-gain inhibition by lactose. *Lancet* 1:954–55, 1977.

Arroyave G: Nutritive values of dietary proteins: For whom. In *Review of Basic Knowledge: Proceedings of the 9th International Conference of Nutrition (Mexico), 1972*, vol. 1. New York: S. Karger, 1975, pp 43–48.

Barr RG, Levine MD, Watkins JB: Recurrent abdominal pain in childhood due to lactose intolerance. *N Engl J Med* 300: 1:1449–52, 1979.

Bowie MD: Effect of lactose-induced diarrhea on absorption of nitrogen and fat. *Arch Dis Child* 50: 363, 1975.

Brown KH, Parry L, Khatun M, Ahmed MG: Lactose malabsorption in Bangladeshi village children: Relation with age, history of recent diarrhea, nutritional status, and breast feeding. *Am J Clin Nutr* 32:1962–69, 1979.

Calloway DH, Chenoweth WL: Utilization of nutrients in milk and wheat-based diets by men with adequate and reduced abilities to absorb lactose: I. Energy and nitrogen. *Am J Clin Nutr* 26:939–51, 1973.

Committee on Nutrition, American Academy of Pediatrics: Should milk drinking by children be discouraged? *Pediatrics* 53:576–82, 1974.

Committee on Nutrition, American Academy of Pediatrics: The practical significance of lactose intolerance in children. *Pediatrics* 62:240–45, 1978.

Food and Nutrition Board: Background information on lactose and milk tolerance. Washington, D.C.: National Academy of Sciences, National Research Council, May 1972.

Garza C, Scrimshaw NS: Relationship of lactose intolerance to milk tolerance in young children. *Am J Clin Nutr* 29:192–96, 1976.

Gilat T: Lactase deficiency: The world pattern today. *Isr J Med Sci* 15: 369–73, 1979.

Harrison M, Walker-Smith JA: Reinvestigation of lactose intolerant children: Lack of correlation between continuing lactose intolerance and small intestinal morphology, disaccharidase activity, and lactose tolerance tests. *Gut* 18: 48–52, 1977.

Haverberg L, Kwon PH Jr, Scrimshaw NS: Comparative tolerance of adolescents of differing ethnic backgrounds to lactose-containing and lactose-free dairy drinks: I. Initial experience with a double-blind procedure. *Am J Clin Nutr* 33: 17–21, 1980.

Jelliffe DB, Jelliffe EF: The volume and composition of human milk in poorly nourished communities: A review. *Am J Clin Nutr* 31: 492–515, 1978.

Kwon PH Jr, Rorick MH, Scrimshaw NS: Comparative tolerance of adolescents of differing ethnic backgrounds to lactose-containing and lactose-free dairy drinks: II. Improvement of a double-blind test. *Am J Clin Nutr* 33: 22–26, 1980.

Lebenthal E, Antonowicz I, Schwachman H: Correlation of lactase activity, lactose tolerance, and milk consumption in different age groups. *Am J Clin Nutr* 28: 595–600, 1975.

Liebman WM: Recurrent abdominal pain in children: Lactose and sucrose intolerance, a prospective study. *Pediatrics* 64: 43–45, 1979.

Mitchell KJ, Bayless TM, Paige DM, Goodgame RW, Huang SS: Intolerance of eight ounces of milk in healthy lactose-intolerant teenagers. *Pediatrics* 56: 718–21, 1975.

Mitchell JD, Brand J, Halbisch J: Weight-gain inhibition by lactose in Australian aboriginal children: A controlled trial of normal and lactose hydrolyzed milk. *Lancet* 1:500–02, 1977.

Newcomer AD, McGill DB, Thomas PJ, Hofmann AF: Tolerance to lactose among lactase-deficient American Indians. *Gastroenterology* 74: 44–46, 1978.

Paige DM, Bayless TM, Dellinger WS: Relationship of milk consumption to blood glucose rise in lactose intolerant individuals. *Am J Clin Nutr* 27: 296–303, 1974.

Paige DM, Bayless TM, Ferry GD, Graham GG: Lactose malabsorption and milk rejection in Negro children. *Johns Hopkins Med J* 129: 163–69, 1971.

Paige DM, Bayless TM, Huang SS, Wexler R: Lactose hydrolyzed milk. *Am J Clin Nutr* 28: 818–22, 1975.

Paige DM, Bayless TM, Mellits ED, Davis L: Lactose malabsorption in preschool black children. *Am J Clin Nutr* 30: 1018–22, 1977.

Paige DM, Leonardo E, Nakashima J, Adriazen B, Graham GG: Response of lactose intolerant children to different lactose levels. *Am J Clin Nutr* 25: 467, 1972.

Prinsloo JG, Wittman W, Pretorius PJ, Kruger H, Fellingham R: Effect of different sugars in diarrhea of acute kwashiorkor. *Arch Dis Child* 44: 593, 1969.

Protein Advisory Group: Ad hoc working group on milk intolerance—nutritional implication. *PAG Bull* 2: 7, 1972.

Sadre M, Karbasi K: Lactose intolerance in Iran. *Am J Clin Nutr* 32: 1948–54, 1979.

Scrimshaw NS: Strengths and weaknesses of the Committee approach: An analysis of past and present recommended dietary allowances for protein in health and disease. *N Engl J Med* 294: 135–42, 1976.

Simoons FJ, Johnson JD, Kretchmer N: Perspective on milk-drinking and malabsorption of lactose. *Pediatrics* 59: 98–109, 1977.

Stephenson LS, Latham MC, Jones DV: Milk consumption by black and white pupils in two primary schools. *J Am Diet Assoc* 71: 258–62, 1977.

Stoopler M, Frazer W, Alderman MH: Prevalence and persistence of lactose malabsorption among young Jamaican children. *Am J Clin Nutr* 27: 728–32, 1974.

Sutton RE, Hamilton JR: Tolerance of young children with severe gastroenteritis to dietary lactose. *Can Med Assoc J* 99: 980, 1977.

Woteki C, Weser E, Young EA: Lactose malabsorption in Mexican-American children. *Am J Clin Nutr* 29: 19–24, 1976.

CHAPTER 16

RECURRENT ABDOMINAL PAIN

ROLE OF LACTOSE INTOLERANCE

John B. Watkins

Physicians commonly are faced with the diagnostic problem of children with recurrent abdominal pain. When Apley (1975) originally published his seminal monograph *The Child with Abdominal Pains* in 1959, he described in considerable detail a syndrome he termed the "recurrent abdominal pain syndrome of childhood." This syndrome is defined by the presence of at least three discrete episodes of pain severe enough to affect and disrupt the child's activities, with the episodes occurring at least three times over a three-month period. These criteria were intended to exclude organic causation as well as trivial or transient episodes of abdominal discomfort regardless of etiology. This chapter focuses on recurrent abdominal pain as defined by Apley, places into perspective the impact of this symptom complex, and assesses the degree to which lactose malabsorption and lactose intolerance may contribute in causing the pain.

PROFILE OF THE SYNDROME

In studies by Apley and others drawn from a variety of social, economic, and ethnic groups, the incidence of attacks of recurrent abdominal pain has been found to vary between 9% and 15% of the general pediatric population (Liebman

Supported in part by a grant (HD-08489) from the National Institutes of Health, a grant from the Wolbach Fund, and a grant from the Shadow Medical Research Foundation.

1978, Bain 1974, Stone and Barbero 1970). Psychogenic factors have been cited most frequently as etiological or triggering mechanisms for the attacks of pain. Organic factors such as peptic ulcer and urinary tract infection have been found to occur only rarely in most large series, accounting for 2% to 10% of cases. In the patients described by Apley, the age of onset was noted to be after 4 years of age, peaking at 6 to 7 years of age. Both sexes were affected equally. The prevalence of the symptom complex decreases slowly after 10 to 12 years of age (Apley 1975).

The school absenteeism rate is reported to be greater than 1 day in 10 in 28% of these children. Two-thirds had sporadic attacks of pain. Past history often reveals a relatively high incidence of neonatal difficulty such as respiratory distress or excessive colic. Infantile colic occurred in 29% of individuals in one series, a rate significantly higher than the 15% incidence in normal premature and full-term infants (Liebman 1978, Myers and Thaler 1971). A high frequency of behavior and personality disorders, together with a history of abdominal pain in other family members, has been observed.

Aside from psychological and environmental factors, recurrent abdominal pain in children also is thought to be due to autonomic dysfunction (Oster 1972). Pallor, headache, and constipation have been noted. An abnormal pupillary response to the cold pressure test with enhanced pupillary dilation and a delay in the recovery phase when compared to an unaffected control group was observed by Rubin et al. (1967). Similarly, an excessive rectosigmoid response to prostigmine methyl sulfate, a parasympathetic agonist, was recorded in 18 patients with recurrent abdominal pain, whereas the baseline colonic contractions were quantitatively and qualitatively similar to the control group (Kopel et al. 1967). Transit time studies also have reflected varying degrees of delay leading to the suggestion that the pain may be due to an abnormality of colonic function or colonic spasm. Nevertheless, the causal or effectual relationships between abdominal pain and emotional upset, environmental or familial factors, and autonomic dysfunction have not been established consistently.

Clearly, the dilemma presented by children with this syndrome is that the symptom complex can be a sign of both psychosomatic and organic disease. However, both prospective and retrospective studies indicate that overt organic disease develops rarely. Only 3 of 161 patients (2%) reported by Stickler and Maryly (1979) developed organic disease over a six- to seven-year follow-up period. Furthermore, in two of the three children who ultimately developed inflammatory bowel disease, the diagnosis could have been suspected at the time of presentation by the presence of anemia and weight loss.

Despite these reassuring statistics, physicians have difficulty in diagnosing recurrent abdominal pain and excluding organic disease. This is illustrated by a recently completed retrospective study of 119 youngsters in whom a large number of diagnostic studies were ordered before the physicians were comfortable with a nonorganic diagnosis (Liebman 1978). Of these children, 99 had upper gastrointestinal series, 52 barium enemas, 34 intravenous pyelograms, 22 fiber optic endoscopy, and 18 had proctoscopy and rectal biopsy. Some authors even have recommended routine upper endoscopy or an exploratory laparotomy (Tedesco et al. 1976, Johnson et al. 1974), despite strong evidence that such procedures are futile.

STUDY RELATING LACTOSE INTOLERANCE AND RECURRENT ABDOMINAL PAIN

The diagnostic and therapeutic confusion demonstrated by these examples stimulated the search for factors unrelated to disease that might be responsible for this symptom complex in children. A factor isolated for study was the genetically predetermined maturational decline in intestinal lactase activity. This occurs normally in many school-age children and was shown in 1971 to be associated with intermittent abdominal pain in five children (Bayless and Huang 1971). The timing of the decline in activity is reported to occur at 5 to 6 years of age in Caucasian children with normal small bowel histology and enzymatically proven isolated lactase deficiency (Lebenthal et al. 1975). The decline could not be suspected by milk-drinking habits for at least up to 4 years of age. Awareness of milk intolerance as well as the amount of milk consumed thereafter appeared to vary among family members.

A similar time course for other Caucasian populations has been observed, but the decline in lactase activity may occur somewhat earlier (e.g., at three years) in both blacks and American Indians (Welsh et al. 1978, Newcomer et al. 1977). The timing for the onset of lactase deficiency in these populations is not reflected in nor accelerated by mucosal damage or acute diarrheal illness, but appears to be an independent phenomenon. The appearance of symptoms and the recognition of lactose intolerance in these studies also did not appear to correlate well with the decrease in intestinal lactase levels or the amount of milk intake. Instead, the recognition of symptoms appeared to correlate best with increasing age. Studies in teenagers and adults indicate a 70% to 75% awareness of lactose intolerance and altered milk consumption (Bayless et al. 1975, Mitchell et al. 1975).

PROSPECTIVE STUDY OF CHILDREN WITH ABDOMINAL PAIN

Having established that there is an association between low lactase levels and the symptoms of lactose intolerance that could result in the symptoms of recurrent abdominal pain (Bayless and Huang 1971), a prospective study was initiated to determine the prevalence of lactose malabsorption in consecutive children with recurrent abdominal pain (Barr et al. 1979). The population consisted of 80 school children 4 to 15 years of age (mean 9.6 years) seen at the Medical Diagnostic Clinic over a 12-month period.

Lactose malabsorption was determined using a noninvasive lactose breath hydrogen test. Lactose malabsorption was diagnosed when there was an increase at 90 to 120 minutes in breath hydrogen concentration of 10 parts per million or greater above the lowest or baseline value after a lactose load of 2 g per kg, with a maximum of 50 g, administered as a 20% solution. These values have been established as diagnostic of lactose malabsorption in individuals with biopsy-proven lactase deficiency (Barr et al. 1980). (This aspect is also discussed in chapters 8 and 9 of this volume.) Symptom scores were recorded for eight hours after the ingestion of lactose to determine whether symptom response to lactose loading was a useful discriminator in children with recurrent abdominal pain (Stephenson and Latham 1974).

Children who were identified as lactose malabsorbers by breath hydrogen testing were given a nonblind six-week diet trial that consisted of a two-week lactose elimination period, a two-week period of their normal diet containing lactose, and then a second lactose elimination period. During the entire six-week period, the children and their parents recorded in a diary pain episodes as well as any diet "breaks." The definition of a pain episode required that there be an asymptomatic period before and after the episode. Finally, each episode was recorded singly, regardless of severity.

Prevalence of Lactose Malabsorption and Symptom Responses.   The results of the study indicated that the prevalence of lactose malabsorption among the 80 patients tested was 40%. Sixteen of 59 white, 12 of 16 black, and 4 of 5 Hispanic children were malabsorbers. These prevalence figures are similar to those obtained from an age-matched, control population without abdominal pain also evaluated by the breath hydrogen test, but using a smaller lactose load (Barr et al. 1978), and to another series of recurrent abdominal pain patients and controls (Liebman 1979).

Questionnaires about the symptom response to the lactose load were completed by the majority of malabsorbers (88%) and absorbers (77%). The symptom scores were higher for lactose malabsorbers, particularly in the most severe categories of diarrhea, gas, and bloating (table 16.1). Symptom response proved to be an unreliable means for identifying lactose malabsorbers because of substantial overlap in reports of symptomatic severity. For example, since symptoms, regardless of severity, represent a positive response, nearly all malabsorbers were included (96%), as well as a high percentage of lactose absorbers (68%). Overlap is reduced only if the "more serious" or intense symptoms of diarrhea and cramps of moderate severity were included; but then, these criteria excluded some malabsorbers, identifying only 75% of the malabsorbers yet still including 27% of the absorbers. The history of milk ingestion, pain frequency, and the presence or absence of diarrhea were not helpful in distinguishing lactose malabsorbers from absorbers. Diarrhea was reported more frequently in malabsorbers (40%) but also appeared in 27% of absorbers.

TABLE 16.1
Symptom scores after lactose ingestion in children with
recurrent abdominal pain

Symptom	Malabsorbers (28 children)	Absorbers (37 children)	Significance
Diarrhea	1.18 ± 1.25	0.19 ± 0.50	P < 0.001
Gas	1.11 ± 1.07	0.59 ± 0.87	P = 0.036
Bloating	0.54 ± 0.88	0.16 ± 0.44	P = 0.029
Cramps	1.32 ± 1.02	0.81 ± 1.08	P = 0.057
Total	4.14 ± 2.90	1.76 ± 1.75	P < 0.001

Source: Barr et al. 1979, reprinted with permission.
Note: Lactose load was 2 g per Kg, maximum 50 g. Figures for malabsorbers and absorbers indicate the mean ± SD.

Symptom scores obtained after lactose ingestion have been recommended and utilized in epidemiological studies of lactose intolerance (Desai et al. 1967). They do not, however, help to identify affected persons who present with abdominal pain as their chief complaint. This lack of specificity may relate to the fact that abdominal pain is the least helpful of all the symptoms in distinguishing lactose malabsorbers from unaffected persons. Also, it may be due to the unreliability of reporting by patients and to parental concern about the cause of symptoms (or both).

History of Abdominal Pain and Milk Drinking. The history of the frequency of abdominal pain episodes varied over a wide range, yet the medians were virtually identical in the two groups. Upon looking at the history of milk ingestion more closely to determine whether a significant difference had been missed (a type II error), we calculated the one-tailed probability that more absorbers than malabsorbers ingested one glass of milk per day; the difference was small (P < 0.061). Since this difference could not be detected from the clinical history sheets, the children are probably similar in this regard. Thus, it appears that the physician cannot rely upon the differences in milk ingestion, pain frequency, or the presence of diarrhea to identify lactose malabsorption even when the symptoms are recorded daily and in a prospective manner.

DIET TRIAL

The possible relationship between the predisposition to lactose malabsorption and the severity of symptoms after lactose or milk consumption must be confirmed clinically by a diet trial. Since most lactase-deficient subjects will show intolerance if given enough lactose, the relevant test situation would appear to be only the response in comparison to the patient's usual lactose-containing diet.

In our study, 28 of 32 patients showing lactose malabsorption on tolerance testing participated in the six-week diet trial described above. Twenty (71%) reported a greater frequency of pain during the lactose phase when compared to the lactose elimination periods. Of the 20 children who completed all three phases of the study (fig. 16.1), 14 confirmed an increase in the number of pain episodes on resuming ingestion of foods containing lactose in their usual amounts, with the increase in pain frequency being highly significant (P < 0.002). The remaining 6 patients did not report an increase in pain frequency during the lactose phase, and 4 of the 6 were without pain by the end of the study. This implies a spontaneous elimination of pain over the six-week period due to factors other than the removal of lactose from the diet.

The inclusion of a double-blind crossover design for the diet trial would have helped eliminate the bias introduced by the possible hope that dietary management would be successful. However, in this study, an additional measure of

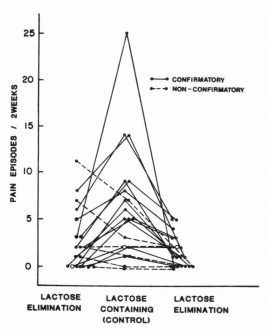

FIGURE 16.1. Symptom response to diet trial in 20 children diagnosed as lactose malabsorbers by breath hydrogen tests. Solid lines represent the 14 subjects whose pain frequency increased during the lactose phase; broken lines indicate the 6 subjects whose pain frequency did not increase. The open circle represents the patient who reduced milk intake during the control period because of increasing pain. Source: Barr et al. 1979, reprinted with permission.

objectivity was achieved by accepting a confirmatory response only when there was an increased pain frequency during the resumption of the regular lactose diet for that child.

VARIATIONS IN SYMPTOMATIC RESPONSE TO LACTOSE

More investigations are needed to determine the factors that combine and contribute to an individual's sensitivity to the symptoms induced by lactose malabsorption. Investigators have implicated the onset of symptoms with changes in the bacterial flora, the administration of antibiotics, or changes in gastric emptying after gastric surgery (Welsh 1970). Secondly, it has been proposed that due to its apical distribution on the villus lactase is more sensitive to damage than the other intestinal disaccharidases (Welsh et al. 1969), or that tolerance may be related to differences in the distribution of enzyme activity along the jejunum among different individuals (Newcomer and McGill 1966). By measuring the amount of nonabsorbed carbohydrate that reaches the terminal ileum, Bond and Levitt (1976) have demonstrated functionally that such a variation in the absorption of lactose exists in normals and in lactase-deficient subjects. Such studies have demonstrated that significant quantities of lactose may reach the colon even with normal lactase levels and that the colonic bacteria metabolize nonabsorbed carbohydrate.

Recent data suggest that incomplete lactose absorption may, indeed, be the norm in newborn infants (Chiles and Watkins 1979, MacLean and Fink 1980). Thus, the colonic bacterial flora and the colonic ecosystem may play major roles in processing nonabsorbed carbohydrate. Much more information is needed concerning the roles of dietary, genetic, or environmental factors in this process.

In terms of colonic motor function, recent studies have demonstrated significant differences in the myoelectrical and motor responses of the colon to feeding in patients with the "irritable bowel syndrome" (Snape et al. 1976). A difference in individual sensitivity to lactose malabsorption may relate to such an underlying irritable bowel symptom complex (Snape et al. 1978), but no objective colonic motility studies have been conducted yet in patients with lactose malabsorption and recurrent abdominal pain to confirm this impression.

In conclusion, the belief that recurrent abdominal pain is always either secondary to organic disease or "psychogenic" is not supported by our studies. Since both lactase insufficiency and continued lactose ingestion occur normally in many school-age children, studies that exclude organic disease but do not control for lactose malabsorption may be unnecessarily biased in favor of a "psychogenic" origin. Numerous factors may combine to produce symptoms of lactose intolerance. The prevalence and clinical indistinctness of symptoms indicate that an objective investigation is needed to determine the presence of lactose malabsorption in children with recurrent abdominal pain before invasive diagnostic procedures are used or before a psychogenic basis is assumed. When lactose malabsorption is present, a trial of lactose elimination, combined with a period on the patient's usual diet, may provide diagnostically significant information. Since lactase insufficiency may be secondary to an intestinal injury or occur independently of an underlying disease, the patient's clinical course must be followed and, if necessary, further diagnostic tests should be performed.

REFERENCES

Apley J: *The Child with Abdominal Pains,* 2nd ed. Oxford: Blackwell Scientific Publications, 1975.

Bain HW: Chronic vague abdominal pain in children. *Pediatr Clin North Am* 21: 991–1000, 1974.

Barr RG, Becker MC, Watkins JB, Heymann PW: Lactose malabsorption, abdominal pain, and lactose ingestion in a multiethnic school population. *Gastroenterology* 74: 1006a, 1978.

Barr RG, Levine MD, Watkins JB: Recurrent abdominal pain of childhood due to lactose intolerance: A prospective study. *N Engl J Med* 300: 1449–52, 1979.

Barr RG, Watkins JB, Perman JA, Boehme C: Mucosal function and breath hydrogen excretion: Comparative studies in the clinical evaluation of children with nonspecific abdominal complaints. *Pediatrics* (in press).

Bayless TM, Huang SS: Recurrent abdominal pain due to milk and lactose intolerance in school-aged children. *Pediatrics* 47: 1029–32, 1971.

Bayless TM, Rothfeld B, Massa C, Wise L, Paige D, Bedine M: Lactose and milk intolerance: Clinical implications. *N Engl J Med* 292: 1156–59, 1975.

Bond JH, Levitt MD: Quantitative measurement of lactose absorption. *Gastroenterology* 70: 1058–62, 1976.

Chiles C, Watkins JB, Barr R, Tsai PY, Goldman DA: Lactose utilization in the newborn: Role of colonic flora. *Pediatr Res* 13: 365a, 1979.

Desai HG, Chitre AV, Jeejeebhoy KN: Lactose loading: A simple test for detecting intestinal lactase: Evaluation of different methods. *Gastroenterol Jpn* 108: 177–88, 1967.

Johnson LF, Vanderhood JA, Black S: The role of exploratory laparotomy for chronic abdominal pain in children. *Nebr Med J* 59: 430–33, 1974.

Kopel FB, Kim IC, Barbero GJ: Comparison of rectosigmoid motility in normal children, children with RAP, and children with ulcerative colitis. *Pediatrics* 39: 539–45, 1967.

Lebenthal E, Antonowicz I, Shwachman H: Correlation of lactase activity, lactose tolerance and milk consumption in different age groups. *Am J Clin Nutr* 28: 595–600, 1975.

Liebman WM: Recurrent abdominal pain in children: A retrospective survey of 119 patients. *Clin Pediatr* (Phila) 17: 149–53, 1978.

Leibman WM: Recurrent abdominal pain in children: Lactose and sucrose intolerance, a prospective study. *Pediatrics* 64: 43–45, 1979.

MacLean WC, Fink BB: Lactose malabsorption by premature infants: Magnitude and clinical significance. *J Pediatr* 97: 383–88, 1980.

Mitchell KJ, Bayless TM, Paige DM, Goodgame RW, Huang SS: Intolerance of eight ounces of milk in healthy lactose-intolerant teenagers. *Pediatrics* 56: 718–21, 1975.

Myers JE, Thaler MM: Colic in low birth weight infants. *Am J Dis Child* 122: 25–27, 1971.

Newcomer AD, McGill DB: Distribution of disaccharidase activity in the small bowel of normal and lactase deficient subjects. *Gastroenterology* 51: 481–88, 1966.

Newcomer AD, Thomas PJ, McGill DB, Hofmann AF: Lactase deficiency: A common genetic trait of the American Indian. *Gastroenterology* 72: 234–37, 1977.

Oster J: Recurrent abdominal pain, headache and limb pains in children and adolescents. *Pediatrics* 50: 429–36, 1972.

Rubin LS, Barbero GJ, Sibinga MS: Pupillary reactivity in children with recurrent abdominal pain. *Psychosom Med* 29: 111–20, 1967.

Snape WJ Jr, Carlson GM, Cohen S: Colonic myoelectric activity in the irritable bowel syndrome. *Gastroenterology* 70: 326–30, 1976.

Snape WJ, Matarazzo SA, Cohen S: Effect of eating and gastrointestinal hormones on human colonic and myoelectrical and motor activity. *Gastroenterology* 75: 373–78, 1978.

Stephenson LS, Latham MC: Lactose intolerance and milk consumption: The relation of tolerance to symptoms. *Am J Clin Nutr* 27: 296–303, 1974.

Stickler G, Maryly DB: Recurrent abdominal pain. *Am J Dis Child* 133: 486–89, 1979.

Stone RT, Barbero GH: Recurrent abdominal pain in childhood. *Pediatrics* 45: 732–38, 1970.

Tedesco FJ, Goldstein PD, Gleason WA, Keating JP: Upper gastrointestinal endoscopy in the pediatric patient. *Gastroenterology* 70: 492–94, 1976.

Welsh JD: Isolated lactase deficiency in humans: Report on 100 patients. *Gastroenterology* 49: 257–77, 1970.

Welsh JD, Poley JR, Bhatia M, Stevenson DE: Intestinal disaccharidase activities in relation to age, race, and mucosal damage. *Gastroenterology* 75: 847–55, 1978.

Welsh JD, Zschiesche OM, Anderson J, Walker A: Intestinal disaccharidase activity in celiac disease (gluten sensitive enteropathy). *Arch Intern Med* 123: 33–38, 1969.

CHAPTER 17

ACQUIRED CARBOHYDRATE
INTOLERANCE IN CHILDREN
CLINICAL MANIFESTATIONS AND
THERAPEUTIC RECOMMENDATIONS

Fima Lifshitz

Carbohydrate intolerance first was recognized at the beginning of this century in infants with lactose intolerance following gastroenteritis (Jacobi 1901, Finkelstein and Meyer 1911). It is now known that carbohydrate intolerance may occur as a secondary complication of several diverse systemic and/or intestinal disorders (Herbst et al. 1969, Johnson et al. 1974, Lifshitz 1977a, 1980). It also may occur when a patient has primary carbohydrate malabsorption or an ontogenetic lactase deficiency (Kretchmer 1971, 1972). Whenever carbohydrate intolerance occurs, it may play an important role in the pathophysiology of the primary disease, as well as in the eventual fate of the patient (Lifshitz et al. 1971a,b, Kumar et al. 1977).

Carbohydrate intolerance is a clinical syndrome characterized by diarrhea with acid stools and carbohydrate in feces; whereas malabsorption of carbohydrates and disaccharidase deficiencies are laboratory findings that may or may not lead to carbohydrate intolerance. Healthy people with the highly prevalent ontogenetic lactase deficiency tolerate up to 15 g lactose without symptoms (Stephenson and Latham 1974). Whereas patients with acquired lactose intolerance cannot tolerate these levels of lactose, diarrheal disease may be more prolonged and severe (Lifshitz et al. 1971 a,b), body weight losses are more marked (Kumar et al. 1977), and dietary treatment is usually necessary for improvement.

PATHOPHYSIOLOGY OF CARBOHYDRATE INTOLERANCE

Carbohydrate Malabsorption. There are three types of carbohydrate malabsorption that could lead to carbohydrate intolerance: ontogenetic, primary, and secondary. All of these may produce malabsorption in one, several, or all dietary carbohydrates by a variety of mechanisms as shown in table 17.1. Ontogenetic carbohydrate malabsorption occurs in humans in the immediate neonatal period and in many ethnic groups beyond 3 to 5 years of age (Kretchmer 1971, 1972). At these times of development, the intestinal absorptive capacity for lactose is low because of the low levels of lactase activity that are determined ontogenetically. Primary carbohydrate malabsorption is the type seen in patients with any one of the rare specific congenital alterations of the intestinal surface oligodisaccharidases or of the capacity to transport glucose. These may appear very early in life or have a late onset in adults (Lifshitz 1980, Welsh 1970). They usually involve a single carbohydrate and the intestinal mucosa remain intact. Secondary carbohydrate malabsorption is associated with several diseases of systemic and/or of intestinal origin (described below). In these patients there is usually acquired mucosal damage that could affect one or all the oligosaccharidases and/or alter the intestinal transport capacity of actively transported solutes such as glucose. At times there may even be interference with intestinal permeability, leading to impaired fructose transport. Secondary carbohydrate malabsorption always should be considered when an individual previously able to tolerate carbohydrates suddenly loses this capacity.

Lactose and Lactase. Selective lactose intolerance is the most frequent clinical problem. This is due to isolated lactase deficiency and lactose malabsorption from any of the above-mentioned types. The ontogenetic lactase deficiency is of high incidence among the majority of healthy individuals throughout the world and it presently is considered the "normal state" after childhood, since the ontogenesis of lactase is such that its activity normally decreases in most humans and in all animal species after weaning (Herbst et al. 1969, Johnson et al. 1974,

TABLE 17.1
Mechanisms of carbohydrate malabsorption

1. Deficiency of mucosal surface oligosaccharidases	Selective lactase
	Generalized
2. Altered transport capacity	Decreased active transport
	Abnormal permeability
3. Reduced exposure for absorption	Decreased time
	Decreased surface

Kretchmer 1971, 1972). In addition, primary lactase deficiency could account for a relatively low number of patients who are lactose intolerant, particularly those of populations who would be expected to tolerate lactose well. An isolated lactase deficiency frequently may result from secondary causes, which may neither alter the other oligodisaccharidases, nor produce other intestinal alterations. This may occur because of the relatively low lactase concentration, the superficial localization of this enzyme on the microvillous brush border, and the rate-limiting characteristics for glucose transport, as compared with other oligodisaccharidases (Gray 1975).

Carbohydrate Intolerance. The presence or absence of carbohydrate intolerance as a consequence of intestinal malabsorption is determined by several factors. These include the level of the intestinal disaccharidase activity; the magnitude of intestinal carbohydrate malabsorption; the amount of the oral carbohydrate load to which the patient is exposed; the gastric emptying time; the colonic reabsorptive capacity, which may compensate for the excess water and solute load coming from the small intestine; and the type of intestinal bacterial flora, which may assist in the hydrolysis of the unabsorbed carbohydrate and alleviate some of the symptoms of carbohydrate intolerance (Gallagher et al. 1974).

The presence of sufficiently active carbohydrate and fermentative products within the lumen is associated with secretion of fluid and electrolytes until osmotic equilibrium is reached (Launiala 1968). In addition, there is a loss of mucosal cells and intestinal disaccharidases (Teichberg et al. 1978). Bacterial fermentation of the unabsorbed carbohydrates produces large quantities of hydrogen gas and organic acids (Ingelfinger 1967). Increased intestinal volume may lead to motility alterations and exacerbate diarrhea (Launiala 1968). Elimination of the unabsorbed carbohydrate results in improvement regardless of the etiology of the primary disease (Burke et al. 1965, Lifshitz et al. 1971 a,b).

CLINICAL DISORDERS ASSOCIATED WITH CARBOHYDRATE INTOLERANCE

The ontogenetic type of carbohydrate malabsorption rarely leads to carbohydrate intolerance, since these people usually are not exposed to sufficient intake of carbohydrate to induce clinical symptoms. Moreover, most children less than 3 years old, except prematures, have adequate lactase levels to allow for milk drinking. This is true even in populations destined to become lactase deficient. Carbohydrate intolerance also may occur as a consequence of the primary carbohydrate malabsorption syndromes. Although they are relatively rare disorders, they play an important role leading to specific carbohydrate intolerances, which persist for the life span of the patient.

Carbohydrate intolerance can result as a temporary acquired complication, secondary to a variety of clinical disorders (Lifshitz 1977a, 1980). Included are diseases of the gastrointestinal tract with intestinal epithelial damage, i.e., malabsorption syndrome, diarrheal disease, and parasites such as in giardia lambia infestation. Systemic alterations also may result in intestinal alterations through a variety of mechanisms, i.e., primary protein-energy malnutrition, hypoxia, drugs (birth control, colchicine), food protein hypersensitivity, and immune deficiency syndromes. In all these instances carbohydrate intolerance improves following recovery from the primary disease.

The most frequent secondary carbohydrate intolerance is that acquired in diarrheal disease of infancy (Lifshitz et al. 1971a). In this case the mechanism of carbohydrate malabsorption may be directly related to the pathogenesis of diarrhea, as well as to complications of the disease such as dehydration and shock. Microorganisms induce diarrhea as a result of contamination of the upper small bowel, through interference with intestinal transport processes by any one or a combination of mechanisms reviewed elsewhere (Lifshitz 1977b). Mucosal damage results from either tissue invasion and destruction of the epithelial cell by enteric pathogens or from cell injury caused by products of bacterial metabolic activity acting upon foodstuffs and host secretions, i.e., deconjugated bile salts, short-chain organic acids, and alcohol (Midtvedt 1974, Binder 1973, Chernov et al. 1972, Barona et al. 1974).

Certain enteric viruses such as rotavirus and Norwalk agent also induce morphological and functional changes in the small intestine by penetration of the enterocyte (Gall 1980, Kapikian et al. 1976). Rotaviruses seem to be the principal cause of diarrhea and carbohydrate intolerance in infancy (Holmes et al. 1976). It has been postulated that intestinal lactase is the receptor and uncoating enzyme for these enteric viruses. Before diarrhea occurs the virus must infect gut epithelium rich in lactase. This hypothesis is consistent with the high prevalence of lactose intolerance in gastroenteritis in infancy (Lifshitz et al. 1971b, Kumar et al. 1977), whereas in adults who usually are not sensitive to infection with this virus, lactose intolerance complicating diarrheal disease is infrequent.

Acquired carbohydrate intolerance also may occur in several disease processes affecting the intestine directly or indirectly via systemic disease. For example, hypoxia has been shown to be an important factor leading to carbohydrate malabsorption in several animal species (Northrop and Van Liere 1941, Guthrie and Questral 1956) as well as in newborn infants (Akesode et al. 1973, Book et al. 1976, Bunton et al. 1977, Tejani et al. 1979) and results from a decreased (Na^+-K^+) adenosine triphosphatase activity in the intestinal mucosa (Lifshitz et al. 1976). In premature infants neonatal hypoxia could lead to carbohydrate intolerance that could hinder the recovery of these patients once the principal illness has improved. Disaccharide intolerance also may lead to severe complications such as monosaccharide intolerance and necrotizing enterocolitis (Akesode et al. 1973, Book et al. 1976, Bunton et al. 1977, Tejani et al. 1979). In other conditions lactose intolerance may be a factor in the symptomatology of the primary disease, i.e., gluten-sensitive enteropathy (Lifshitz et al. 1965) and irritable bowel disorders (Chalfin and Holt 1967). However, lactose intolerance has not been confirmed in other conditions such as cystic fibrosis, where initially it was suspected to be a frequent complication (Antonowicz et al. 1978).

CLINICAL CONSEQUENCES OF CARBOHYDRATE INTOLERANCE

The clinical consequences of carbohydrate intolerance are listed in table 17.2. The severity and the frequency of these problems are directly related to the degree of impaired carbohydrate absorption, to the dose of the oral carbohydrate load, and to the other variables described above. The most prevalent complications of carbohydrate intolerance are dehydration and electrolyte deficits. The volume of water excreted by patients with carbohydrate intolerance may be up to three times that of an isotonic solution of the sugar present in the bowel (Launiala 1968). In addition, there may be other small molecules of high osmotic pressure (such as organic acids), which result from carbohydrate fermentation and which contribute to increased fluid losses. Carbohydrate intolerance also can lead to metabolic acidosis, which is a prominent feature of severe diarrhea. It has been shown that the most important source of excess hydrogen ions in children with diarrhea is from bacterial carbohydrate fermentation (Lugo-de-Rivira et al. 1972). In addition, the presence of organic acids within the intestinal lumen may stimulate secretion and loss of large quantities of bicarbonate from serum to neutralize the luminal acid load.

The duration of the diarrheal disease may be related more often to carbohydrate intolerance than to the primary agent that triggered the initial illness. For example, diarrhea in acute gastroenteritis may persist for as long as lactose is present in the diet; when this carbohydrate is eliminated a prompt recovery may ensue (Burke et al. 1965, Lifshitz et al. 1971b). In fact, in infantile gastroenteritis a lactose-free diet may diminish the duration and the severity of diarrhea as compared with a diet of cow's milk (Dagan et al. 1980).

The general nutritional status of an infant may be profoundly affected by carbohydrate intolerance. Even when diarrhea is mild, the presence of lactose

TABLE 17.2
Clinical consequences of carbohydrate intolerance

1. Altered stools	Increased volume
	Prolonged duration
2. Systemic effects	Metabolic acidosis
	Malnutrition
3. Bacterial proliferation	Aggravation of intestinal malabsorption
	Pneumatosis intestinalis
4. Macromolecular absorption	Protein hypersensitivity
	Toxemia
	Sepsis

intolerance is associated with more marked body weight losses (Kumar et al. 1977). Fifty percent of the total calorie requirements of children are derived from dietary carbohydrates. Therefore, losses of carbohydrates account for considerable calorie deficits. The presence of unabsorbed carbohydrates in the intestinal lumen also enhances protein and nitrogen losses (Darrow 1946). In addition, it may lead to dilution of bile acid concentrations below the critical micellar level for efficient fat absorption (Ringrose et al. 1972). The association of disaccharidase deficiencies, carbohydrate intolerance, and steatorrhea long has been recognized (Lifshitz and Holman 1964).

Enteric Bacteria. The presence of unabsorbed carbohydrates and of fermentative products in the small bowel lumen may facilitate the further colonization and proliferation of enteric bacteria in the upper segments of the intestine (Coello-Ramirez and Lifshitz 1972). Nonspecific bacterial proliferation of fecal and colonic bacteria occurs frequently in infants with diarrhea as a secondary complication due to several factors (Lifshitz 1977b). The disturbed intestinal motility and the presence of free carbohydrates within the lumen may be important factors influencing enteric bacterial proliferation. This may lead to a further deterioration of intestinal function because enteric bacteria proliferating in the upper bowel generate metabolites such as deconjugated bile salts, hydroxy fatty acids, and alcohol that are injurious to the proximal portions of the small intestine. Clinically, this may result in aggravation of the diarrhea and worsening of the dietary intolerances. A patient with lactose intolerance may become intolerant to other disaccharides (Lifshitz et al. 1971a,b) and if the diarrhea persists for a longer period, then monosaccharide intolerance may ensue (Lifshitz et al. 1970).

Continuing dietary intolerance and nutrient losses not only impair the infant's ability to recover from the initial illness, but also may increase the susceptibility to other conditions, i.e., pneumatosis intestinalis, sepsis, and food protein hypersensitivity. The source of gas in pneumatosis intestinalis may be the hydrogen produced by bacterial fermentation of the unabsorbed carbohydrate. It is of interest that this condition can occur in infants with lactose intolerance secondary to diarrheal disease (Coello-Ramirez et al. 1970) and as a sequela of lactose intolerance secondary to neonatal hypoxia (Akesode et al. 1973, Book et al. 1976, Bunton et al. 1977, Tejani et al. 1979).

Intestinal Permeability. It long has been known that macromolecular permeability might be altered in gastroenteritis since there is measurable absorption of egg albumin and there are frequently milk protein antibodies present in serum following diarrhea (Gruskay and Cooke 1955). Increased macromolecular absorption may lead to the development of hypersensitivity and allergy to foodstuffs in the susceptible host. This process could be related to carbohydrate intolerance. There is a frequent association between carbohydrate intolerance and protein-sensitive enteropathy in children with gastroenteritis (Iyngkaran et al.

1979). Milk protein allergy can be associated with lactose intolerance and a secretory IgA deficiency (Harrison et al. 1976). Soy protein hypersensitivity apparently acquired during the course of gastroenteritis also has been recognized (Ament and Rubin 1972) and found to be associated with monosaccharide intolerance (Goel et al. 1978).

In experimental studies it has been shown that under certain conditions of pathophysiologic stress the normal barriers to the intestinal transport of macromolecules may be functionally and structurally altered, leading to an increased leakage of intact protein across the intestinal epithelium (Teichberg 1980). In diarrheal disease there are several alterations that may promote an increased passage of macromolecules across the intestine, including luminal hyperosmolar gradients (Cooper et al. 1978), cellular disruption by pathogens (Block et al. 1979), increased levels of deconjugated bile salts, and lactose intolerance (Teichberg 1980). An increased passage of intact macromolecules across the intestine may lead to production of circulating reaginic (IgE) antibodies to ovalbumin in rats infected with *Bordetella pertussis* (Bazin and Platteau 1976). Therefore, one may hypothesize that a child with gastroenteritis and lactose intolerance may become sensitive to food proteins. As shown in fig. 17.1, this could result in a vicious cycle leading to chronic diarrhea. After improvement, the patient may recover the capacity to tolerate dietary carbohydrates with persistence of protein hypersensitivity (Goel et al. 1978).

However, in an infant with diarrhea and carbohydrate intolerance, it may be difficult to ascertain whether cow's milk protein hypersensitivity is the result or the cause of the disease. Cow's milk protein enteropathy itself may induce intestinal mucosal damage leading to disaccharidase deficiencies and carbohydrate intolerance (Lubos and Gerrard 1967, Iyngkaran et al. 1979). Milk protein sensitivity in a genetically susceptible host may follow early exposure to cow's milk formula in infancy (Stintzing and Zetterstrom 1979). At this time in life the intestinal penetration of macromolecules is increased since the epithelial barrier is not fully developed (Walker 1980, Teichberg 1980), thereby permitting an en-

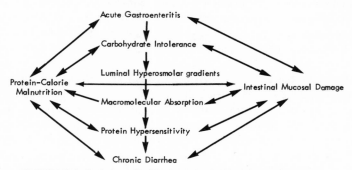

FIGURE 17.1. Pathogenesis of food protein sensitive enteropathy in acute gastroenteritis with carbohydrate intolerance.

hanced absorption of intact protein. Thus, further studies remain to be done to ascertain whether lactose intolerance in milk-intolerant infants is primary (Sunshine and Kretchmer 1964, Lifshitz and Holman 1964, Burke et al. 1965) or secondary to milk protein hypersensitivity (Liu et al. 1967).

THERAPEUTIC CONSIDERATIONS

The presence of carbohydrate intolerance is a primary indication for dietary treatment. As soon as the diagnosis is made the offending carbohydrate should be eliminated from the diet. This usually results in prompt improvement of diarrhea. The dietary treatment of carbohydrate intolerance has been described elsewhere (Lifshitz 1973). However, it should be pointed out that dietary treatment of carbohydrate malabsorption may not be required if malabsorption is not accompanied by clinical intolerance. It has been considered inappropriate to discourage milk drinking among individuals with ontogenetic lactase deficiency solely because of fear of lactose intolerance (Committee on Nutrition 1974). Indeed, the milk-drinking habits of healthy populations who are lactose malabsorbers are modified by the individuals themselves, reducing the intake of large quantities of milk without influencing intermediate patterns of milk consumption (Paige et al. 1972, Stephenson et al. 1977, Lisker et al. 1978).

Another important consideration pertains to the dietary treatment of infants with acute gastroenteritis. These patients have a high frequency of carbohydrate intolerance (Lifshitz et al. 1971a). The Committee on Nutrition of the American Academy of Pediatrics has recommended that a lactose-free diet be the initial feeding of malnourished children with severe diarrhea (Barness 1979). Others have shown that these types of feedings, as the initial choice for infants less than 1 year of age with acute gastroenteritis, significantly reduce the duration and severity of diarrhea (Dagan et al. 1980). A diet containing sucrose is more efficient and promotes more weight gain than one containing lactose, even after recovery from diarrhea (Strickland et al. 1979). The elimination of carbohydrates from the diet of these patients should be for a brief period, since carbohydrate tolerance is recovered rapidly once there is improvement of the disease (Lifshitz et al. 1971b). Moreover, the elimination of dietary carbohydrates for prolonged periods may in itself perpetuate altered carbohydrate absorption (Pergolizzi et al. 1977).

These dietary recommendations should be limited to infants receiving cow's milk formulas. Infants fed human milk have a decreased incidence and severity of diarrhea and of carbohydrate intolerance (Woodbury 1922, Mata and Urrutia 1971, Okuni et al. 1972, Brown et al. 1979). This is evident even though there is a relatively higher lactose content in human milk (approximately 7%) than in cow's milk (approximately 4%). Human milk contains other factors such as the biffidus factor activity (György et al. 1953, 1963) in concentrations 50 to 100 times higher than cow's milk. Thus, this may account for a better lactose tolerance of human milk than that observed with cow's milk feedings, both in health and in disease states. Moreover, human milk provides other immunological advantages that may help in the treatment of infectious diarrhea and in necrotizing enterocolitis (Coello-Ramirez et al. 1977, Barlow et al. 1974). Therefore such feedings should be encouraged even during diarrheal disease.

However, there may be intolerance to human milk in diarrheal disease (King 1972), and there also may be necrotizing enterocolitis in infants fed breast milk exclusively (Moriartey et al. 1979). Therefore, the pediatrician must weigh carefully the use of milk and sugars other than lactose in individuals who exhibit carbohydrate intolerance and should permit consumption in accordance with clinical courses.

REFERENCES

Akesode F, Lifshitz F, Hoffman M: Transient monosaccharide intolerance in a newborn infant. *Pediatrics* 51: 891–97, 1973.

Ament ME, Rubin GE: Soy protein—another cause of the flat intestinal lesion. *Gastroenterology* 62: 227–34, 1972.

Antonowicz I, Lebenthal E, Schwachman H: Disaccharidase activities in small intestinal mucosa in patients with cystic fibrosis. *J Pediatr* 92: 214–19, 1978.

Barlow B, Santulli TV, Heird WC, Pitt N, Blanc WA, Schullinger UN: An experimental study of acute neonatal enterocolitis: The importance of breast milk. *J Pediatr Surg* 9: 587–95, 1974.

Barness L (ed): *Pediatric Nutrition Handbook*. Evanston, Ill.: American Academy of Pediatrics, 1979, p 385.

Barona E, Pirola RC, Lieber CS: Small intestinal damage and changes in cell population produced by ethanol ingestion in the rat. *Gastroenterology* 66: 226–34, 1974.

Bazin H, Plateau B: Production of circulating reaginic (IgE) antibodies by oral administration of ovalbumin to rats. *J Immunol* 30: 679–83, 1976.

Binder HJ: Fecal fatty acids—mediators of diarrhea? *Gastroenterology* 65: 847–50, 1973.

Block KJ, Block DB, Stearns M, Walker WA: Intestinal uptake of macromolecules: VI. Uptake of protein antigen *in vivo* in normal rats and in rats infected with *Nippostrongylus brasiliensis* or subjected to mild systemic anaphylaxis. *Gastroenterology* 77: 1039–44, 1979.

Book LS, Herbst JJ, Jung AL: Carbohydrate malabsorption in necrotizing enterocolitis. *Pediatrics* 57: 201–04, 1976.

Brown KH, Parry L, Khatun M, Ahmed MG: Lactose malabsorption in Bangladeshi village children: Relation with age, history of recent diarrhea, nutritional status and breast feeding. *Am J Clin Nutr* 32: 1962–69, 1979.

Bunton GL, Durbin GM, McIntosh N, Shaw DG, Taghizadeh A, Reynolds EOR, Rivers RPA, Urman G: Necrotizing enterocolitis: Controlled study of three years experience in a neonatal intensive care unit. *Arch Dis Child* 52: 772–77, 1977.

Burke V, Kerez KR, Anderson CM: The relationship of dietary lactose to refractory diarrhoea in infancy. *Aust Paediatr J* 1: 147–60, 1965.

Chalfin D, Holt PR: Lactase deficiency in ulcerative colitis, regional enteritis and viral hepatitis. *Am J Dig Dis* 12: 81–87, 1967.

Chernov AJ, Doe WF, Compertz D: Intrajejunal volatile fatty acids in the stagnant loop syndrome. *Gut* 13: 103–06, 1972.

Coello-Ramírez P, García-Cortés MJ, Díaz-Bensussen S, Domingues-Camacho C, Zuniga V:

Tratamiento con calostro humano a niños con gastroenteritis infecciosa prolongada. *Bol Med Hosp Inf* 34: 487–506, 1977.

Coello-Ramírez P, Gutierrez-Topete G, Lifshitz F: Pneumatosis intestinalis. *Am J Dis Child* 120: 3–9, 1970.

Coello-Ramírez P, Lifshitz F: Enteric microflora and carbohydrate intolerance in infants with diarrhea. *Pediatrics* 49: 233–42, 1972.

Committee of Nutrition, American Academy of Pediatrics: Should milk drinking by children be discouraged? *Pediatrics* 53: 576–82, 1974.

Cooper M, Teichberg S, Lifshitz F: Alterations in rat jejunal permeability to a macromolecular tracer. *Lab Invest* 38: 447–54, 1978.

Dagan R, Gorodischer R, Moses S, Margolis C: Lactose free formula for infantile diarrhea. *Lancet* 1: 207, 1980.

Darrow DC: The retention of electrolytes during recovery from severe dehydration due to diarrhea. *J Pediatr* 28: 515–39, 1946.

Finkelstein H, Meyer LF: Zur technile und indikation der einahrung mit eiweissmilch. *Munch Med Wochenschr* 58: 340–45, 1911.

Gall DG: Viral gastroenteritis. In *Clinical Disorders in Pediatric Gastroenterology and Nutrition*, F Lifshitz (ed). New York: Marcel Dekker, 1980, pp 293–99.

Gallagher CR, Molleson AL, Caldwell JH: Lactose intolerance and fermented dairy products. *J Am Diet Assoc* 65: 418–19, 1974.

Goel K, Lifshitz F, Kahn E, Teichberg S: Monosaccharide intolerance and soy protein hypersensitivity in an infant with diarrhea. *J Pediatr* 93: 617–19, 1978.

Gray GM: Carbohydrate digestion and absorption: Role of the small intestine. *N Engl J Med* 292: 1225–30, 1975.

Gruskay FL, Cooke RE: The gastrointestinal absorption of unaltered protein in normal infants and in infants recovering from diarrhea. *Pediatrics* 16: 763–69, 1955.

Guthrie JE, Questral JH: Absorption of sugars and amino acids from isolated surviving intestine after experimental shock. *Arch Biochem Biophys* 62: 485–96, 1956.

György P: A hitherto unrecognized biochemical difference between human milk and cow's milk. *Pediatrics* 11: 98–108, 1963.

György P, Noris RF, Rose CS: Biffidus factor: I. A variant of lactobacillus biffidus requiring a special growth factor. *Arch Biochem Biophys* 48: 193–201, 1953.

Harrison M, Kilby A, Walker-Smith JA, Frace NE, Wood CBS: Cow's milk protein intolerance: A possible association with gastroenteritis, lactose intolerance and IgA deficiency. *Br Med J* 1: 1501–04, 1976.

Herbst JJ, Sunshine P, Kretchmer N: Intestinal malabsorption in infancy and childhood. In *Advances in Pediatrics*, I Schulman (ed). Chicago: Year Book Medical Publishers, 1969, pp 11–64.

Holmes IH, Schnagi RD, Rodger S, Ruck BJ, Gust ID, Bishop RF, Barnes GL: Is lactase the receptor and uncoating enzyme for infantile enteritis (rota) viruses? *Lancet* 1: 1387–88, 1976.

Ingelfinger FJ: Malabsorption: The clinical background. *Fed Proc* 26: 1388–90, 1967.

Iyngkaran N, Abdin Z, Davis K, Boey CG, Prathrap K, Yadar M, Lam SK, Puthucheary SD: Acquired carbohydrate intolerance and cow's milk protein-sensitive enteropathy in young infants. *J Pediatr* 95: 373–78, 1979.

Jacobi A: Milk-sugar in infant feeding. *Trans Am Pediatr Soc* 13: 150–60, 1901.

Johnson JD, Kretchmer N, Simoons FJ: Lactose malabsorption: Its biology and history. *Adv Pediatr* 21: 197–237, 1974.

Kapikian AZ, Kim HW, Wyatt RG, Cline WL, Auobio JO, Brandt CO, Rodriguez WJ, Sack DA, Chanock RM, Parrott RH: Human reovirus-like agent as the major pathogen associated with winter gastroenteritis in hospitalized infants and young children. *N Engl J Med* 294: 965–72, 1976.

King F: Intolerance to lactose in mother's milk. *Lancet* 2: 335, 1972.

Kretchmer N: Memorial lecture: Lactose and lactase—a historical perspective. *Gastroenterology* 61: 805-13, 1971.

Kretchmer N: Lactose and lactase. *Sci Am* 227: 70-78, 1972.

Kumar V, Chandrasekaran R, Bhaskar R: Carbohydrate intolerance associated with acute gastroenteritis. *Clin Pediatr* (Phila) 16: 1123-27, 1977.

Launiala K: The effect of unabsorbed sucrose and mannitol on the small intestinal flow rate and mean transit time. *Scand J Gastroenterol* 3: 665-71, 1968.

Lifshitz F: Current therapy of the malabsorption syndrome and intestinal disaccharidase deficiencies. In *Current Therapy*, 6th ed, S Gillis, BM Kagan (eds). Philadelphia: Saunders, 1973, pp 236-47.

Lifshitz F: Carbohydrate problems in pediatric gastroenterology. *Clin Gastroenterol* 6: 415-29, 1977a.

Lifshitz F: The enteric flora in childhood disease—diarrhea. *Am J Clin Nutr* 30: 1811-18, 1977b.

Lifshitz F: Carbohydrate malabsorption. In *Clinical Disorders in Pediatric Gastroenterology and Nutrition*, F Lifshitz (ed). New York: Marcel Dekker, 1980, pp 229-47.

Lifshitz F, Coello-Ramirez P, Contreras-Gutierrez MD: The response of infants to carbohydrate oral loads after recovery from diarrhea. *J Pediatr* 79: 612-17, 1971b.

Lifshitz F, Coello-Ramirez P, Gutierrez-Topete G: Monosaccharide intolerance in infants with diarrhea: I. Clinical course of 23 infants. *J Pediatr* 77: 595-603, 1970.

Lifshitz F, Coello-Ramirez P, Gutierrez-Topete G, Cornado-Cornet MC: Carbohydrate intolerance in infants with diarrhea. *J Pediatr* 79: 760-67, 1971a.

Lifshitz F, Holman GH: Disaccharidase deficiencies with steatorrhea. *J Pediatr* 64: 34-44, 1964.

Lifshitz F, Klotz AP, Holman GH: Intestinal disaccharidases in gluten-sensitive enteropathy. *Am J Dig Dis* 10: 47-57, 1965.

Lifshitz F, Wapnir RA, Pergolizzi R, Teichberg S, Lipkin A: Alterations in intestinal transport and Na^+ K^+ ATPase in hypoxia. *Fed Proc* 35: 464, 1976.

Lisker R, Aguilar L, Zavala C: Intestinal lactase deficiency and milk drinking capacity in the adult. *Am J Clin Nutr* 31: 1499-1503, 1978.

Liu H-Y, Tsao MJ, Moore B, Giday Z: Bovine milk protein-induced intestinal malabsorption of lactose and fats in infants. *Gastroenterology* 54: 27-34, 1967.

Lubos MC, Gerrard JW, Buchan DJ: Disaccharidase activities in milk sensitive and celiac patients. *J Pediatr* 70: 325-33, 1967.

Lugo-de-Rivira C, Rodriguez H, Torres-Pinedo R: Studies on the mechanisms of sugar malabsorption in infantile infectious diarrhea. *Am J Clin Nutr* 25: 1248-53, 1972.

Mata LJ, Urrutia JJ: Intestinal colonization of breast fed children in a rural area of low socioeconomic level. *Ann NY Acad Sci* 176: 93-109, 1971.

Midtvedt T: Microbial bile acids transformation. *Am J Clin Nutr* 27: 1341-47, 1974.

Moriartey RR, Finer NN, Cox SF, Phillips HJ, Therman A, Stewart AR, Ulan OA: Necrotizing enterocolitis and human milk. *J Pediatr* 94: 295-96, 1979.

Northrup DW, Van Liere EJ: Effect of anoxia on absorption of glucose and glycine from small intestine. *Am J Physiol* 134: 288-91, 1941.

Okuni M, Okinaga K, Baba K: Studies on reducing sugars in stools of acute infantile diarrhea, with special reference to differences between breast fed and artificially fed babies. *Tohoku J Exp Med* 107: 395-402, 1972.

Paige DM, Bayless TM, Graham GG: Milk program helpful or harmful to Negro children? *Am J Public Health* 62: 1486-88, 1972.

Pergolizzi R, Lifshitz F, Teichberg S, Wapnir RA: Interaction between dietary carbohydrates and intestinal disaccharidases in experimental diarrhea. *Am J Clin Nutr* 30: 482-89, 1977.

Ringrose RE, Thompson JB, Welsh JD: Lactose malabsorption and steatorrhea. *Am J Dig Dis* 17: 533-38, 1972.

Stephenson LS, Latham MC: Lactose intolerance and milk consumption: The relation of tolerance to symptoms. *Am J Clin Nutr* 27: 296-303, 1974.

Stephenson LS, Latham MC, Jones DV: Milk consumption by black and by white pupils in two primary schools. *J Am Diet Assoc* 71: 258–62, 1977.

Stintzing G, Zetterstrom R: Cow's milk allergy: Incidence and pathogenetic role of early exposure to cow's milk formula. *Acta Paediatr Scand* 68: 383–87, 1979.

Strickland A, Garza C, Nichols B: Formula effects on growth after diarrhea. *Am J Clin Nutr* 32: 937, 1979.

Sunshine P, Kretchmer N: Studies of small intestine during development: III. Infantile diarrhea associated with intolerance to disaccharidases. *Pediatrics* 34: 38–50, 1964.

Teichberg S: Penetration of epithelial barriers by macromolecules: The intestinal mucosa. In *Clinical Disorders in Pediatric Gastroenterology and Nutrition*, F Lifshitz (ed). New York: Marcel Dekker, 1980, pp 185–202.

Teichberg S, Lifshitz F, Pergolizzi R, Wapnir RA: Response of rat intestine to a hyperosmotic feeding. *Pediatr Res* 12: 720–25, 1978.

Tejani N, Lifshitz F, Harper RG: The response to an oral glucose load during convalescence from hypoxia in newborn infants. *J Pediatr* 94: 792–96, 1979.

Walker WA: Intestinal defenses in health and disease. In *Clinical Disorders in Pediatric Gastroenterology and Nutrition*, F Lifshitz (ed). New York: Marcel Dekker, 1980, pp 99–119.

Welsh JD: Isolated lactase deficiency in humans: Report on 100 patients. *Medicine* 41: 257–77, 1970.

Woodbury RM: The relation between breast and artificial feeding and infant mortality. *Am J Hyg* 2: 668–87, 1922.

CHAPTER 18

MILK SUPPLEMENTATION

FOR CHILDREN IN THE TROPICS

Kenneth H. Brown

Rehabilitation of severely malnourished patients and supplementary feeding of children at risk for undernutrition traditionally have been accomplished with milk-based formulas. These formulas can be the sources of satisfactory energy and high-quality protein intakes in a variety of clinical and field situations. However, the use of milk-based formulas as rehabilitation foods in poorer tropical countries has become the focus of controversy, both in scientific journals and in lay publications (Simoons et al. 1977). The controversy is based in part on the fact that many children from some ethnic groups with primary low lactase activity develop diarrhea following the consumption of high doses of milk; but social, economic, and political issues also are involved. Unfortunately, there is limited scientifically derived information available regarding the nutritional consequences of milk ingestion by known lactose malabsorbers.

The value of milk supplementation was of particular interest for nutrition planners in Bangladesh, where childhood undernutrition is common and high rates of primary low lactase activity and secondary lactose malabsorption might be expected. To determine the nutritional efficacy of milk supplementation for that population, two sets of studies were undertaken. The first attempted to define the prevalence of lactose malabsorption among village children and to identify selected clinical conditions associated with malabsorption (Brown et al. 1979). The second measured the nutritional consequences of milk supplementation for known lactose malabsorbers by means of metabolic balance studies (Brown et al. 1980).

The field studies were carried out in two villages of Matlab Thana, the field station of the Cholera Research Laboratories. A random sample of 234 children previously stratified according to age and nutritional status, as defined by percentage of expected weight for age, was examined for lactose malabsorption using the breath hydrogen test (Solomons et al. 1977). Lactose malabsorption was defined as a rise of breath hydrogen concentration of at least 20 ppm above the baseline value following the ingestion of 2 g per kg of lactose as a 10% aqueous solution. Malabsorption also was assumed when there were moderately severe or severe signs of lactose intolerance within 24 hours of the test, regardless of the results of the breath hydrogen test.

The age-related prevalences of lactose malabsorption and intolerance, as presented graphically in figure 18.1, indicate that at least 80% of all children older than 36 months malabsorbed lactose. All infants under 6 months of age absorbed the sugar completely, and children between 6 months and 37 months of age showed intermediate rates of lactose malabsorption.

The relationship between the history of recent diarrhea and malabsorption rates is shown in figure 18.2. The high rates of lactose malabsorption in older children precluded a meaningful analysis of whether malabsorption is associated with diarrhea in those age groups. However, there was a tendency towards greater frequency of malabsorption in association with recent diarrhea in all the younger age groups and there was a significantly higher prevalence of lactose malabsorp-

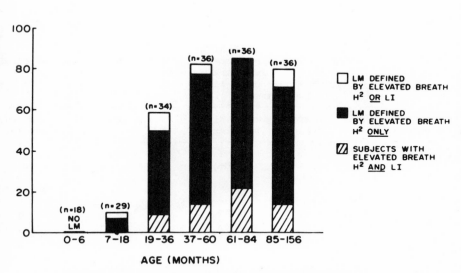

FIGURE 18.1. Age-related prevalences of lactose malabsorption (LM) and lactose intolerance (LI). Source: Brown et al. 1979, reprinted with permission.

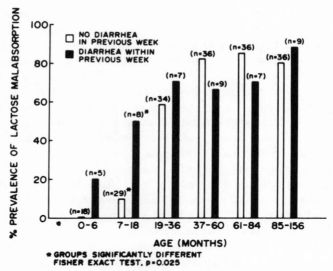

FIGURE 18.2. Relationship between recent history of diarrhea and malabsorption rates. Source: Brown et al. 1979, reprinted with permission.

tion among children aged 7 months to 18 months who had a positive history of diarrhea.

Diarrhea-free children were classified as either well nourished or poorly nourished according to their percentages of both expected weight for age and weight for height. The rates of lactose malabsorption are given in tables 18.1 and

TABLE 18.1

Percentage expected weight for age and prevalence of lactose malabsorption among well nourished and poorly nourished subjects

Age in months	N	Well nourished		N	Poorly nourished	
		Weight for age*	No. and (%) with malabsorption		Weight for age*	No. and (%) with malabsorption
7 to 18	15	74.6% (1.6)	3 (20.0%)	14	59.1% (1.4)	0 (0.0%)
19 to 36	19	73.6% (1.3)	10 (52.6%)	15	59.7% (1.3)	10 (66.7%)
37 to 60	19	74.1% (1.2)	17 (89.5%)	17	58.2% (1.1)	13 (76.5%)
61 to 84	19	75.1% (0.7)	16 (84.5%)	17	56.5% (1.0)	15 (88.2%)
85 to 156	20	74.5% (1.3)	18 (90.0%)	16	52.5% (0.9)	13 (81.2%)
Total	92	74.3% (0.5)	64 (69.6%)	79	57.1% (0.6)	51 (64.6%)

*Mean percentage expected weight for age, compared with U.S. reference data (National Center for Health Statistics 1977). Numbers in parentheses represent the standard errors ± 1.

18.2 for the two systems of classification. There was no difference in rates of lactose malabsorption when the results were analyzed on the basis of children's expected weight for age. However, when the children were compared on the basis of expected weight for height, there was significantly more malabsorption in the poorly nourished subjects aged 19 months to 36 months.

The effect of continuing breast feeding was examined in the weanling age group, which was defined as the age range encompassing both the youngest child not breast feeding at all and the oldest child still breast feeding. Breast-fed children experienced significantly lower rates of lactose malabsorption than did fully weaned children of similar age and nutritional status (table 18.3).

These studies, though geographically limited, indicate that lactose malabsorption is probably extremely common in the relatively homogeneous population of Bangladesh. Furthermore, those children who have a history of recent diarrhea, those who are weaned early, and possibly those who are acutely malnourished, are more likely to malabsorb lactose.

To learn whether the supplements of protein and energy from milk consumed by a lactose malabsorber more than offset the potential increases in fecal excretion of nutrients induced by lactose ingestion, the second set of studies was undertaken. Twelve healthy, but mildly undernourished, boys between 5 and 7 years of age were admitted to the metabolic ward of the Children's Nutrition Unit in Dacca. The subjects had been diagnosed as lactose malabsorbers by both the breath hydrogen test and a modified lactose tolerance test (table 18.4). During

TABLE 18.2

Percentage expected weight for height and prevalence of lactose malabsorption among well nourished and poorly nourished subjects

Age in months	Well nourished			Poorly nourished		
	N	Weight for height*	No. and (%) with malabsorption	N	Weight for height*	No. and (%) with malabsorption
7 to 18	14	87.4% (1.0)	1 (7.1%)	14	79.9% (0.6)	2 (14.3%)
19 to 36	16	89.4% (1.1)	6† (37.5%)	16	79.6% (1.2)	13† (81.2%)
37 to 60	18	90.0% (1.1)	16 (88.9%)	18	80.1% (0.8)	14 (77.8%)
61 to 84	17	93.7% (1.4)	15 (88.2%)	17	79.0% (1.0)	14 (82.4%)
85 to 156	18	93.6% (1.0)	14 (77.8%)	18	82.4% (0.9)	17 (94.4%)
Total	83	90.0% (1.1)	52 (62.6%)	83	79.2% (0.5)	60 (72.3%)

Note: Children with percentage expected weight for height above the median for each age group were considered "well nourished" and those below were classified as "poorly nourished."
*Compared to U.S. reference data (National Center for Health Statistics 1977). Numbers in parentheses represent the standard errors ± l.
†Groups significantly different by Fisher Exact Test, P = 0.01.

TABLE 18.3
Prevalence of lactose malabsorption in breast-fed and nonbreast-fed children in weanling age group

	Breast-fed children		Children no longer breast-fed	
	Lactose absorbers	Lactose malabsorbers	Lactose absorbers	Lactose malabsorbers
No. of children	15	11	1	10
(% of breast-fed or % of nonbreast-fed)	(57.7%)	(42.3%)*	(9.1%)	(90.9%)*
Mean age in months	29.3	29.5	22.0	32.7
(± 1 S.E.)	(1.7)	(2.0)	—	(2.1)
Mean percentage of expected wgt for age	68.9	68.8	76.4	64.2
(± 1 S.E.)	(2.1)	(2.5)	—	(2.9)
Mean percentage of expected wgt for hgt	84.4	82.5	85.2	79.2
(± 1 S.E.)	(1.8)	(1.5)	—	(2.7)

Source: Brown et al. 1979, reprinted with permission.
Note: The weanling age group was defined as the age range encompassing both the youngest child not breast feeding at all and the oldest child still breast feeding.
*Rates of malabsorption significantly different by Fisher Exact Test, $P = 0.007$.

TABLE 18.4
Clinical characteristics of study subjects

Study #	Percentage expected ht/age*	Percentage expected wt/ht*	Max. blood glucose rise (mg/dl)†	Signs of lactose intolerance‡	Lowest lactose dose with breath hydrogen rise > 20 ppm (g/ kg body weight)
E-19	90.7	81.0	18	++	0.5
E-20	91.4	90.1	8	++	2.0
E-21	80.0	96.2	5	0	2.0
E-22	86.2	81.7	18	++	1.0
E-23	84.7	80.9	5	++	0.5
E-24	82.9	108.0	0	++	1.0
E-25	91.6	93.5	3	++	0.5
E-26	86.2	96.7	15	++	1.0
E-27	84.7	85.4	0	±	0.5
E-28	82.4	73.9	0	++	1.0
E-29	81.7	94.0	8	++	1.0
E-30	81.2	89.9	5	+	1.0
Mean	85.3	89.3	7		

Source: Brown et al. 1980, reprinted with permission.
*Compared to NCHS reference data (National Center for Health Statistics 1977).
†Lactose dose 2 g per kg body weight.
‡0 = no signs of intolerance;
  ± = questionable signs (mild cramping);
  + = mild/moderate signs (1 loose bowel movement and/or flatus or severe cramping);
  ++ = severe signs (more than 1 liquid bowel movement).

the initial 12-day study period they were fed a "baseline" rice and vegetable diet designed to approximate common consumption patterns in rural Bangladesh (Institute of Nutrition and Food Science 1977). The diet provided 95 kcal per kg per day with 6% of energy as protein, 16% as fat, and the remainder as carbohydrate.

During the second and third study periods the baseline diets were supplemented with one of two simulated milks (casein, vegetable oil, and glucose or casein, vegetable oil, and lactose in water) twice daily at breakfast and lunch using a dose of 12.5 ml per kg body weight at each feeding (table 18.5). The evening meal remained unchanged. The dosage and timing of the milk supplements were planned to provide the additional nutrient intakes with only moderate lactose burdens at each meal, and to conform to a schedule that might be feasible for a field-based feeding program. If totally absorbed, the total milk supplement of 25 ml per kg body weight per day would provide an additional 16 kcal and 0.875 g of reference protein per kg body weight per day (equivalent to approximately 17% and 87% of suggested daily energy and protein intakes, respectively, for this age group) (FAO/WHO Ad Hoc Expert Committee 1973).

Urine and feces were collected quantitatively for the last 7 days of the study periods. The apparent absorption of nitrogen, fat, energy, and carbohydrate and the apparent retention of nitrogen were measured by standard techniques. In addition, a breath hydrogen test was performed before and after breakfast on two occasions during each diet period.

The children's weight gains, nutrient absorption levels, and relative intestinal transit times are presented for each diet in table 18.6. The subjects gained significantly more weight while consuming the supplemented diets than during the baseline period (P < 0.001), but there was no difference between the effects of the glucose and the lactose milk supplements. Since the supplemented diets were neither isocaloric nor isonitrogenous with the baseline diet, the increased nitrogen retention on the supplemented diets was expected. The similar apparent

TABLE 18.5
Food and estimated nutrient contents of simulated milk formulas

Food	Amount (g/100 ml)	Energy (kcal/100 ml)	Protein (g/100 ml)	Fat (g/100 ml)	Carbohydrate (g/100 ml)
Casein powder	4.07	14	3.50	—	—
Vegetable oil	3.50	31.5	—	3.50	—
Lactose or glucose	5.00	20	—	—	5.00
Total nutrients		65.5	3.50	3.50	5.00
Percentage of energy			21	48	31

Source: Brown et al. 1980, reprinted with permission.
Note: Dosage of 25 ml per kg body weight per day was calculated to provide 87% of recommended protein intake and 17% of recommended energy intake for the age group in question (FAO/WHO Ad Hoc Expert Committee 1973).

TABLE 18.6
Effect of study diets on subjects' weight gain, nutrient absorption, and
relative intestinal transit time

Diet	Wt. gain g/kg body wt/day	Fecal energy kcal/ day	Fecal energy % of intake	Fecal nitrogen g/day	Apparent nitrogen Absorp. % of intake	Apparent nitrogen Retent. % of intake
Rice/vegetable mean	0.98[a]	104	9.0	1.278	55.8*	4.5*
(SE)	(0.48)	(13)	(1.3)	(0.073)	(2.3)	(2.9)
Rice/vegetable, glucose milk mean	3.39[b]	106	7.2	1.340	73.2*	18.4*
(SE)	(0.56)	(9)	(0.4)	(0.067)	(1.3)	(1.7)
Rice/vegetable + lactose milk mean	3.98[c]	130	8.6	1.471	71.0*	21.6*
(SE)	(0.51)	(28)	(1.3)	(0.097)	(1.1)	(2.1)

Diet	Fecal fat g/day	Fecal fat % of intake	Fecal carbohydrate g/day	Fecal carbohydrate % of intake	Fecal wet wt. g/day	Post-prandial breath H_2 rise ppm	Intestinal transit time Hrs
Rice/vegetable mean	1.69	8.3	11.8	5.7	117	2.1[d]	19.0[g]
(SE)	(0.40)	(2.5)	(3.0)	(1.5)	(13)	(0.7)	(1.5)
Rice/vegetable, glucose milk mean	1.38	4.1	11.9	5.1	125	2.3[e]	16.2
(SE)	(0.18)	(0.5)	(2.1)	(0.7)	(11)	(0.5)	(1.5)
Rice/vegetable + lactose milk mean	1.40	4.3	17.8	7.1	167	6.4[f]	12.6[h]
(SE)	(0.13)	(0.5)	(7.2)	(2.4)	(25)	(1.0)	(1.6)

Source: Brown et al. 1980, reprinted with permission.
Note: Levels of significance obtained by paired t-tests: [a] = different from [b] and [c], $P < 0.001$; [d] and [e] different from [f], $P < 0.001$; [g] different from [h], $P < 0.025$.
*Rice/vegetable diet not compared statistically with milk-supplemented diets because intakes were not isocaloric and isonitrogenous.

absorption and retention of nitrogen with the lactose and glucose milks is noteworthy, though. Given the individual variation in nitrogen absorption and retention detected for the two supplemented diets, a difference between diets of as little as 3% would have been identified.

Although the children tended to have increased fecal energy and carbohydrate excretion while consuming the diet containing lactose, the differences between the supplemented diets were not statistically significant. The increased variances of those parameters during the lactose diet period indicate that there was greater heterogeneity of responses to the lactose diet than to the lactose-free diet. The type of milk supplement had no effect on fecal fat excretion or apparent fat absorption.

The postprandial breath hydrogen test performed during each of the diet periods showed a significant increase of hydrogen excretion related to lactose consumption ($P < 0.025$) (table 18.6). However, there was no significant correlation between individual subjects' breath hydrogen excretion and fecal energy or carbohydrate losses.

There was a strong correlation between mean daily fecal wet weight and fecal energy and carbohydrate excretion for individual subjects during each diet study period ($P < 0.001$) (figs. 18.3 and 18.4). This correlation is potentially useful to health auxiliaries supervising feeding programs. If fecal weight increases excessively on a diet containing lactose, increased energy losses will be likely. On the other hand, if fecal excretion is not increased markedly, usual nutrient absorption can be assumed.

On the basis of evidence from this study it appears that milk can be tolerated and utilized well by young lactose malabsorbers when it is provided in relatively low doses and with additional food sources. However, it is suggested that milk not be delivered as the single source of energy in a supplemental feeding program in the tropics. Instead, it should be mixed with the traditionally consumed weaning and children's foods to bolster their protein and energy density. The milk should be introduced into the diet slowly and fecal excretion patterns should be monitored to determine how well the supplement is absorbed. Used in this way, milk can provide an important nutritional supplement even in settings where lactose malabsorption is common.

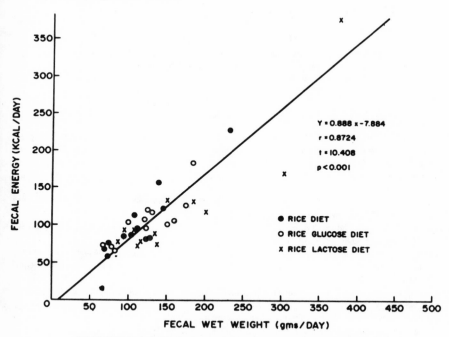

FIGURE 18.3. Individual subjects' fecal energy excretion and mean daily fecal wet weight during each diet study period. Source: Brown et al. 1980, reprinted with permission.

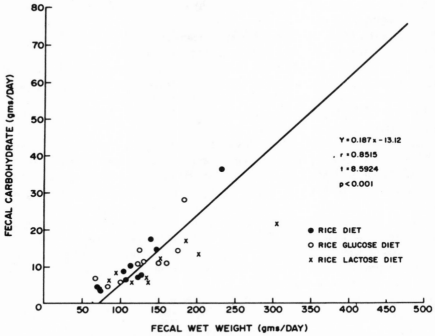

FIGURE 18.4. Individual subjects' fecal carbohydrate excretion and mean daily fecal wet weight during each diet study period. Source: Brown et al. 1980, reprinted with permission.

REFERENCES

Brown KH, Khatun M, Parry L, Ahmed MG: Nutritional consequences of low dose milk supplements consumed by lactose-malabsorbing children. *Am J Clin Nutr* 33: 1054–63, 1980.

Brown KH, Parry L, Khatun M, Ahmed MG: Lactose malabsorption in Bangladeshi village children: Relation with age, history of recent diarrhea, nutritional status, and breast feeding. *Am J Clin Nutr* 32: 1962–69, 1979.

FAO/WHO Ad Hoc Expert Committee: *Energy and Protein Requirements,* WHO Technical Report Series, no. 522. Geneva: World Health Organization, 1973.

Institute of Nutrition and Food Science, University of Dacca: *Nutrition Survey of Rural Bangladesh, 1975–76.* Dacca: University of Dacca, Dec. 1977.

National Center for Health Statistics: *NCHS Growth Curves for Children Birth–18 Years, United States,* DHEW Publication no. (PHS) 78-1650. Hyattsville, Md.: U.S. Department of Health, Education and Welfare, 1977.

Simoons FJ, Johnson JD, Kretchmer N: Perspective on milk-drinking and malabsorption of lactose. *Pediatrics* 59: 98–109, 1977.

Solomons, NW, Viteri FE, Hamilton LH: Application of a simple gas chromatographic technique for measuring breath hydrogen. *J Lab Clin Med* 90: 856–62, 1977.

CHAPTER 19

LACTOSE DIGESTION

BY PREMATURE INFANTS

HYDROGEN BREATH TEST RESULTS VERSUS

ESTIMATES OF ENERGY LOSS

William C. MacLean, Jr., and Beverly B. Fink

BACKGROUND

The premature infant presents a unique opportunity to study a human organism with low intestinal lactase that habitually consumes large quantities of lactose with apparently few symptoms. As such the premature infant may be a paradigm for the symptomatic adaptations that take place in those of the world's population with low levels of intestinal lactase who continue to drink milk. Fifteen years ago, Auricchio et al. (1965) were able to examine disaccharidase activity in the intestines of 27 fetuses and newborns who died shortly after birth. Sucrase and maltase activities were present in substantial amounts by four to six months in utero. Lactase concentrations, in contrast, increased only during the last eight weeks, reaching peak values near term. Some of the infants studied by Auricchio had been fed one or more days prior to succumbing. There was a suggestion that these infants had higher levels of intestinal lactase than infants not fed, a fact that

This study was supported by Research Grant RO1 HD 11172 from the National Institutes of Health, U.S.P.H.S. The authors acknowledge the technical assistance of Mr. Robert P. Placko. Dr. E. David Mellits aided in the statistical analysis of the data. This study would not have been possible without the continued cooperation of the medical and nursing staffs of the Infant Special Care Unit and the Newborn Nursery (Nelson 2) of The Johns Hopkins Hospital.

caused him to speculate that feeding of the prematurely born infant might induce an early postnatal rise in lactase and that this increase might account for the ability of the premature infant to tolerate large lactose loads.

Based on the tissue.concentration of lactase and the length of the small intestine in individual infants, Auricchio calculated the amount of lactose that could be hydrolyzed per 24 hours if the entire small intestine were assumed to be acting maximally. These calculations are shown in table 19.1. Because it is highly unlikely that a maximal rate of hydrolysis would be maintained 24 hours per day, these estimates err on the high side. Also shown in table 19.1 are mean weights for gestational age, based on the intrauterine growth curve, and the daily lactose intakes for infants of different gestational ages, assuming a total energy intake of 120 kcal per kg body weight per day from human milk or formula. When Auricchio's estimates of maximal hydrolysis are combined with these projected intakes one concludes that nearly all the lactose ingested by a premature infant in the 800 g to 1,000 g range would pass into the colon. Depending on the individual lactase concentration, an infant in the 1,300 g to 1,400 g range would be expected to malabsorb 60% to 70% of ingested lactose. Even the infant near term might lose substantial amounts of lactose.

Auricchio concluded that the large lactose load of the breast-fed full-term infant probably exceeds the ability of the small intestine to hydrolyze this sugar. Although at first it seems unreasonable to suggest that the full-term infant may malabsorb substantial quantities of the only source of carbohydrate in its natural diet, evidence is accruing in increasing amounts that this is the case. Significant amounts (0.5% to 2.0%) of reducing substance, as well as glucose, galactose, and lactose itself, have been detected in the stools of infants being breast-fed or fed modified cow milk formulas (Davidson and Mullinger 1970). A recent study demonstrated that substantial quantities of hydrogen were being excreted in the breath of full-term infants by 7 days of age (Chiles et al. 1979). The peak values were 55 ± 15 ppm (mean $\pm$ SEM) while consuming lactose loads of 1.8 ± 0.2 g per kg at each feeding. Breath hydrogen values in this range are considered indicative of substantial lactose malabsorption in older children and adults (Perman et al. 1978). Nevertheless, all infants were asymptomatic and growing well.

TABLE 19.1
Calculated maximal in vitro hydrolysis of lactose by the entire neonatal small intestine

Gestational age (lunar months)	N	Lactose hydrolysis* (g/24 hrs)		Mean† wt. (g)	Lactose intake at 120 kcal/kg/day (g)	Estimated percentage malabsorbed
		< day	> day			
6	1	0.3	—	875	10.8	97
7–8	6	3.8	6.4	1,375	16.9	62–78
8–9	8	5.8	23.4	2,100	25.8	9–22

*Auricchio et al. 1965.
†Based on intrauterine growth curve.

TABLE 19.2
Gestational ages and birth weights of premature infants studied

Gestational age	No. of infants	No. of studies	Birth weight (g)*
29 weeks	1	7	1,010
30–32 weeks	5	21	1,571 ± 190
34–38 weeks	16	51	1,731 ± 474

Source: MacLean and Fink 1980, table 2, reprinted with permission.
*Mean birth weight ± SD.

CURRENT STUDIES

Studies in the pediatrics unit at Johns Hopkins for the past several years have focused on the adaptations that allow the premature infant with low intestinal lactase levels to consume large quantities of lactose with apparent impunity. The work of Bond and Levitt (1976) suggested the possible importance of the colonic microflora as a second intestinal enzyme system in this adaptation. As part of a larger study of lactose digestion by premature infants, breath hydrogen excretions have been measured as an index of carbohydrate malabsorption. Twenty-two infants with uncomplicated neonatal courses have been studied thus far.* Descriptive data on the infants studied are listed in table 19.2. Seventy-nine individual studies have been carried out during the first seven weeks of life. All infants were consuming a standard infant formula containing lactose. All were being managed in accord with usual nursery routines. Feeding frequency was every two, three, or four hours, depending on the size and tolerance of the infant. Each infant was studied as soon after reaching an intake of 50 kcal per kg per day as possible, and then weekly thereafter until the time of discharge. Breath samples were obtained preprandially and then postprandially at one-half hour and then at hourly intervals through five hours, regardless of whether the infants were fed subsequently.

Accurate determination of hydrogen concentration requires the collection of end-expiratory air. Other investigators have reported the use of a small nasal cannula in children too young to cooperate (Perman et al. 1978). In the present studies, collection through a small feeding tube in the posterior nasal pharnyx was found to be more reliable. Once the tube is taped into place, the infant generally becomes quiet quite soon thereafter. About 0.5 ml to 1.0 ml of air then is aspirated into a syringe at the end of each expiration in synchronization with the infant's respiration. All samples are taken in duplicate and run in duplicate.

Breath hydrogen concentration has been determined using a Quintron Model S Gas Chromatograph modified as suggested by Solomons et al. (1977). The carrier gas is argon. Room air with a known concentration of hydrogen (52.5 ppm) is used to calibrate the instrument. The precision of this measurement in

---

*The protocol and consent form for these studies were approved by the Joint Committee on Clinical Investigation of The Johns Hopkins Medical Institutions.

our laboratory has been found to be ± 4 ppm, in close agreement with the data reported by others using the same instrument (Solomons et al. 1978).

RESULTS

Seventy-five percent of the infants studied were excreting substantial amounts of hydrogen, more than 8 ppm, by 2 weeks of age; and all were excreting hydrogen in amounts indicative of lactose malabsorption by 3 weeks of age. The slight delay in the onset of hydrogen excretion by these premature infants relative to full-term infants may possibly be explained by the slower introduction of oral feeding in premature infants. There could also be a slower development of colonic flora capable of fermenting lactose.

Energy intake (kcal per kg per day), lactose intake per feeding (g per kg per feeding), and the rate of weight gain for the infants studied are shown graphically in fig. 19.1. By the end of the first week, the mean energy intake was approximately 80 kcal per kg per day. By the third to fourth weeks, intakes were as high

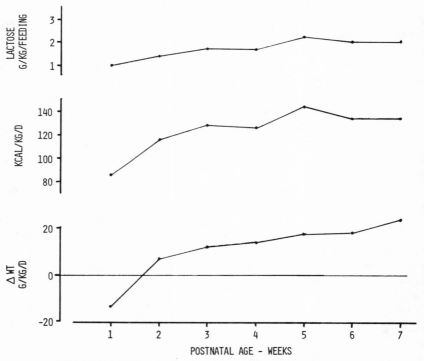

FIGURE 19.1. Lactose and energy intakes and rates of weight gain during the seven weeks of study.

as 140 kcal per kg per day. Lactose intakes during these weeks were approximately 2 g per kg per feeding, tantamount to performing a modified lactose tolerance test at each feeding. The expected weight loss during the first week was replaced by adequate rates of weight gain during the second and subsequent weeks.

The values for preprandial and peak concentrations of breath hydrogen (mean ± SEM) are shown in fig. 19.2. The preprandial value frequently was not the lowest value during the five-hour study. Commonly, breath hydrogen concentration fell during the first 30 to 60 minutes after eating, rising again subsequently. This lack of synchronization between feeding and hydrogen rise is not surprising, since the time at which lactose from the previous feeding would reach the colon and begin fermenting would not necessarily relate to the time of the next feeding. There was considerable variation in the pattern obtained with different infants. This problem was overcome to a large extent by using the five-hour mean value for breath hydrogen excretion (fig. 19.3).

Regression analysis was used to look for effects of gestational age, postnatal age, and the early introduction of lactose on lactose tolerance by the infants, as indicated by breath hydrogen excretion. Preprandial, peak, and five-hour mean hydrogen excretions were used as dependent variables. Gestational age, post-

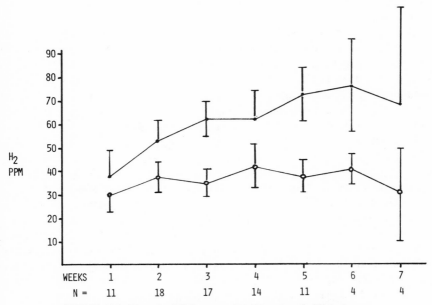

FIGURE 19.2. Mean (± SEM) preprandial (O) and peak (●) hydrogen concentrations in prematures during the seven weeks of study. The number of studies during each week also is shown.

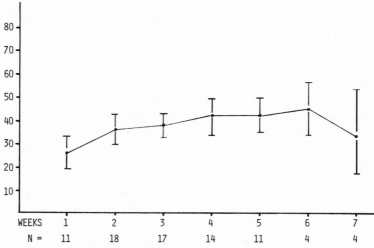

FIGURE 19.3. Mean (± SEM) value for the five-hour mean breath H_2 concentration in prematures during the seven weeks of study.

natal age, lactose intake (both as g per kg per day and as g per kg per feeding), and the frequency of feeding were used as independent variables. Nonlinear correlations were looked for but none of significance were found.

Peak hydrogen concentration was not significantly related to gestational age. There was a significant linear correlation between peak hydrogen concentration and increasing postnatal age in the 79 observations carried out on the 22 subjects (r = 0.248, P < 0.05). Lactose intake, however, also increased significantly with increasing postnatal age. When multiple regression analysis was carried out daily lactose intake remained significantly related to peak hydrogen concentration (r = 0.373, P < 0.001). Daily lactose intake also was the variable most significantly related to the five-hour mean hydrogen concentration (r = 0.345, P < 0.01).

Variations in Breath Hydrogen Excretion. Data from three additional patients are presented in table 19.3 to illustrate the range of responses in breath H_2 excretion seen and the possible effect of parenteral antibiotics on this. Patient number 34 was an infant of 36 weeks gestational age. Breath H_2 excretion was markedly elevated by 6 days of age, and then decreased during the second and third weeks of life. Clinical course was uncomplicated throughout. These data are compatible with the hypothesis that large amounts of lactose were reaching the colon and being fermented by the microflora early on. Less lactose was being fermented during the second two studies, suggesting either that with increasing postnatal age intestinal lactase was playing a larger role, with less lactose reaching the colon, or that the predominant fecal flora had changed. The latter seems

TABLE 19.3
Patterns of breath H_2 response in three selected premature infants

Patient (gestational age)	Age (days)	Weight (g)	Diet		Feeding frequency	Breath H_2 (ppm)	
			Source	Kcal/kg/day		Peak	Mean
No. 34	6	1,730	Enfamil	113	Q 3 hr.	91	49
(36 wks.)	13	1,920	Enfamil	125	Q 4 hr.	31	16
	20	2,100	Enfamil	113	Q 4 hr.	27	14
Comment: Generally uncomplicated course.							
No. 32	6	960	Enfamil	60	Q 2 hr.	5	3
(29 wks.)	10	1,040	Enfamil	120	Q 2 hr.	3	2
	15	1,080	Enfamil	106	Q 2 hr.	40	28
	22	1,160	Enfamil	116	Q 2 hr.	63	34
Comment: Parenteral penicillin and Kanamycin—days 1 to 9.							
No. 31	9	1,500	HM*-Enfamil	53	Q 2 hr.	6	5
(34 wks.)	26	1,370	HM	117	Q 2 hr.	8	7
	32	1,530	HM	131	Q 4 hr.	125	66
Comment: NPO first 4 days. PDA ligated D14. NPO + antibiotics D14-21. Loose stools D26. Normal stools D32.							

*HM = human milk.

less likely since the infant had not received antibiotics and stool pattern was unchanged.

Effects of Antibiotics. Patient number 32 received parenteral penicillin and kanamycin for the first nine days of life. Breath H_2 excretions were very low on days 6 and 10. Six days after stopping antibiotics peak breath H_2 concentration had increased to 40 ppm. During the subsequent week breath H_2 concentrations increased even further. One cannot be certain if antibiotic treatment retarded development of the fecal flora in this infant since 25% of infants not receiving antibiotics also did not excrete H_2 in breath during the first two weeks of life. That antibiotics retarded development of the fecal flora is certainly a possibility. A similar situation was observed in infant number 31, who was excreting less than 8 ppm H_2 at 9 days of age and who then received one week of antibiotics from day 14 to day 21. On restudy at day 26, peak breath H_2 concentration was still only 8 ppm and the infant's stools were loose. Six days later breath H_2 had risen to 125 ppm; stool pattern was normal.

DISCUSSION

The breath hydrogen excretion data in the infants studied to date suggest that malabsorption of lactose by premature infants is the rule. Despite breath concentrations of hydrogen in ranges that are associated with symptomatic lactose intolerance in older children and adults, these infants were symptom-free and gaining weight rapidly. These seemingly paradoxical pieces of information raise the question of the nutritional significance of lactose malabsorption by these infants.

The importance of lactose malabsorption should relate in some degree to the magnitude of the phenomenon. Several approaches were used in an attempt to quantitate the malabsorption of lactose in these infants. A modification of the formula of Solomons et al. (1978) was used to calculate the total amount of hydrogen excreted during a five-hour study using the values obtained by interval sampling. A respiratory rate of 40 and a tidal volume of 6 mg per kg were assumed (Dawes 1968). The mean value for hydrogen excretion for all 79 studies was estimated to be 2.75 ml H_2 per kg per five hours. Published values for the amount of breath hydrogen excreted per gram of lactulose, and the relative amount of hydrogen produced in vitro when lactose rather than lactulose is fermented, were used to estimate the amount of lactose available for fermentation in the colons of the infants studied (Bond and Levitt 1972, Solomons et al. 1978). Depending on the assumptions that were made, an average of 8.3 g to 13.9 g lactose per kg per day was estimated to have passed the ileocecal valve and to have been fermented. The corresponding mean lactose intake for all studies was 12.5 g per kg per day.

A more direct means of arriving at the magnitude of lactose malabsorption was possible using the regression of five-hour mean hydrogen excretion on lactose intake per day (fig. 19.4). A mean lactose intake of 4.5 g per kg per day or less was not associated with abnormal breath hydrogen excretion. Lactose intakes beyond 4.5 g per kg per day resulted in a linear increase in the amount of hydrogen excreted. The difference between the mean amount of lactose ingested (12.5 g per kg per day) and the mean intake that was associated with no significant hydrogen production (4.5 g per kg per day) is an estimate of the amount of lactose malabsorbed (8.0 g per kg per day), approximately 64% of intake. Clearly some infants were malabsorbing less than this; presumably many were malabsorbing more.

Lactose malabsorption of this degree represents a potential energy loss to the infant of great significance and yet all infants were gaining weight well. Stool collections were carried out in 29 of these infants during the days they were studied. Mean stool weight was 6 g per day. Even if it were assumed that 20% of the stool were dry matter and that all of this were carbohydrate, fecal energy loss would be estimated to be approximately 4.9 kcal or 3.1 kcal per kg per day, about 2.5% of total energy intake. Since the premature infant is known to malabsorb fat and has obligatory stool nitrogen losses, this figure is probably an overestimation of carbohydrate loss in the stool. The inference to be drawn from these findings is that the volatile fatty acids that are an end-product of fermentation are most likely being absorbed in the colon. Although there is an energy loss by carrying out the initial steps of hexose metabolism without adenosine triphosphate production, the absorption of volatile fatty acids could salvage between 65% and 80% of the potential useful energy in carbohydrate lost into the colon, depending on the type of fermentation occurring.

Both full-term and premature infants appear to malabsorb variable but significant quantities of lactose. Is there any potential benefit to the infant of this physiological malabsorption? The answer to this question is purely speculative. The colonic microflora of the breast-fed infant differs substantially from that of the bottle-fed infant, although some of this change must be attributed to difference in protein intake (Bullen et al. 1976, Bullen et al. 1977). A fecal flora of predominantly lactose fermenters, as opposed to putrefactive bacteria, may favor colonization with organisms that tend to be less pathogenic to the infant.

The presumption of lactase insufficiency in the premature infant had led physicians caring for these infants to rely progressively on formulas in which part or all of the lactose has been replaced by other carbohydrates. One must ask whether there is any potential danger in removing lactose from the diet of these infants. Lactose is present uniquely in milk and has been shown to facilitate the absorption of calcium in experimental animals, even in those with low intestinal lactase (Leichter and Tolensky 1975). A preliminary report suggests that this is true in the human infant as well (Ziegler and Fomon 1980). One also should take note of the increased incidence of rickets that has been recorded in premature infants being fed lactose-free soy-based formulas.

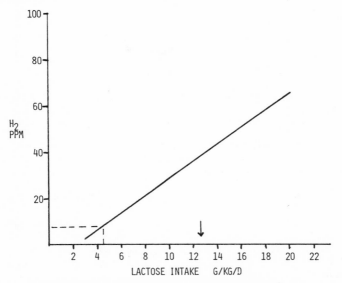

FIGURE 19.4. Regression of five-hour mean H_2 concentration on lactose intake per day. Source: MacLean and Fink 1980, reprinted with permission.

CONCLUSIONS

The lessons learned thus far from the study of lactose absorption in the premature infant should cause investigators to rethink some of the concepts concerning lactose intolerance in older children and adults. The premature infant provides a human model for lactase insufficiency. It has been argued that lactose malabsorption by children and adults with low intestinal lactase levels also prejudices the absorption of other nutrients. This has been used as an argument for the removal of milk from the diets of these individuals, even if they are asymptomatic. The excellent growth and development and the lack of micronutrient deficiencies in premature infants raised on formulas containing lactose suggest that if there is a negative effect of lactose malabsorption on the absorption of other micronutrients its magnitude must be quite small. Finally, although breath hydrogen excretions in the range seen in these infants are certainly indicative of lactose malabsorption, there is no reason to equate them with clinical lactose intolerance. Breath hydrogen excretions in these ranges by older children and adults following standard lactose tolerance testing frequently result in the diagnosis of lactose intolerance and the subsequent removal of all lactose from the diet. There are many individuals with demonstrated low intestinal lactase levels who are able to consume lactose without significant symptoms. The experience with full-term and premature infants suggests that the decision to remove lactose from the diet should be based on symptoms rather than on the results of lactose tolerance testing.

REFERENCES

Auricchio S, Rubino A, Mürset G: Intestinal glycosidase activities in the human embryo, fetus, and newborn. *Pediatrics* 35: 944–54, 1965.

Bond JH, Levitt MD: Use of pulmonary hydrogen (H_2) measurements to quantitate carbohydrate absorption: Study of partially gastrectomized patients. *J Clin Invest* 51: 1219–25, 1972.

Bond JH, Levitt MD: Fate of soluble carbohydrate in the colon of rats and man. *J Clin Invest* 57: 1158–64, 1976.

Bullen CL, Tearle PV, Stewart MG: The effect of "humanized" milks and supplemented breastfeeding on the faecal flora of infants. *J Med Microbiol* 10: 403–13, 1977.

Bullen CL, Tearle PV, Willis AT: Bifidobacteria in the intestinal tract of infants: An in-vivo study. *J Med Microbiol* 9: 325–33, 1976.

Chiles C, Watkins JB, Barr RG: Lactose utilization in the newborn: Role of colonic flora. *Pediatr Res* 13: 365, 1979.

Davidson AGF, Mullinger M: Reducing substances in neonatal stools detected by Clinitest. *Pediatrics* 46: 632–35, 1970.

Dawes GS: *Foetal and Neonatal Physiology*. Chicago: Yearbook Medical Publishers, 1968.

Leichter J, Tolensky AF: Effect of dietary lactose on the absorption of protein, fat and calcium in the postweaning rat. *Am J Clin Nutr* 28: 238–41, 1975.

MacLean WC Jr, Fink BB: Lactose malabsorption by premature infants: Magnitude and clinical significance. *J Pediatr* 97: 383–88, 1980.

Perman JA, Barr RG, Watkins JB: Sucrose malabsorption in children: Noninvasive diagnosis by interval breath hydrogen determination. *J Pediatr* 93: 17–22, 1978.

Solomons NW, Viteri FE, Hamilton LH: Application of a simple gas chromatographic technique for measuring breath hydrogen. *J Lab Clin Med* 90: 856–62, 1977.

Solomons NW, Viteri FE, Rosenberg IH: Development of an interval sampling hydrogen (H₂) breath test for carbohydrate malabsorption in children: Evidence for a circadian pattern of breath H₂ concentration. *Pediatrics* 12: 816–23, 1978.

Ziegler EE, Fomon SJ: Lactose and mineral absorption in infancy. *Pediatr Res* 14: 513, 1980.

CHAPTER 20

CLINICAL IMPLICATIONS
OF CHILDHOOD LACTOSE INTOLERANCE

Lewis A. Barness

At least six different forms of lactose intolerance have been documented: premature, congenital, acquired, developmental, and two forms of galactose intolerance. Lactase deficiency in the prematurely born infant is described by MacLean and Fink (chapter 19). The congenital hereditary form of lactose intolerance, which is symptomatic in infancy, is very rare, as pointed out by Welsh (chapter 6). An acquired form occurring after an episode of diarrhea is very common, and usually resolves spontaneously in days or weeks (see chapter 17). A late developmental form, also genetic, is recognized in different populations; it appears with symptomatic onset between 5 and 14 years of age. The usual symptomatology of these four forms of lactose intolerance includes diarrhea and abdominal pain. Some specific deficiencies related to malabsorption have been suggested.

The other forms of lactose intolerance are related to the hydrolytic products of lactose digestion. These are uridylyl transferase deficiency and galactokinase deficiency. Both of these are inherited as autosomal recessive diseases and even small amounts of galactose or lactose can lead to disastrous consequences. In children with the transferase deficiency, cirrhosis, cataracts, and mental retardation may occur. Children with galactokinase deficiency develop fewer symptoms but may develop cataracts later in life.

Lactase deficiency with lactose intolerance may be suspected in children with persistent diarrhea or otherwise unexplained chronic abdominal pain. This is distinct from lactase deficiency following an episode of diarrhea. Lactase defi-

214

ciency can be diagnosed by biopsy of the intestinal mucosa and direct measurement for the enzyme. It may be suspected if reducing substances are present in the stool and subsequently identified as lactose or by observation of the patient who develops persistent diarrhea following ingestion of lactose. With lactose intolerance due to lactase deficiency, glucose does not rise in the blood after a lactose tolerance test. More recently the use of hydrogen excretion through the lungs has been reported to be an accurate indicator of lactose intolerance due to lactase deficiency. While this test has received enthusiastic acclaim for accuracy, experience with it for specificity still is limited.

Some studies have indicated that premature infants may grow more rapidly when a different sugar such as sucrose is substituted for lactose in the diet. Such substitution is thought to be effective due to the late development of lactase in the gut of the fetus (Committee on Nutrition 1978). Other sugars appear to be easily absorbed in those with lactose intolerance. Although lactose intolerance has been suggested in children who develop abdominal pain following the ingestion of milk, there may be other factors in the milk that produce similar symptomatology. While abdominal pain may be a sign of lactose intolerance it is not diagnostic of lactose intolerance (Liebman 1979).

Over the past 20 years there has been a dramatic increase in the use of formula for American babies. Expansion of the infant formula industry has required tremendous amounts of lactose. Such formulas attempt to duplicate as closely as possible the chemical composition of human milk in an effort to improve on the old evaporated milk formulas. Lactose for formula presently is available in sufficient quantities, especially from milks. If formulas continue to be used in large quantities, the availability of lactose may be decreased and its price may skyrocket. No substitute yet is available for this sugar. Although it has been synthesized chemically, the process remains expensive.

Lactose may have certain benefits for the young infant. Because of the slower digestability of lactose, it is hydrolyzed far down the gut, favoring the development of an acid stool and gram positive flora. Lactose itself is not able to maintain the flora; it must be consumed in conjunction with a low protein diet and low fiber foods. A mixed diet almost invariably leads to gram negative flora in the intestinal tract (György et al. 1953, Cornely et al. 1957).

Lactose in the diet also is said to favor absorption of calcium and fat, perhaps due to the acid medium of the stool. Similarly, ingestion of lactose is said to lead to softer stools. It is well known that milk is a convenient source of protein. It is also a rich source of energy, B vitamins, and fat, although its fat content is largely saturated or monounsaturated rather than polyunsaturated. Polyunsaturated fats are important precursors of prostaglandins.

Lactose-free diets generally imply low-dairy diets. In the absence of all dairy foods, other sources must be found for needed protein, fat, energy, calcium, and B vitamins. Partially fermented milks, such as the cheeses, can be used in these diets. But, the biological value of casein is not as high as that of other types of animal proteins, nor is cheese an inexpensive source of protein. Still, many substitutes are available for whole milk so that those children who do not like milk or are made ill by milk need not be required to drink milk.

Recent observations on calcium requirements indicate that as protein is increased in a diet, more calcium is required to maintain calcium balance. While the calcium in milk is not well absorbed, meat proteins do favor absorption of calcium in a diet. Meats available today, especially the processed meats that are mechanically deboned, contain more than adequate amounts of calcium. Many vegetables, fish, nuts, and legumes also are rich in calcium. Thus, milk need not be considered essential to supply this nutrient.

In light of recent research on lactose intolerance, the Committee on Nutrition of the American Academy of Pediatrics (1978) has reexamined the symptomatology of lactose intolerance as well as the use of milk, particularly in the school lunch program. On weighing present evidence of milk benefits and intolerance, the committee adheres to its position that it would be inappropriate to discourage supplemental milk feeding programs targeted at children, merely on the basis of primary lactose intolerance. The committee continues to encourage the development of equally nutritious and acceptable supplementary foods in areas where milk production is inefficient and uneconomical. In the refeeding of malnourished children, milk use should not be discouraged as long it continues to provide the best and cheapest source of high quality protein, except in cases of severe diarrhea. Some of these children will require lactose-free diets if recovery is to be achieved with minimal complications. Further studies are needed to understand better the needs, the uses, and the improper uses of lactose in the diet of infants and children.

REFERENCES

Committee on Nutrition, American Academy of Pediatrics: The practical significance of lactose intolerance in children. *Pediatrics* 62: 240–45, 1978.

Cornely DA, Barness LA, Gyorgy P: Effect of lactose on nitrogen metabolism and phenol excretion in infants. *J Pediatr* 51: 40–45, 1957.

György P, Mello MI, Torres FE, Barness LA: Growth promotion in rats by crude concentrates of the bifidus factor. *Proc Soc Exp Biol Med* 84: 464–65, 1953.

Liebman WM: Abdominal pain: Lactose and sucrose intolerance. *Pediatrics* 64: 43–45, 1979.

VII

DEVELOPMENT OF LOW-LACTOSE
PRODUCTS

CHAPTER 21

ENZYME TECHNOLOGY AND THE DEVELOPMENT

OF LACTOSE-HYDROLYZED MILK

Arthur G. Rand, Jr.

Milk is considered a significant source of at least eight essential nutrients; it provides 10% or more of the recommended daily allowance for protein, riboflavin, calcium, vitamin D, niacin, vitamin B_{12}, phosphorous, and iodine (Phillips and Briggs 1975). The American dairy industry has effectively promoted the use of this nutritious and valuable food, and it is available in a wide variety of processed and preserved dairy products. Milk also has found increased use as an effective functional ingredient in an amazing range of food products. This wide availability and dependence on milk products in the American diet can create serious problems for those who are milk intolerant due to intestinal lactase deficiency. For such individuals, the risk of serious discomfort limits the utility of milk as a vehicle for supplying essential nutrients.

FOOD ENZYME TECHNOLOGY

Milk intolerance is a problem that is potentially soluble through food enzyme technology. An obvious step would be addition of a food grade lactase (beta-galactosidase) to a milk product, followed by incubation to predigest the lactose

The author would like to acknowledge the contributions of Dr. James A. Hourigan, Mr. Thomas P. Maculan, Mrs. Mary Anne DeAngelis, and Mr. Kevin J. Finnie, whose innovative research made this manuscript possible. This work was supported by the Rhode Island Agricultural Experiment Station, Hatch Act Funds, and the Shadow Medical Research Foundation, Inc. Contribution number 1947 of the Rhode Island Agricultural Experiment Station.

and hydrolyze the milk sugar into the component monosaccharides—glucose and galactose. This approach takes advantage of two unique properties of enzymes: (1) their narrow specificity, which guarantees that only the desired reaction will occur in the product, thereby maintaining the nutritional integrity of the food; and (2) their catalytic function, which implies that very little enzyme is needed to produce a very large effect.

At the present, only two enzymes have met the exacting regulatory and commercial standards of purity, specificity, activity, and durability, while also conforming to the pH and temperature optima for treating milk products. One is the lactase from *Kluyveromyces lactis* (Maxilact), which has been used for hydrolysis of lactose in milk at both 4°C and 35°C in the pH range of 6 to 7 (Kosikowski and Wierzbicki 1973, Turner et al. 1976). The other is a lactase from *Aspergillus niger* (formerly known as Lactase LP, now Lactase N), which has a pH optimum of 4 to 5 at 55°C and has been used primarily to hydrolyze lactose in whey (Ford 1975), but also has been used for milk (Rand and Linklater 1973).

The effectiveness of food enzyme technology as a solution to clinical symptoms and low blood glucose rises associated with milk intolerance has been verified in numerous short-term experiments (Paige et al. 1975, Jones et al. 1976, Turner et al. 1976). Recent studies also have established the long-term acceptance of lactase-produced, low-lactose milk (Reasoner et al. 1981, Cheng et al. 1979). Thus, lactose-hydrolyzed milk offers milk-intolerant persons a dietary alternative to ceasing milk consumption, and can minimize the possibility of dangerously low intake levels for calcium, phosphorous, vitamin D, and riboflavin (Birge et al. 1967, Phillips and Briggs 1975).

Why, then, has the North American diary industry been reluctant to provide lactose-hydrolyzed milk? Part of the answer probably lies in confusion over the exact size of the population that is merely lactose intolerant versus the proportion that is actually both lactose and milk intolerant. However, the expense and availability of the required enzyme is also an important factor, and these drawbacks are compounded further by costly product inhibition that occurs during the reaction. The problems of enzyme cost and availability can be addressed by increased production and recovery/reuse of lactase through immobilization. Product inhibition is a more difficult problem, one that cannot be solved by immobilization per se. In the most severe cases of milk intolerance, the desired degree of lactose hydrolysis is so high (95%) that it may be impossible to achieve this level in commercial practice, unless complete elimination of product inhibition can be realized.

MILK PROCESSING

The fungal lactase from *A. niger* is an enzyme with exceptional thermal stability (fig. 21.1). The enzyme has a temperature optimum very close to 63°C, a significant temperature in dairy processing since it is one of the pasteurization

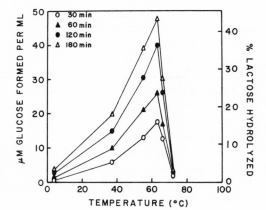

FIGURE 21.1. Temperature optimum for fungal lactase. The substrate was 4% lactose in 0.1 M sodium phosphate buffer at pH 6.5, and the enzyme concentration was 8 mg/10 ml. Source: Rand and Linklater 1973, reprinted with permission.

temperatures that have been used for milk. If milk is heated to this temperature and held for 30 minutes, the milk can be legally pasteurized.

Figure 21.2 illustrates the possible use of fungal lactase to process milk. If the fungal lactase is added to milk in the cold, the enzyme is heat activated as the temperature rises to 63°C for pasteurization, and hydrolysis of the lactose in the milk will occur during the 30- to 60-minute holding period. The hydrolysis process then occurs while growth of the pathogenic microorganisms is minimized. Thus, dairy plants could batch pasteurize milk and accomplish lactose hydrolysis in one operation.

The common pasteurization conditions employed for milk now avoid heating for such long times. The usual process is high temperature short time, in which the milk is heated to at least 72°C and held for not less than 15 seconds. This is not sufficient time to accomplish lactose hydrolysis, which is a relatively slow process. However, enzymatic hydrolysis of lactose in milk has been adapted to

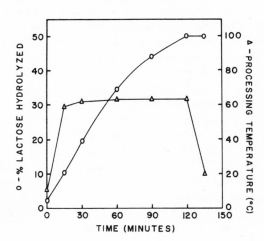

FIGURE 21.2. Processing of lactose-hydrolyzed skim milk with fungal lactase. The enzyme concentration was 0.33%. Source: Rand and Linklater 1973, reprinted with permission.

this process. It is possible to employ the fungal lactase, again, by addition to the milk in the cold, and to rely on the thermal stability of the enzyme to survive pasteurization and then hydrolyze the lactose in the milk, after the milk is put into cold storage (Finnie 1980). While 30% of the *A. niger* enzyme did survive an exposure of 73°C for 16 seconds, this fungal lactase requires heat activation and the resulting lactose hydrolysis reached only 8% to 10% during cold storage of milk. An enzyme that is active at refrigeration temperatures, such as the yeast lactase from *K. lactis,* would be required to accomplish lactose hydrolysis in cold milk. Unfortunately, yeast lactase does not have the heat stability to survive milk pasteurization. However, Dahlquist et al. (1977) have developed a method that circumvents this problem. Yeast lactase can be cold sterilized by ultrafiltration and injected into cooled milk following heat processing.

The alternate approach would be to accomplish lactose hydrolysis in milk prior to pasteurization. This process also requires yeast lactase that can be added to cold milk and that will accomplish up to 90% hydrolysis of lactose overnight at about 4°C to 6°C (Hourigan and Rand 1977). It is a normal operation at many dairy plants to receive milk late in the day and then hold it overnight at 4°C to 6°C for processing the next morning. Therefore, it is possible to hydrolyze the lactose and then process the hydrolyzed milk within a normal high temperature short time dairy operation. All enzyme treatments that would be utilized for processing lactose-hydrolyzed milk must be designed realistically, and must be processes that would minimize any additional treatment, steps, or equipment. The goal must be to hold the cost to a minimum so that the only additional expense would be that of the added enzyme.

PRODUCT INHIBITION

The problem that limits the use of enzyme-hydrolyzed low-lactose milk most severely is competitive product inhibition. Lactase enzymes used in milk processing are restricted by accumulation of the end product, galactose.

The effects of product inhibition on lactose hydrolysis in milk are illustrated in fig. 21.3. It is apparent that the lactose hydrolysis in milk in this case can be separated into two reaction groups. One occurs in milk with no sugar added or in which only glucose has been added. The second type occurs in milk samples to which galactose has been added. A comparison of the reaction times at 15 minutes and 30 minutes illustrates that the galactose is reducing the hydrolysis of lactose in the milk by about 50%. Hourigan (1976) made a direct comparison between the kinetics and inhibition of the two major food grade lactases in milk. The results are summarized and compared to previous results in table 21.1. Both enzymes are affected by galactose, but a comparison of the kinetic ratios reveals that the yeast enzyme, Maxilact ($K_m/K_i = 7.45$), is less severely inhibited in skim milk than the fungal enzyme, Lactase LP ($K_m/K_i = 13.5$).

Obviously, reduction of product inhibition during lactose hydrolysis by lactase enzymes will maximize enzyme efficiency. Hourigan (1976) proposed several

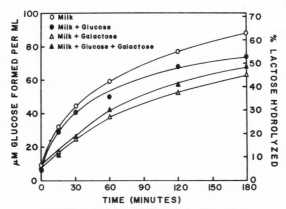

FIGURE 21.3. Lactose hydrolysis in skim milk at 63°C with fungal lactase in the presence of added glucose and galactose. The enzyme concentration was 0.25%. Source: Rand and Linklater 1973, reprinted with permission.

approaches that might be effective. Selection of lactase enzymes that have the highest affinity for lactose and the lowest affinity for the galactose inhibitor, or a low K_m/K_i ratio, can maximize the efficiency. Since lactases are essentially beta-galactosidases, product inhibition can be reduced by removing the beta-galactose product. Altering the mutarotation equilibrium to shift the beta form to the alpha form, would eliminate the specific form of the galactose that will combine with the enzyme. Enzymatic modification of the galactose to a form that would not complex with the enzyme could be another approach. The most common strategy would be to maintain much higher concentrations of the lactose (substrate) than of the galactose (product) in the vicinity of the enzyme. Since this is a competitive inhibition process, if the substrate can be replaced constantly in the vicinity of the enzyme, the product will be displaced and inhibition reduced.

TABLE 21.1
Inhibition of food grade lactase enzymes by galactose

Enzyme	Conditions*	K_m (app.) (mM)	K_i (app.) (mM)	K_m/K_i	Reference
Maxilact (*K. lactis*)	pH 7.0 phosphate buffer at 25°C	16.0	42.00	0.38	Woychik et al. 1974
Maxilact (*K. lactis*)	reconstituted skim milk at 35°C	63.7	8.55	7.45	Hourigan 1976
Lactase LP (*A. niger*)	pH 4.5 sodium phosphate buffer at 60°C	~50	3.90	13.00	Weetall et al. 1974
Lactase LP (*A. niger*)	reconstituted skim milk at 50°C	32.9	2.44	13.50	Hourigan 1976

*The substrate was lactose; galactose was a competitive inhibitor.

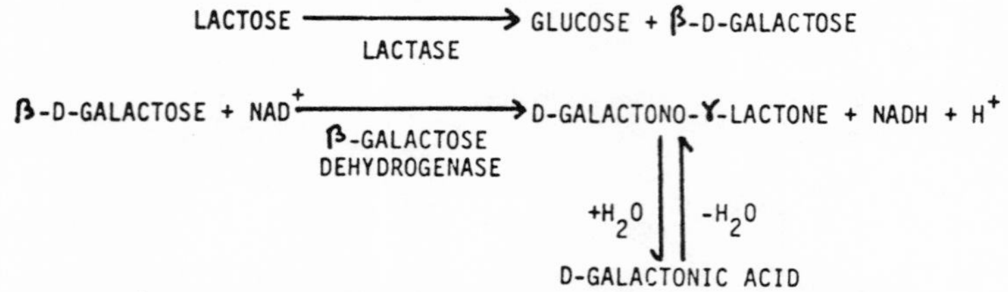

LACTOSE $\xrightarrow[\text{LACTASE}]{}$ GLUCOSE + β-D-GALACTOSE

β-D-GALACTOSE + NAD$^+$ $\xrightarrow[\substack{\text{β-GALACTOSE}\\\text{DEHYDROGENASE}}]{}$ D-GALACTONO-Υ-LACTONE + NADH + H$^+$

$+H_2O$ $\quad$ $-H_2O$

D-GALACTONIC ACID

FIGURE 21.4. The coupled enzyme system for β-galactose reduction of lactose hydrolysis.

LACTASE PRODUCT MODIFICATION

Enzymatic conversion of the products resulting from lactose hydrolysis by lactase is one approach with the potential to reduce inhibition and generate new products (Finnie et al. 1979). Figure 21.4 illustrates one process in which this theory can be tested. Coupling beta-galactose dehydrogenase, an enzyme specific for beta-galactose, with lactase can remove the competitive inhibitor by conversion to the corresponding lactone, which subsequently will hydrolyze to galactonic acid.

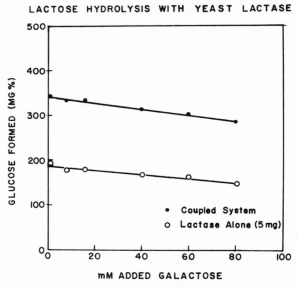

FIGURE 21.5. Coupled lactose hydrolysis with *K. lactis* lactase at 25°C in the presence of added galactose. The substrate was 2.7% lactose in 0.05 M Tris buffer at pH 6.5; lactase concentration was 0.4 units/ml; beta-galactose dehydrogenase concentration was 0.11 units/ml; and NAD concentration was 0.17 mg/ml; ●——● coupled, ○——○ lactase only.

Implementation of this enzyme system with the food grade lactases is shown in figs. 21.5 and 21.6. The beta-galactose dehydrogenase enzyme, when tried with the commercially available yeast lactase from *K. lactis* in milk, with concentrations of added galactose, shows a slight decline in activity (fig. 21.5). However, the coupled enzyme system virtually doubles the actual production of glucose compared to lactase alone, indicating that much greater hydrolysis of the lactose occurs when this product is removed.

A comparison of the coupled enzyme system with fungal lactase illustrates the significantly different K_i for this enzyme, when compared under the same conditions of added galactose in milk (fig. 21.6). The inhibitor binds very quickly to the fungal lactase at low galactose levels in milk, and activity declines rapidly before the coupled enzyme system can have any effect. Finally, at the higher galactose levels, the coupling system begins to exert a positive effect, shifting the equilibrium toward galactonic acid, and producing an increase in lactose hydrolysis.

Coupled enzymatic reactions for efficient conversion of the lactose in milk to acid is a process with the potential for development of new dairy products (Rand and Hourigan 1975). Enzymes that can convert both glucose and galactose to acid could provide an alternative method for milk acidification and yield efficient lactose hydrolysis processes. This method has been tested with two enzymes that react with both glucose and galactose. Figure 21.7 shows the acidification reaction in milk with the enzyme hexose oxidase from a marine red alga (Rand 1972). Figure 21.8 illustrates the formation of acid in skim milk when catalyzed by lactose dehydrogenase, an enzyme separated from cells of *Pseudomonas graveolens* (Wright and Rand 1973). In the presence of yeast lactase, a rapid drop in pH occurs as the monosaccharides are converted to acid. While there is some reaction in both cases with lactose, the acid development is greatly en-

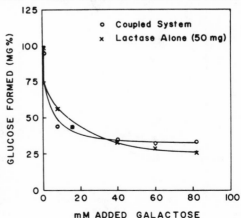

LACTOSE HYDROLYSIS WITH FUNGAL LACTASE

FIGURE 21.6. Coupled lactose hydrolysis with *A. niger* lactase at 25°C in the presence of added galactose. The substrate was 2.7% lactose in 0.05 M Tris buffer at pH 6.5; lactase concentration was 0.7 units/ml; beta-galactose dehydrogenase concentration was 0.11 units/ml; and NAD concentration was 0.17 mg/ml; O——O coupled, X——X lactase alone.

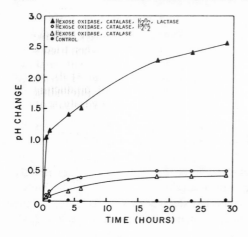

FIGURE 21.7. Acidification of lactose-hydrolyzed skim milk at 30°C by hexose oxidase. The yeast lactase concentration was 0.13%; hexose oxidase concentration was 0.1 unit/ml; catalase concentration was 20 units/ml; and hydrogen peroxide concentration was 0.1%. Source: Rand 1972, copyright © by Institute of Food Technologists, reprinted with permission.

hanced by lactase. The type of food product produced has a distinctive taste due to the bland thickened milk solids and to a mild aldonic acid souring. Products similar to yogurt can be produced quickly and easily, but they have a low lactose content. Additional possibilities for coupled enzymatic acidification include cottage and pizza-type cheeses, soured creamed products, and gelled dessert-type products.

LACTASE PRODUCT REMOVAL

The most common approach to decreasing end product inhibition has been to maintain a substrate concentration at a higher level than the inhibitor in the vicinity of the enzyme. This is perhaps one way in which the mammalian small

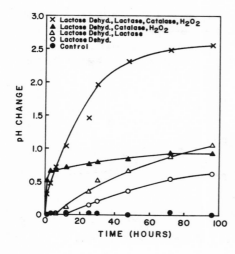

FIGURE 21.8. Formation of acid in lactose-hydrolyzed skim milk at 25°C by lactose dehydrogenase. The yeast lactase concentration was 0.25%; lactose dehydrogenase concentration was 9 units/ml; catalase concentration was 9 units/ml; and hydrogen peroxide concentration was 0.1%. Source: Wright and Rand 1973, copyright © by Institute of Food Technologists, reprinted with permission.

TABLE 21.2
Variation of lactose flow and glucose production due to changes in
pressure for a localized lactase reactor

Pressure (psig)*	Flow rate		Permeate glucose (mg/dl)	Glucose production	
	(ml/min)	(ml/hr)		(mg/hr)	(mg/min)
2.5	0.87	52.2	345	180	3.00
5.0	1.72	103.2	172	178	2.96

Note: Conditions were 30°C and 1,000 μg enzyme/cm^2.
*psig = gauge pressure.

intestine deals with this problem of galactose inhibition for the lactase, which is
effectively an immobilized enzyme on the apical surface of the small intestine.
This system is capable of rapid hydrolysis and absorption of lactose in individuals who are not lactase deficient (Gray 1975). While mammalian lactase is
subject to product inhibition (Wallenfels and Malhotra 1961), the combined
process of hydrolysis and absorption is controlled by the rate of the absorptive
process (Gray 1975). Thus, intestinal lactose hydrolysis is more efficient than it
would be in milk, which is conventionally a batch system in which there is no
way of removing the end products, which simply accumulate. A system with
lactase localized adjacent to a membrane would provide rapid removal of products through the membrane and maintain substrate concentration near the enzyme
much greater than the product concentration.

A membrane lactase reactor has been developed by localizing the *K. lactis*
lactase on the lumen side of a hollow fiber in a pressure-induced flow regime
(Maculan et al. 1978). The dependence of glucose production on flow rate in this
type of reactor is shown in table 21.2. Pressure-induced variations in the flow rate
produced proportional changes in glucose production. Increasing the pressure
twofold effectively doubled the flow rate, and the glucose production was pro-
portionately decreased to one-half. Table 21.3 shows the effect of enzyme concentration in the reactor at constant pressure and flow rates. Glucose production was
proportional to the localized enzyme concentration, since a threefold increase
virtually tripled the glucose production. Guy and Bingham (1978), in a study

TABLE 21.3
Variation of glucose production with lactose hydrolysis at different enzyme
concentrations in a localized lactase membrane reactor

Flow rate (ml/min)	Enzyme concentration (μg/cm^2)	Glucose production (mg/dl)
1.31	1,000	98
1.37	3,000	289

Note: Conditions were 25°C and 5 psig.

describing the properties of soluble *K. lactis* lactase, were unable to obtain a proportionate increase in lactose hydrolysis with increasing enzyme concentrations added to milk. This was due to competitive product inhibition, which restricted the ability of the soluble lactase. Thus, it appears that forcing the substrate through the enzyme layer in a membrane reactor kept the substrate concentration much greater than the product concentration in the vicinity of lactase and tended to promote hydrolysis.

LACTASE CAPSULES

The major efforts to overcome the consequences of milk intolerance have been directed mainly at enzyme processing of milk. An alternate method would be to supply the deficient lactase enzyme to the intolerant person just prior to consumption of the food containing the lactose.

DeAngelis et al. (1979) developed an immobilized lactase as a dose form. The *K. lactis* lactase was encapsulated in algin beads and enterically coated to deliver the enzyme to the site of lactose digestion and absorption, the small intestine. This approach permitted lactose hydrolysis to occur under conditions of product removal to minimize inhibition, while protecting lactase from protease degradation. A small clinical study involving six milk-tolerant and six milk-intolerant volunteers was utilized to establish the efficacy of this approach. Each of these volunteers was screened for symptoms with 240 ml skim milk on day one. The immobilized lactase-algin beads were administered as a capsule on subsequent days just prior to the same level of milk consumption, and the symptoms and severity for bloating, cramps, flatulence, and diarrhea were monitored by each subject. Table 21.4 shows the effect of this product on the average number of symptoms and the average severity reported per person. Only one person in the control group reported any symptoms with milk, while the milk-intolerant people had an average of 7.2 symptoms. A placebo algin bead capsule produced essentially the same result. One lactase capsule reduced the symptoms by 58%, and two capsules reduced symptoms by over 75%.

TABLE 21.4
Effect of lactase dose treatments on milk intolerance symptoms

Treatment	Average degree of severity/person*	
	Milk tolerant	Milk intolerant
Milk	1.2	7.2
1 Lactase capsule	0.0	3.0
2 Lactase capsules	0.0	1.7
1 Placebo capsule	0.0	7.3

*Includes four symptoms—bloating, cramps, flatulence, and diarrhea. Severity rated as: 1 = mild, 2 = moderate, 3 = severe.

CONCLUSIONS

Lactose-hydrolyzed milk is a viable product of enzyme technology, but the manufacture must be conducted optimally in terms of adaptation to milk processing and lactase efficiency. The enzyme efficiency is dependent on product inhibition, which appears to be a common problem for lactases. To obtain economically high degrees of conversion for the product-inhibited enzymatic hydrolysis of lactose in milk, industrial processes incorporating removal or conversion of the end products may be necessary. A lactase dose form can be an alternative approach to overcoming the product inhibition of these enzymes.

REFERENCES

Birge SJ, Keutmann HT, Cuatrecasas P, Whedon GD: Osteoporosis, intestinal lactase deficiency and low dietary calcium intake. *N Engl J Med* 276: 445–48, 1967.

Cheng AHR, Brunsor O, Espinoza J, Fones HL, Monckeberg F, Chichester CO, Rand AG, Hourigan JA: Long-term acceptance of low-lactose milk. *Am J Clin Nutr* 32: 1989–93, 1979.

Dahlquist A, Asp N-G, Burvall A, Rausing H: Hydrolysis of lactose in milk and whey with minute amounts of lactase. *J Dairy Res* 44: 541–48, 1977.

DeAngelis MA, Lausier JM, Rand AG: Development of a lactase dose form by microencapsulation. *IFT 79 Program Abstr* 39: 129, 1979.

Finnie KJ: Continuous processing of low lactose milk to minimize lactase product inhibition. Master's thesis, University of Rhode Island, Kingston, 1980.

Finnie KJ, Hourigan JA, Rand AG: Reduction of product inhibition during enzymatic lactose hydrolysis. *IFT 79 Program Abstr* 39: 101, 1979.

Ford JR: Immobilized lactase: A review and engineering analysis. *Enzyme Technol Dig* 4: 23–29, 1975.

Gray GM: Carbohydrate digestion and absorption: Role of the small intestine. *N Engl J Med* 292: 1225–30, 1975.

Guy EJ, Bingham EW: Properties of beta-galactosidase of *Saccharomyces lactis* in milk and milk products. *J Dairy Sci* 61: 147–51, 1978.

Hourigan JA: Kinetic studies of the enzymic hydrolysis of lactose. Ph.D. thesis, University of Rhode Island, Kingston, 1976.

Hourigan JA, Rand AG: The production and use of low-lactose milk. *Proc Nutr Soc Aust* 2: 72, 1977.

Jones DV, Latham MC, Kosikowski FV, Woodward G: Symptom response to lactose-reduced milk in lactose-intolerant adults. *Am J Clin Nutr* 29: 633–38, 1976.

Kosikowski FV, Wierzbicki LE: Lactose hydrolysis of raw and pasteurized milks by *Saccharomyces lactis* lactase. *J Dairy Sci* 56: 146–48, 1973.

Maculan TP, Hourigan JA, Rand AG: Application of a localized enzyme membrane reactor for the hydrolysis of lactose. *J Dairy Sci* 61 (Suppl. no. 1): 114, 1978.

Paige DM, Bayless TM, Huang SS, Wexler R: Lactose intolerance and lactose hydrolyzed milk. In *Physiological Effects of Food Carbohydrates*, A Jeanes, J Hodge (eds). ACS Symposium Series no. 15. Washington, D.C.: American Chemical Society, 1975, pp 191–206.

Phillips MC, Briggs GM: Milk and its role in the American diet. *J Diary Sci* 58: 1751–63, 1975.

Rand AG: Direct enzymatic conversion of lactose to acid: Glucose oxidase and hexose oxidase. *J Food Sci* 37: 698–701, 1972.

Rand AG, Hourigan JA: Direct enzymatic conversion of lactose in milk to acid. *J Dairy Sci* 58: 1144–50, 1975.

Rand AG, Linklater PM: The use of enzymes for the reduction of lactose levels in milk products. *Aust J Dairy Technol* 28: 63–67, 1973.

Reasoner J, Maculan TP, Rand AG, Thayer WR: Clinical studies with low-lactose milk. *Am J Clin Nutr* 34: 54–60, 1981.

Turner SJ, Daly T, Hourigan JA, Rand AG, Thayer WR: Utilization of a low-lactose milk. *Am J Clin Nutr* 29: 739–44, 1976.

Wallenfels K, Malhotra OK: Galactosidases. In *Advances in Carbohydrate Chemistry,* ML Wolfrom, RS Tipson (eds). New York: Academic Press, 1961, 16: 239.

Weetall HH, Havewala NB, Pitcher WH, Detar CC, Vann WP, Yaverbaum S: Preparation of immobilized lactase, continued studies on the enzymatic hydrolysis of lactose. *Biotechnol Bioeng* 16: 689–96, 1974.

Woychik JH, Wondolowski MV, Dahl KJ: Preparation and application of immobilized beta-galactosidase of *Saccharomyces lactis.* In *Immobilized Enzymes in Food and Microbial Processes,* AC Olson, CL Cooney (eds). New York: Plenum Publishing, 1974, pp 41–49.

Wright DG, Rand AG: Direct enzymatic conversion of lactose to acid: Lactose dehydrogenase. *J Food Sci* 38: 1132–35, 1973.

CHAPTER 22

POTENTIAL APPLICATIONS

FOR LACTOSE-HYDROLYZED MILK AND WHEY

FRACTIONS IN DAIRY FOODS

V. H. Holsinger

The potential for the enzymatic modification of the lactose in dairy products has been recognized since the early 1950s. With the commercial development of effective lactases (β-galactosidases) isolated from microbial sources, the widespread production of lactose-modified dairy products became possible. At present, lactose-modified beverage milk may be purchased in some local supermarkets and in some dairy stores.

AVAILABLE ENZYMES

The two lactase enzymes of commercial significance are isolated from the yeast *Saccharomyces lactis* (*S. lactis*) and the fungus *Aspergillus niger* (*A. niger*). These lactases vary widely in their properties, particularly in pH and temperature optima. Lactase from *S. lactis* has a pH optimum of 6.8 to 7.0, a pH stability of 6.0 to 8.5, and a temperature optimum of 35°C. The lack of stability below pH 6.0 precludes the use of *S. lactis* lactase in treating acid whey (pH 4.5), although it is well suited for treating milk (pH 6.6) and sweet whey (pH 6.2). However, *A. niger* lactase, with a pH optimum of 4.0 to 4.5, wide pH stability (pH 3.0 to 7.0), and a temperature optimum of 55°C, is available for the enzymatic modification of acid whey (Woychik and Holsinger 1977).

Purity, activity, and cost of the lactases must be considered in the development of any large-scale enzymatic manufacturing process for lactose hydrolysis. The simplest method is to add the soluble enzyme directly to the milk; however, batch operations of this type are expensive because the enzyme is not recoverable for reuse.

Immobilized enzyme technology has been evaluated with lactases to improve the economics of lactose hydrolysis. A detailed discussion of the physical and chemical methods available for lactase immobilization is outside the scope of this chapter, but the subject has been reviewed (Wondolowski 1976). A satisfactory immobilized system has not been developed with *S. lactis* lactase because of a lack of stability after immobilization (Woychik et al. 1974). *A. niger* lactase, however, has proven adaptable to immobilized systems, although some operating difficulties still exist (Olson and Stanley 1973, Hustad et al. 1973, Hasselburger et al. 1974).

Applications.   Hydrolysis of the lactose in milk or whey results in changes in several physical and chemical properties of interest to the dairy manufacturer. Benefits include reduction of lactose content, prevention of lactose crystallization, increase in solubility and sweetness, and more readily fermentable sugars. Applications are obvious, not only for modifying functional characteristics, but also for providing low lactose dairy products for the lactase-deficient or lactose-intolerant individual.

Test Products.   Evaluation of lactase in product manufacture was conducted by preparing a series of dairy products from lactase-treated milk with 28% to 90% of the lactose converted to monosaccharides (Guy et al. 1974). The enzyme used was isolated from *S. lactis* as a colorless free-flowing powder; the enzyme is also available in fluid form in a glycerol carrier. Lactose hydrolysis was carried out in

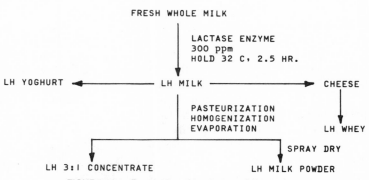

FIGURE 22.1. Preparation of low-lactose dairy products.

a batch operation by incubating fresh pasteurized whole or skimmed milk pre-heated to 32°C with 300 ppm lactase for 2.5 hours with continuous agitation (fig. 22.1) or by treating milk held in the silo at 4°C with 150 ppm for 16 to 18 hours (Thompson and Brower 1976). After treatment in this manner, the fluid milk could be used directly as a beverage or processed further into other products (fig. 22.1).

MODIFIED MILK APPLICATIONS

When the organoleptic qualities of lactase-treated milk were evaluated, some difficulties were encountered because hydrolysis of lactose to the constituent monosaccharides glucose and galactose resulted in a marked increase in sweetness intensity of the milk. An objective sweetness scale, developed to simplify reporting the changes brought about by lactose hydrolysis, permitted the results of lactase action to be equated with the addition of sucrose to untreated milk. Hydrolyzing 30%, 60%, and 90% of the lactose present had almost the same effects on flavor as adding 0.3%, 0.6%, and 0.9% sucrose, respectively, to the milk (Guy et al. 1974).

Although the only flavor change detected in lactase-treated beverage milk was the increased sweetness, there was some question as to whether this change would be acceptable to the consumer. In a study carried out at The Johns Hopkins University, Paige et al. (1975) reported that Negro adolescents, a target population for low-lactose milk, found milk with 90% of its lactose in the hydrolyzed form was acceptable to drink even though 56% of the respondents judged it to be sweeter than an untreated control.

Frozen 3:1 Concentrates. A highly attractive way of preserving milk with minimal flavor change is in the form of a frozen 3:1 concentrate. Unfortunately, such concentrates thicken and coagulate during storage because of the crystallization of lactose, which is brought to the saturation point by concentration of the milk.

Early research had shown that lactose hydrolysis led to improved physical stability of concentrated milks during storage (Tumerman et al. 1954). However, when milk with 90% of its lactose hydrolyzed by lactase was concentrated and frozen, storage stability was increased by only one month over that of an untreated control (fig. 22.2). Further examination of Tumerman's work has shown that the samples had been heated above pasteurization requirements. Subsequently, samples that were postheated at 71°C for 30 minutes after being canned showed only a moderate rise in viscosity after the nine months of storage (fig. 22.2). There was no significant difference in flavor score of the reconstituted concentrate containing 90% hydrolyzed lactose and an untreated fresh control with added sucrose (Guy et al. 1974, Holsinger and Roberts 1976).

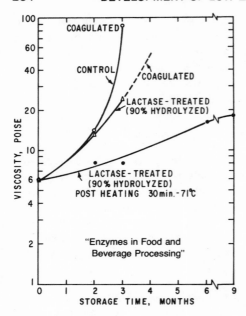

FIGURE 22.2. Effect of storage on viscosity of frozen 3:1 pasteurized whole milk concentrates. Source: Woychik and Holsinger 1977, p. 72, reprinted with permission.

Dried Products. Some problems were encountered in spray drying skim and whole milk concentrates. Because of the lactose hydrolysis, the powder, especially the skim powder, had a tendency to stick to the hot metal surfaces of the spray dryer. The powder also lumped in the cone and star valve unless cooled with forced dry air as it left the cone. When the sticking properties of low-lactose nonfat dry milk were investigated, it was found that the "sticking" temperature was lowered 10 to 15 degrees by the lactose treatment as compared with that of an untreated skim powder of comparable moisture content (table 22.1).

For efficient spray drying, the surfaces of the powder collecting apparatus should be held at temperatures below 60°C. Drying temperatures should be reduced to a minimum, and the powder should be cooled rapidly after collection to avoid clumping.

TABLE 22.1
"Sticking" temperatures of low-lactose nonfat dry milk

Sample	Percentage lactose hydrolyzed	Sticking point (°C)
Control	0	75.4
Low-lactose A	80	59.2
Low-lactose B	87	64.6

Source: Guy et al. 1974, table 10, reprinted with permission.

Cultured Products. Cultured products always have been of interest to the lactase-deficient individual because of the fermentation of the lactose. Cultured products manufactured from lactase-treated milk include buttermilk, yogurt, and cottage and cheddar-type cheeses.

Low-lactose cultured buttermilk has been prepared readily from lactase-treated milk. However, the increased sweetness brought about by lactose hydrolysis was objectionable to most consumers even though the coagulation time was reduced (Gyuricsek and Thompson 1976).

Yogurt, particularly the fruit-flavored types, is enjoying a rapidly increasing popularity. Yogurt generally has been thought to contain low levels of lactose because of the utilization of lactose during the fermentation process. However, only about 15% to 20% of the lactose is utilized during fermentation, and the practice of fortifying yogurt with nonfat milk results in appreciable amounts of added lactose. Lactose values of 3.3% to 5.7% have been reported in commercial yogurts, amounts comparable to that found in fluid milk (Goodenough 1975).

Lactase treatment of milk prior to yogurt manufacture resulted in accelerated acid development, which may be due to the more rapid utilization of total available carbohydrate when free glucose is present. For example, from a starting lactose concentration of 7.11%, only about 26% of the lactose was utilized, yielding a lactose concentration of 5% in a control (table 22.2). Yet when the milk was lactase-treated before being cultured, the sugar utilization pattern was quite different; the galactose was not utilized at all by the organisms and an appreciable amount of the lactose was still present (table 22.2) (O'Leary and Woychik 1976).

The manufacture of yogurt from lactase-hydrolyzed milk also made plain yogurt more acceptable to the consumer. On a nine point hedonic scale (Peryam and Pilgrim 1957), lactase-treated yogurt was rated 6.1 compared to 4.9 for the control (Holsinger 1978). The acid flavor appeared to be reduced by the lactase treatment, and consumers in the United States generally prefer less acid yogurts.

TABLE 22.2
Sugar concentrations in control and
lactase-treated yogurts

Sugar	Percentage	
	Control	Lactase-treated
Lactose	5.0	1.5
Glucose	0.0	1.6
Galactose	0.2	2.1

Source: O'Leary and Woychik 1976, table 1, copyright © Institute of Food Technologists, reprinted with permission.

The manufacture of cheddar and cottage cheeses from lactase-treated milk has been described (Thompson and Brower 1976, Gyuricsek and Thompson 1976). In the case of cheddar cheese manufacture, lactose prehydrolysis is advantageous from an economic standpoint; there is virtually no lactose present in aged cheese. Cheddaring time is reduced, and, more important, the ripening time is accelerated so the cheese can be marketed more quickly. Set time is reduced when cottage cheese is made from lactase-hydrolyzed milk, and, in some cases, increased yields have been found.

WHEY APPLICATIONS

A spin-off of the manufacture of cheddar and cottage cheeses from lactase-treated milk is that the whey produced contains hydrolyzed lactose. Economic whey disposal is a problem that has plagued the dairy industry for many years. In 1978, 37.9 billion pounds of whey were produced in the United States, only about 60% of which was utilized (Crop Reporting Board 1979). Because of stringent antipollution regulations, whey is finding its way into more and more food products instead of being disposed of in streams and municipal sewage systems. Modification of the whey by lactase treatment offers considerable potential for new avenues of utilization.

Whey is the greenish-yellow fluid drained from the vat after the casein portion of the milk has been coagulated during cheese manufacture. Its solids contain about 50% of the nutrients of milk (Holsinger et al. 1973); although small amounts of high quality protein equivalent to that of egg are present, fluid whey is essentially a crude solution of lactose (table 22.3).

The increased sweetness brought about by lactose hydrolysis suggests that lactase-modified whey might be useful as an ingredient in sweet foods. The low sweetness level of unhydrolyzed lactose in solution relative to sucrose and other sweeteners does not permit its use as a sweetener, but both glucose and galactose are sweeter than the lactose (table 22.4). In addition, the increase in solubility brought about by treatment with lactase permits the manufacture of noncrystalliz-

TABLE 22.3
Composition of whey solids

Component	Sweet whey	Acid whey
Total protein	11.5%	11.4%
Lactose	74.4%	66.8%
Ash	7.4%	10.2%
Lactic acid	<1.0%	9.6%
Fat	2.7%	<1.0%
pH	6.5	4.7

Source: Holsinger 1976, table 1, reprinted with permission.

TABLE 22.4
Relative sweetness of sugars

Concentration to give equivalent sweetness (percentage)

Sucrose	Glucose	Fructose	Lactose	Galactose
1.0	1.8	0.8	3.5	2.1
5.0	8.3	4.2	15.7	8.3
10.0	13.9	8.6	25.9	15.0

Source: Holsinger 1976, table 3, reprinted with permission.

ing high solids syrups for use in beverages, ice creams, and in other foods (table 22.5).

Whey Beverages.   The use of whey and its fractions for beverage manufacture has been studied extensively, especially in Europe (Holsinger et al. 1974). Such beverages include alcoholic and snack drinks, milk analogues, and liquid breakfasts with protein contents ranging from less than 0.5% to more than 3.5% (table 22.6).

Wines.   The consumption of table wines is increasing rapidly in the United States. In 1978, 2.81 gallons per capita were consumed, representing a market value of more than $2 billion (1979 Market Index 1979). A major problem, however, in utilizing whey as a fermentation substrate has been that relatively few organisms can ferment lactose, *Kluyveromyces fragilis* being the most efficient (O'Leary et al. 1977a). These organisms are also much less alcohol tolerant than glucose fermenting wine yeasts such as *Saccharomyces cerevisiae*.

The availability of lactase-hydrolyzed wheys and whey permeates prepared by ultrafiltration led O'Leary et al. (1977a, 1977b) to compare alcohol production in these media with *S. cerevisiae* and *K. fragilis*. A diauxic fermentation pattern was found in the lactase-treated media, with glucose being fermented before galactose; although *S. cerevisiae* produced alcohol from glucose more rapidly

TABLE 22.5
Solubility of sugars in water at room temperature

Sugar	Solubility
Sucrose	67.9%
Glucose	45.4%
Fructose	80.3%
Lactose	18.0%
Galactose	40.6%

Source: Holsinger 1976, table 2, reprinted with permission.

TABLE 22.6
Types of whey beverages

Beverage use	Percentage protein
Alcoholic beverages	
Kwas, beer,	<0.5
kefir, wine	
Snack beverages	
Soft drinks	0.5–1.0
Drink powders	
Imitation milks	1.0–1.5
Liquid breakfast, dietary supplements	2.5–3.5

Source: Holsinger et al. 1974, reprinted with permission.

than did *K. fragilis*, galactose was fermented only when *S. cerevisiae* was pregrown on galactose. With *S. cerevisiae*, alcohol yields as high as 6.5% were obtained in lactase-treated permeates condensed to 30% to 35% total solids before inoculation; maximum yield with *K. fragilis* was 4.5% at 20% total solids. It was concluded from these studies that, although prehydrolysis of the lactose in wheys and whey permeates is advantageous in that microbial species unable to ferment lactose may be used, commercial processes must consider diauxic problems and must efficiently convert galactose to alcohol.

Researchers at Oregon State University demonstrated the possibility of making a whey wine using a wine yeast. As an extension of this work, the Foremost Food Company,* under an EPA grant, investigated the technical and economic feasibility of whey wine production under commercial conditions.

After the whey protein was removed by ultrafiltration, the whey permeate was given an infusion of glucose, inoculated with wine yeasts, and fermented for 8 to 12 days; 8% to 12% alcohol developed in the mixture. After this was racked, demineralized, and decolorized, a crystal clear product was obtained that then could be processed further into a lightly carbonated ''pop'' wine (fig. 22.3). All of the lactose was still intact and present in this wine. Processing with a lactose fermenting organism was not practical because lactose fermentation is more time consuming, and thus more costly (Palmer and Marquardt 1978).

Nonalcoholic Beverages.   Carbonated beverages of the soft drink type containing whey components are available commercially. Probably the best known of these is Rivella, which appeared on the market in Switzerland in 1952 (Holsinger et al. 1974). Rivella is a sparkling, crystal clear, herbal infusion of deproteinized whey, promoted as something of a therapeutic tonic. This product contains about 9.7% total solids, 45.5% of which are lactose.

*Reference to brand or firm name does not constitute endorsement by the U.S. Department of Agriculture over others of a similar nature not mentioned.

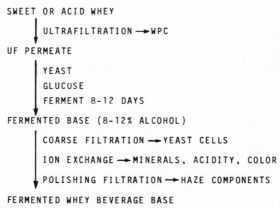

SWEET OR ACID WHEY

  | ULTRAFILTRATION →WPC

UF PERMEATE

  | YEAST
  | GLUCOSE
  | FERMENT 8-12 DAYS

FERMENTED BASE (8-12% ALCOHOL)

  | COARSE FILTRATION →YEAST CELLS
  | ION EXCHANGE →MINERALS, ACIDITY, COLOR
  | POLISHING FILTRATION →HAZE COMPONENTS

FERMENTED WHEY BEVERAGE BASE

FIGURE 22.3. Process flow chart for whey wine production. Source: Palmer and Marquardt 1978, p. 31, reprinted with permission.

A lactase-hydrolyzed whey permeate has been used to develop a prototype snack-type soft drink, "Lactofruit," projected to be cheaper to produce and sell than other whey beverages because of the unique process employed (Fresnel and Moore 1978). The process involves ultrafiltration of the whey, followed by lactose hydrolysis by enzymatic electrocatalysis. Enzymatic electrocatalysis is advantageous in that it is able to counterbalance the loss of enzyme activity with time; the current is regulated continuously so that local pH variations are compensated for and enzyme activity is maintained at a constant level. The basic composition of Lactofruit shows that, in spite of lactase treatment, only 50% hydrolysis was attained; some lactose does remain in the beverage (table 22.7). However, since the drink is not fermented, the taste quality is sweet and different from that of most other whey beverages.

The soft drink market in the United States is enormous; in 1978, 7.6 billion gallons, sufficient to supply 369 12-ounce bottles per capita per annum and

TABLE 22.7
Proximate composition of Lactofruit

Component	g/liter
Glucose	12.5
Galactose	12.5
Lactose	25.0
Ash	4.0–5.0
Nitrogenous components	2.0
Sucrose + flavorings	20.0

Source: Fresnel and Moore 1978, p. 45, reprinted with permission.

representing an estimated wholesale value of $12 billion, were produced (1979 Market Index 1979). Consequently, the whey producers would be very interested in penetrating this market. At the present time, Rivella is undergoing test marketing. Therefore, it is a good possibility that soft drinks containing various levels of lactose, glucose, and galactose soon may be available in the United States; they are already widely available in Europe.

High Protein Beverages. An example of a high protein beverage containing significant amounts of lactose is whey-soy drink mix, a milk analogue designed for use in child feeding programs in developing countries (Holsinger et al. 1977). The formulation, containing 41.3% whey solids, yields a finished product containing about 50% carbohydrate, the bulk of which is lactose.

Because the product was designed for preschool children, no problems with lactose intolerance were anticipated. However, it has been shown that as much as 50% of the population could be lactase deficient by 3 years of age in developing countries, where whey-soy drink mix was distributed (Paige et al. 1972); it seemed advisable to investigate lactose-modified whey-soy drink mix. After trial production runs and storage tests were made with whey with 90% of its lactose hydrolyzed, it was concluded that no production difficulties existed. An additional benefit was conferred by lactase treatment, since consumers preferred the hydrolyzed lactose whey-soy drink mix because of the noticeably sweeter taste (Holsinger and Roberts 1976).

Frozen Desserts. Ice cream and other frozen desserts represent a large outlet for milk. In 1978, 1.20 billion gallons were produced (Crop Reporting Board 1979).

Present ice cream standards permit whey to be used in ice cream up to a level of 25% of the milk-solids-not-fat. Because there had been plans to alter these standards, Guy (1980) evaluated the use of lactase-treated whey as an ingredient in ice cream. Formulation with lactase-treated whey permitted a reduction of 10% or more in the concentration of the cane sugar without loss of quality (table 22.8). This suggests that lactase-treated whey might be used effectively as an ingredient in calorie-reduced sweet foods. Unfortunately, reduction of the milk-solids-not-fat with increasing levels of whey amounted to a 30% increase in the ash and a 20% decrease in the protein content of an ice cream prepared with 11% whey solids.

Another possibility for utilization of lactase-treated whey is as an ingredient in novelty water ices on a stick. According to Guy et al. (1966), cottage cheese whey could be incorporated into water ices at a 2.3% solids level. This is advantageous in that addition of acid whey permits the manufacture of less acid water ice; the calcium and phosphate present in the whey also are present in the ice pop and could be beneficial in reducing dental cavities (Wagg et al. 1965). With only slight formula modifications, lactase-hydrolyzed whey also could be used in water ices.

TABLE 22.8
Formulation of ice creams

	Percentage	
Whey solids*	Milk-solids-not-fat	Cane sugar
0.00	11.00	15.00
2.75	9.50	13.75
5.50	8.00	12.50
8.25	6.50	11.25
11.00	5.00	10.00

Source: Guy 1980, table 2, copyright ©
Institute of Food Technologists, reprinted with permission.
Note: Based on 12% fat and 0.14%
stabilizer.
*67% or 79% hydrolyzed lactose.

Sherbet formulations containing whey solids also have been developed; whey is added at the 5% level (Whittier and Webb 1950). Lactase-treated whey might be a suitable ingredient for sherbet manufacture with only minor formula alterations.

Syrups. Clear, noncrystallizing high solids syrups may be prepared from hydrolyzed-lactose or lactase-treated whey for use as food ingredients. A syrup may be prepared readily with *S. lactis* lactase by treating a lactose solution at pH 6.4 for 6 hours at 30°C. After being heated to inactivate the enzyme, the low-lactose mixture is then decolorized, filtered, demineralized with ion exchange resins, and condensed to 60% total solids (fig. 22.4) (Guy 1978).

At high concentrations, hydrolyzed-lactose syrups are just as sweet as equiva-

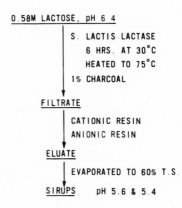

FIGURE 22.4. Process flow chart for enzyme-processed syrups. Source: Guy and Edmondson 1978, p. 544, reprinted with permission.

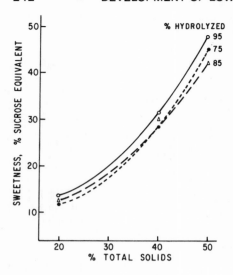

FIGURE 22.5. Sweetness equivalence to sucrose for hydrolyzed-lactose syrups. Source: Guy and Edmondson 1978, p. 546, reprinted with permission.

lent solutions of sucrose (fig. 22.5). Although these syrups cannot compete economically with corn syrups in the United States, in Europe lactase-hydrolyzed syrups from lactose or whey are finding a market as ingredients in some sweet foods.

Confections. Whey has been used for many years as an ingredient in candy. Webb (1966) described a variety of confections in which whey has been used successfully as an ingredient (table 22.9). At present, whey finds its greatest use in caramel manufacture (Alikonis 1973).

Guy (1978) evaluated lactase-hydrolyzed whey and hydrolyzed-lactose syrups as humectants in caramels. Caramels prepared without humectant showed much more sugar crystallization and shrinkage than those containing hydrolyzed-

TABLE 22.9
Candy from whey

Variety	Whey as percentage of total candy solids
Wheyfers	40
Whipped fudge	14
Caramel	21
Taffy	26
Fudge	20

Source: Webb 1966, table 2, reprinted with permission.

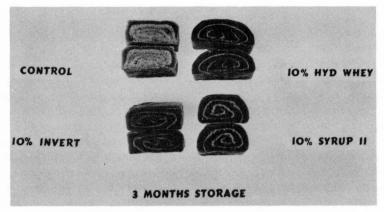

FIGURE 22.6. Physical appearance of caramels after three months of storage at 23°C. Source: Guy 1978, p. 983, copyright © Institute of Food Technologists, reprinted with permission.

lactose syrup or whey (fig. 22.6). After six months of storage, the caramels that contained hydrolyzed-lactose syrups had lost significantly less moisture than had the controls. The sample with the best taste quality was a caramel prepared with the hydrolyzed-lactose syrup.

Presently, whey is not permitted to be added to chocolate because it is not an optional ingredient within the chocolate standards (U.S., Office of Federal Register 1973). However, a successful chocolate formulation containing whey has been developed (O'Connell 1975). The particular whey was 25% demineralized and was used not only as a sucrose replacement but also as a replacement for part of the chocolate liquor (table 22.10). No examples of the lactase-hydrolyzed whey being used in this type of application are currently available; however, if the price of cacao keeps rising, economic factors may bring about the addition of whey to chocolate as well.

TABLE 22.10
Chocolate formulation from whey

Ingredient	Percentage	
	Control	Experimental
Chocolate liquor	12.5	10.0
Whole milk solids	18.0	18.6
Cocoa butter	21.0	21.6
Sucrose	48.0	35.9
Whey solids	—	13.3
Lecithin and vanillin	0.5	0.5

Source: O'Connell 1975, p. 116, reprinted with permission.

SUMMARY AND CONCLUSIONS

Possibilities for widespread production of lactose-modified dairy products have been opened up by the development of commercial sources of the enzyme lactase (β-galactosidase). Low-lactose fluid milk is commercially available. Such milk, when condensed, may be used to manufacture frozen 3:1 concentrates that do not thicken and coagulate during storage. Lactose-modified nonfat dry milk may be manufactured for use as a food ingredient. Cultured products such as yogurt also may be prepared successfully from lactase-treated milk.

Antipollution regulations have brought about the increased use of cheese whey in foods. Lactose-modified whey may be condensed to high solids noncrystallizing syrups for use in soft drinks and confections. Some traditional wine yeasts will ferment low-lactose whey for the manufacture of whey wine. Lactase-treated whey, when added as an ingredient in ice cream, permits a 10% sucrose reduction. Use of lactase-treated products may lead to production efficiencies and permit monetary savings as well as provide nutritional advantages to the lactase-deficient segment of the population.

The dairy industry today has the technology available for the enzymatic hydrolysis of the lactose in milk and milk products. Lactose-modified milks and dairy products may be used with confidence by the lactose-intolerant or lactase-deficient individual. Because of the increased sweetness, some lactase-treated products could be utilized in calorie-reduced sweet foods. Whey production is increasing every year and raises special utilization problems. However, application of lactase enzyme technology offers new opportunities for innovative whey processing into more profitable outlets.

REFERENCES

Alikonis JJ: Whey solids increasing use in confections. In *Proceedings of the Whey Products Conference*, Chicago, Ill., 14–15 June 1973. Philadelphia, Pa.: USDA, ERRC pub. no. 3779, 1973, pp 57–60.

Crop Reporting Board: *Dairy Products Annual Summary 1978*. DA 2-1(79), June. Washington, D.C.: Statistical Reporting Service, USDA, 1979.

Fresnel JM, Moore KK: Swiss scientists develop soft drink from whey. *Food Prod Develop* 12: 45, 1978.

Goodenough E: Carbohydrate content of yogurt: Effects of viable microflora upon digestion of the lactose by laboratory rats. Ph.D. dissertation, Rutgers University, New Brunswick, N.J., 1975.

Guy EJ: Evaluation of milk caramels containing hydrolyzed lactose. *J Food Sci* 43: 980–84, 1978.

Guy EJ: Partial replacement of nonfat milk solids and cane sugar in ice cream with lactose hydrolyzed sweet whey solids. *J Food Sci* 45: 129–33, 1980.

Guy EJ, Edmondson LF: Preparation and properties of sirups made by hydrolysis of lactose. *J Dairy Sci* 61: 542–49, 1978.

Guy EJ, Tamsma A, Kontson A, Holsinger VH: Lactase-treated milk provides base to develop products for lactose-intolerant populations. *Food Prod Develop* 8(8): 50–54, 1974.

Guy EJ, Vettel HE, Pallansch MJ: Use of foam-spray dried cottage cheese whey in water ices. *J Dairy Sci* 49: 1156–57, 1966.

Gyuricsek DM, Thompson MP: Hydrolyzed lactose cultured dairy products: II. Manufacture of yoghurt, buttermilk and cottage cheese. *Cultured Dairy Prod J* 11: 12–13, 1976.

Hasselburger FX, Allen B, Paruchuri EK, Charles M, Coughlin RW: Immobilized enzymes: Lactase bonded to stainless steel and other dense carriers for use in fluidized bed reactors. *Biochem Biophys Res Commun* 57: 1054–62, 1974.

Holsinger VH: New dairy products for use in candy manufacture. *Manufacturing Confectioner* 56(1): 25–28, 1976.

Holsinger VH: Applications of lactose-modified milk and whey. *Food Technol* 32: 35–40, 1978.

Holsinger VH, Posati LP, DeVilbiss ED: Whey beverages: A review. *J Dairy Sci* 57: 849–59, 1974.

Holsinger VH, Posati LP, DeVilbiss ED, Pallansch MJ: Variation of total and available lysine in dehydrated products from cheese wheys by different processes. *J Dairy Sci* 56: 1498–1504, 1973.

Holsinger VH, Roberts NE: New products from lactose-hydrolyzed milk. *Dairy and Ice Cream Field* 159(3): 30–32, 1976.

Holsinger VH, Sutton CS, Vettel HE, Edmondson LF, Crowley PR, Berntson BL, Pallansch MJ: Production and properties of a nutritious beverage base from soy products and cheese whey. In *Proceedings of the IV International Congress of Food Science and Technology,* Madrid, Spain, 23–27 September 1974, vol. V. Valencia, Spain: Instituto de Agroquímica y Tecnología de Alimentos, 1977, pp 25–33.

Hustad GO, Richardson T, Olson NF: Immobilization of β-galactosidase in an insoluble carrier with a polyisocyanate polymer: I. Preparation and properties. *J Dairy Sci* 56: 1111–17, 1973.

1979 Market Index. *Beverage World* 98(1264): 48–78, 1979.

O'Connell RT: Whey in chocolate confections. In *Proceedings of the Whey Products Conference,* Chicago, Ill., 18–19 September 1974. Philadelphia, Pa.: USDA, ERRC pub. no. 3996, 1975, pp 116–18.

O'Leary VS, Green R, Sullivan BC, Holsinger VH: Alcohol production by selected yeast strains in lactose-hydrolyzed acid whey. *Biotechnol Bioeng* 19: 1019–35, 1977a.

O'Leary VS, Sutton C, Bencivengo M, Sullivan B, Holsinger VH: Influence of lactose hydrolysis and solids concentration on alcohol production by yeast in acid whey ultrafiltrate. *Biotechnol Bioeng* 19: 1689–1702, 1977b.

O'Leary VS, Woychik JH: A comparison of some chemical properties of yogurts made from control and lactase-treated milks. *J Food Sci* 41: 791–93, 1976.

Olson AC, Stanley WL: Lactase and other enzymes bound to a phenol-formaldehyde resin with glutaraldehyde. *J Agric Food Chem* 21: 440–45, 1973.

Paige DM, Bayless TM, Huang SS, Wexler R: Lactose intolerance and lactose-hydrolyzed milk. In *Physiological Effects of Food Carbohydrates,* A Jeanes, J Hodge (eds). Washington, D.C.: American Chemical Society, Symposium ser. no. 15, 1975, pp 191–206.

Paige DM, Leonardo E, Cordano A, Nakashima J, Adrianzen TB, Graham GG: Lactose intolerance in Peruvian children: Effect of age and early nutrition. *Am J Clin Nutr* 25: 297–301, 1972.

Palmer GM, Marquardt RF: Modern technology transforms whey into wine. *Food Prod Develop* 12: 31–34, 1978.

Peryam DR, Pilgrim FJ: Hedonic scale method for measuring food preference. *Food Technol* 11(9): Insert 9–14, 1957.

Thompson MP, Brower DP: Hydrolyzed lactose cultured dairy products: I. Manufacture of cheddar cheese. *Cultured Dairy Prod J* 11: 22–23, 1976.

Tumerman L, Fran H, Cornely KW: The effect of lactose crystallization on protein stability in frozen concentrated milk. *J Dairy Sci* 37: 830–39, 1954.

U.S., Office of Federal Register, *Food Regulations: Cacao Products,* Code of Federal Regulations Title 21, part 14, 1 April 1973, p 8.

Wagg BJ, Friend JV, Smith GS: Inhibition of the erosive properties of water ices by the addition of calcium and phosphate. *Br Dent J* 119: 118–23, 1965.

Webb BH: Whey—a low-cost dairy product for use in candy. *J Dairy Sci* 49: 1310–13, 1966.

Whittier EO, Webb BH: *Byproducts from Milk.* New York: Reinhold, 1950, p 223.

Wondolowski MV: Preparation and application of immobilized lactases: A review. In *Proceedings of the International Biodeterioration Symposium, 3rd,* JM Sharpley, AM Kaplan (eds). Barking, Essex, England: Applied Science Publishers, 1976, pp 1033–41.

Woychik JH, Holsinger VH: Use of lactase in the manufacture of dairy products. In *Enzymes in Food and Beverage Processing,* RL Ory, AJ St. Angelo (eds). Washington, D.C.: American Chemical Society, Symposium ser. no. 47, 1977, pp 67–79.

Woychik JH, Wondolowski MV, Dahl KJ: Preparation and application of immobilized β-galactosidase of *Saccharomyces lactis.* In *Immobilized Enzymes in Food and Microbial Processes,* AC Olson, CL Cooney (eds). New York: Plenum, 1974, pp 41–49.

CHAPTER 23

NUTRITIONAL CONSIDERATIONS IN DEVELOPING

LOW-LACTOSE PRODUCTS

AN INDUSTRY PERSPECTIVE

David G. Guy

The role of the food industry in health care is to meet the nutritional needs of patients as defined by the clinician. As new information on nutritional needs becomes available, new directions in product development are charted. The perspective of an industry such as ours can be seen best by a review of the development of products with an emphasis on lactose and protein.

INFANT FORMULAS

Infant formulas are designed to meet the nutritional needs of infants who are not fed human milk. The first infant formulas were cow's milk to which carbohydrate was added to reduce the protein and ash content to a level appropriate for the infant. Although lactose was known to be the carbohydrate of human milk it was not readily available for use in infant feeding since the dairy industry did not have economical means to isolate lactose from whey. The first product developed by this company was Dextri Maltose®, an enzymatic digest of cornstarch to be used as a source of calories in cow's milk formulas. Sufficient lactose was available for commercial use in the 1950s, by which time advances in food technology made it possible to manufacture sterile liquid infant formulas containing nonfat milk, additional lactose, various blends of well-digested vegetable oils, as well as levels of vitamins and minerals recognized to be needed by the infant.

In the 1920s, certain infants were identified who were unable to tolerate formula based on cow's milk. A powdered formula based on full fat soy flour was developed to meet this need. Fortuitously, the soy products contained a readily absorbed fat (soy oil) and no lactose. In the 1920s, many infants with lactose intolerance were diagnosed as "milk allergic" since they developed symptoms when fed milk-based formulas. The early soy-based products were not very elegant and liquid formulas based on terminal sterilization were dark and viscous. Commercial availability of isolated soy protein enabled the development of methionine-supplemented soy protein-based liquid formulas that are a nutritional equivalent to the cow's milk-based formulas. Lactose never was added to the soy protein isolate formulas because commercially available lactose contains trace amounts of milk protein.

In the 1940s, a casein hydrolysate powder was developed as a protein source for parenteral nutrition. This work stimulated the development of protein hydrolysate infant formulas. The original formula, Nutramigen®, contained casein hydrolysate, Dextri Maltose, vitamins, minerals, and vegetable oils. The formula was very useful for feeding sick infants with allergic or gastrointestinal problems unable to digest intact protein. Neonatologists, gastroenterologists, and others recognized a broad spectrum of indications for this product. Special infant formulas are now available that contain hydrolyzed protein, supplemental amino acids, simple carbohydrates, medium-chain triglycerides, and vegetable oils. Recently, osmolality has been identified as a factor that affects intestinal tolerance of these formulas. Originally, the osmolality of some products was high because of the glucose content. This led to development of an isotonic protein hydrolysate formula containing corn syrup solids that clinically is readily digested and absorbed by the infant with gastrointestinal problems. Protein hydrolysate availability allowed the development of specialized products for the nutritional management of inborn errors of amino acid metabolism.

Sophisticated formulas have been developed for low birth weight and premature infants with relatively normal gastrointestinal development. Since lactase is often deficient in the premature infant, the lactose is limited in these formulas. Additionally, part of the fat used in these formulations is medium-chain triglyceride, which is well absorbed by such patients. Easily digested vegetable oils are included to provide essential fatty acids.

ADULT NUTRITIONAL PRODUCTS

Presently, a variety of products is available to the clinician to help meet the nutritional needs of adults for whom conventional diets are inadequate because of reduced intake, elevated needs, or the inability to digest but not ingest food. This latter condition may occur as a result of short bowel syndrome, pancreatitis, or lactose intolerance. Development of nutritional products for adults follows a similar history as that for the infant formulas.

Among the first specialized nutritional products for patients unable to feed themselves was the blenderized hospital diet. It generally was based on milk because milk is a nutrient-dense fluid to which other ingredients can be added to produce a balanced liquid diet. Vegetables were added for vitamins and minerals and occasionally meat was added. Sucrose and corn syrup were added for carbohydrates and calories.

The first tube feeding product developed by this company was Sustagen®, a milk-based powder that could be mixed easily with water to provide the desired caloric density. This product, made from powdered skim milk and added carbohydrate to supply calories and taste acceptability, has a high protein and moderately high lactose content. It is low in fat because of better tolerance and the difficulty of making a high fat powdered product that, when reconstituted as a liquid, would flow through a nasogastric feeding tube.

As with the blenderized hospital diet, a number of problems were experienced with powdered products, among them marginal taste, poor mixability, the possibility of environmental contamination, and the fact that these products are labor intensive. Also, the high lactose content of these early powdered products resulted in gastrointestinal symptoms in the lactose-intolerant patient.

Lactose intolerance also was experienced with the original Portagen® developed for patients with fat malabsorption. All the ingredients were selected, on the basis of the best knowledge then available, as being readily digested. These included skimmed milk (containing lactose), medium-chain triglycerides, and maltodextrins. Nevertheless, some early users experienced diarrhea. This problem eventually was identified as being due to lactose intolerance. Reformulation with the removal of the lactose resulted in one of the first lactose-free products developed for adults.

Environmental contamination and high labor cost as noted above are a negative feature of powdered products. Experience with infant formulas and the fact that Sustagen was being used as an oral beverage led to development of a nutritionally complete liquid oral supplement. This supplement, Sustacal®, is formulated to satisfy the altered nutritional needs of a broad range of patients by providing a generous level of protein, relatively low fat, and balanced amounts of vitamins and minerals while maintaining excellent taste acceptability. The original product used skim milk as a protein source. It became evident that formulas containing lactose were often inappropriate for the lactose-intolerant hospitalized patient. To fill the need for a low-lactose formula, the level of skim milk in Sustacal was reduced to the marginal amount necessary to provide the excellent organoleptic qualities of milk. The remainder of the protein was supplied by casein and soy isolate. Sucrose and corn syrup solids were used to replace the lactose and maintain the oral acceptability of the product. Clinical tests carried out by Dr. Bayless at Johns Hopkins indicated that the ingestion of 240 ml of low-lactose Sustacal did not elicit gastrointestinal symptoms or increases in breath hydrogen in 3 white and 1 black healthy lactose-intolerant volunteers.

These same subjects were symptomatic and had a breath hydrogen rise following the consumption of an equal quantity of skim milk. Further product development had led to the complete elimination of lactose. This product has been extensively tested and found to be accepted as well as supplements containing lactose. This is an important consideration for an oral food.

FUNCTION OF THE MAJOR DIETARY CONSTITUENTS

Two types of considerations go into the selection of the nutrients used in commercially prepared oral products: nutritional adequacy and food technology capability.

Complete nutritional products contain protein for the body's use in synthesis of structural, carrier, immunological, oncotic, enzymatic proteins, and other functional proteins. They contain fat for energy, membrane integrity, environmental protection; and act as precursors for prostaglandins. Carbohydrate is added for energy, protein sparing, immunity, detoxification, matrixing, and genetic duplication.

The human lacks the ability to form certain essential nutrients. These must be obtained from the diet. They are, of course, the vitamins, essential amino acids, and essential fatty acids. There are no essential carbohydrates. All dietary carbohydrates are converted to glucose by the body since glucose is the primary fuel for the body. For the other essential functions of carbohydrate, glucose is converted in the body to ribose, galactose, glucuronides, and substituted sugars. Thus, removal of lactose from a nutritional product will not cause a deficiency as would removing protein or polyunsaturated fat.

FUNCTIONALITY AND FOOD TECHNOLOGY

Functionality, a major consideration in food technology, is the ability of one ingredient to interact with others to result in a final form. An example might be the ability of certain proteins to remain hydrophilic in the presence of heat, salts, or acids and thereby to remain in a water-based solution. Functionality is one of the factors in the decision to use a certain nutrient source. The others are nutritional quality, taste, and medical sequelae. Any ingredient, whether used as a source of protein, carbohydrate, fat, or minerals, must meet these four criteria.

Few would deny that the taste of milk is very acceptable and that the protein quality is excellent. Milk is highly functional, being heat stable and able to remain in solution in the presence of fats, minerals, and water. Unfortunately, milk can produce medical complications for some subjects because it contains lactose. Egg, in particular egg white, certainly has excellent nutritional quality, produces minimal medical complications, and has little taste. However, its functionality is poor since products containing egg cannot be vigorously mixed or terminally sterilized without becoming solid.

Commercially available soy proteins have good nutritional quality, especially when supplemented with certain essential amino acids. The functionality of soy protein is very good, and can be made into both liquid and solid products. Furthermore, it is hypoallergenic and the medical complications are minimal. Finally, soy has a fair taste acceptance, although some object to the beany taste.

Animal proteins vary in nutritional quality from excellent for the flesh protein to poor for connective proteins such as collagens and gelatins. The functionality of these proteins varies from fair to poor. Meat can be blenderized, but it cannot be heat sterilized and kept functional as a fluid. Collagen, or gelatin, has fair functionality and tends to be acid stable. Medical complications with animal protein are limited; however, some animal proteins are allergenic. The taste is fair to poor. Protein isolated from beef muscle has a poor taste; it is the beef fat and the processing that make meat taste good.

Finally, there are the hydrolysates and the purified amino acids. They have fair functionality in that they are acid soluble unlike most other proteins. Unfortunately, they do not have the ability to bind other nutrients. In a high fat formula product, for example, hydrolysates will separate into two layers; whereas milk, egg, and soy proteins will bind fats and water resulting in a homogeneous product. The major medical complication of hydrolysates and amino acids is their high osmolality with the potential for diarrhea; and the taste is unacceptable to most people.

Thus, in developing oral nutritional products, when the decision is one of what protein to use, because of its excellent nutritional quality, taste, and functionality, milk remains the protein source of choice in many situations. However, because of the problem of lactose intolerance, the isolated milk protein free of lactose must be used. Until recently, that protein has been primarily casein. Whey protein is now available in different forms. A demineralized form can be used to develop a low ash infant formula with lactose. A lactose-free high ash whey can be used for adult nutritional products. Whey protein is fairly functional, but is not exceptionally heat stable. Thus, the functional quality of whey is not as good as whole or skimmed milk.

To date, in order to respond to medical demand for lactose-free products, this company has chosen to rely on casein, soy proteins, and casein hydrolysates in order to achieve an optimal balance among nutritional quality, taste, functionality, and medical sequelae. A similar rationale has gone into the choice of the source of the carbohydrate, fat, vitamins, and minerals used in our nutritional products. However, with advances in food technology, as well as advances in nutritional science, new sources of nutrients or new means of adjusting the functionality of traditional nutrient sources may result in products that have little resemblance to those presently available.

CHAPTER 24

DEVELOPMENT OF
LACTOSE-REDUCED MILK PRODUCTS

Alan E. Kligerman

Efforts are underway to increase the availability of dairy-modified lactose-reduced milk. Plans call for offering dairy products made from enzyme-modified milk.

LACTASE ENZYME DEVELOPMENT AND MARKETING

Product development first involved obtaining an exclusive license for a lactase enzyme manufactured by the Dutch firm, Gist Brocades. The enzyme is a beta-galactosidase from *Kluyveromyces lactis* yeast. The safety and efficacy of the enzyme then were analyzed thoroughly and a Generally Recognized as Safe (GRAS) Affirmation Petition was filed. Initially the enzyme was offered in dry powdered form in individual dosage packets. The enzyme was suspended in an anhydrous glucose diluent; this was considered the most innocuous diluent, since lactose itself is converted to glucose as one-half its breakdown product. Each dosage packet modified one quart of milk to approximately a 70% lactose hydrolysis level in 24 hours. Levels of 90% or 100% hydrolysis could be achieved easily by adding more lactase enzyme or by waiting longer than 24 hours.

Recently the lactase enzyme instead has been marketed in a liquid form that has greater stability and is easier to use. The liquid enzyme is available in 30-quart, 12-quart, and 4-quart treatment sizes. Since the liquid has proven more practical to use and has a longer shelf life, the powdered form of the enzyme has been phased out. The enzyme currently is available through drugstores, specialty food stores, and via direct mail. At approximately \$5.98 for the 30-quart size, it costs the customer 20¢ to modify one quart of milk, or slightly less than 5¢ per glass (225 ml).

Preliminary marketing of the enzyme itself began in 1976 with a market test for product acceptability. The announcement of the enzyme's availability in June 1976 resulted in a large number of inquiries. At first, product requests were filled through direct mail, then the enzyme began to be carried in drug and specialty or health food stores. Sales continue to expand at a brisk pace, with thousands of customers still buying directly by mail. The volume of mail order sales has enabled the firm to evaluate purchasing habits by undertaking periodic customer surveys.

DAIRY-MODIFIED MILK

The efforts to date are preliminary to the marketing of a dairy-modified ready-to-drink lactose-reduced milk. One of the drawbacks to modifying the milk at home is that the user must wait 24 hours for the lactase enzyme to act. Although surveys indicate that some customers may prefer to modify milk at home themselves rather than to purchase it in ready-to-drink form, for most, dairy-modified milk should be more convenient. Not only is it ready to drink at the time of purchase, it also costs less than its home-modified counterpart (10¢ less per quart, or 2½¢ less per glass).

Dairy-modified milk may be processed using either a 24-hour batch holding method or a continuous method. Both have been tested thoroughly. In the batch holding method, the dairy isolates the raw fluid milk and adds the enzyme. The milk is held at 40°F and at the end of 24 hours is checked for hydrolysis. The continuous method utilizes an automatic electric syringe, which adds the enzyme to the milk at the time the carton is filled. The machine is relatively small in size and is actuated by a photoelectric eye. The first filling machine stop station occurs at the point where the carton bottom is formed. The enzyme is added at this point, followed less than a second later by the milk, which mixes thoroughly with the lactase enzyme. The carton then is sealed and moves to the refrigerator. As long as the milk takes 24 hours to reach the consumer (which it almost always does), the milk will be hydrolyzed to at least a 70% lactose removal level. The hydrolysis proceeds further when this method is used. There have been no spoilage problems and no bacterial problems with the milk using either method, i.e., adding the enzyme prior to or after pasteurization.

The hydrolysis level may be checked easily with a cryoscope. The freezing point of milk descends by 0.0275°C for each 10% hydrolysis (Keeney and Kroger 1974). Alternatively, the dairy could use a faster but less exact method, a Lilly Testape (normally used to check for glucose in the urine). The upper limit of the tape corresponds to an 80% hydrolysis level in milk.

Dairy-modified milk was made available beginning in July 1979 in a few test locations in the eastern United States. Informing consumers about the rationale and availability of such a product is a complex matter, but according to our observations, once informed, consumers begin purchasing and continue to purchase extremely reliably. The initial market test of dairy-modified milk was in the Allentown, Bethlehem, and Wilkes-Barre, Pennsylvania areas. The market tests were supported with consumer-directed radio and newspaper advertising as well as with publicity in all media, including television. The test campaign used 1,000 radio spots and 1,000-line newspaper advertisements. Two separate ads were run; one emphasized how nice it was for someone to be able truly to enjoy milk again, and the other gave facts about the product itself.

THE MARKET FOR MODIFIED MILK

The market for modified milk originally had been envisioned as being almost exclusively black and Oriental, with reduced but strong demand in the central European and Mediterranean ethnic groups. This estimate has been modified somewhat as experience has been gained and purchasers have been canvassed.

Age now appears to be the dominant characteristic among users of the lactase enzyme. Thus far, approximately 66% of the enzyme's sales to men and 68% of the sales to women are to those over 55 years of age. The lowest levels of use are among those in their teens and twenties, with a rise at the lower age scale, among infants and children under 12 years of age. Only 13.8% of sales are to people 18 years of age and under.

A recent mail survey of 200 customers brought a 70% response rate. Analysis of those responses indicates that over half of the product's users are of northern European origin, including individuals of Scandinavian, English, and Scotch-Irish backgrounds. Any of several factors may account for this seemingly anomalous result, e.g., the greater inclination of some people to try new products, to acknowledge a problem such as lactose intolerance, and to respond to a mail survey.

While there are other approaches to dealing with lactose intolerance, primarily through the use of nonlactose milk analogues, it is felt that using milk itself, either in its lactose-reduced form or modified at home by adding the lactase enzyme, is superior. These approaches cause the least change in the milk's original state, form, and taste as well as in its mode of consumption. The fact that enhanced calcium utilization is associated with lactose absorption supports this choice. By adding the lactase enzyme, milk retains its native carbohydrate, whereas the nonlactose milk analogues remove the carbohydrate and replace it with another sugar.

FUTURE PRODUCTS AND POLICY CONSIDERATIONS

The third phase of product development will involve offering other dairy products made from the modified milk—canned milk, cottage cheese, puddings, and frozen concentrated milk. An excellent frozen concentrated milk has been developed already. It reconstitutes in a ratio of 4 to 1, like most frozen orange juice, and has superior taste and stability. Successful pilot runs of canned milk, cottage cheese, yogurt, and ice cream also have been made. The company expects its GRAS Affirmation Petition to be approved for most uses contemplated, and possibly for all uses after additional data requested by the U.S. Food and Drug Administration have been submitted.

Efforts to interest government agencies in specifying the enzyme-modified milk for publicly funded feeding programs have been received politely but thus far have not resulted in substantive action. The company would like to see government menu planners recognize the need for lactose-hydrolyzed milk for certain high risk population groups. A government publication, *Nutrition Canada* (1973), notes that calcium is a nutrient in chronic shortage in the Canadian diet and that when milk is excluded from the diet alternate sources of calcium are not utilized satisfactorily. The availability of lactose-reduced milk could do much to alleviate this problem.

What is called for now is recognition on the part of the dairy trade associations that the problem of lactose intolerance does exist, that it can pose a nutritional threat, and that offering a lactose-reduced milk product will lead to higher, not lower, consumption of milk. Widespread use of modified milk appears unlikely, however, unless the dairy industry can be convinced of the need for it.

Producing lactose-hydrolyzed milk can only help the dairy industry, which is now experiencing a decline in the volume of fluid milk consumption while the consumption of other drinks such as sodas, juice, beer, and coffee is growing. Milk companies represented at the 1979 Dairy Convention in Chicago did express appreciable interest in the lactase enzyme product, but in general the industry appears to perceive the marketing of a lactose-reduced milk as a threat. Since most milk sold today is in fact "modified" (skimmed, homogenized, partially skimmed with solids added, flavored), it is difficult to understand such objections.

In an effort to contribute further to an understanding of the lactase enzyme and to evaluate the need for it, the company has funded several studies of its usefulness in modifying milk for the following groups: infants with colic; lactose-intolerant children of primary school age; children with cystic fibrosis; adult patients undergoing pelvic radiation; and lactose-intolerant adults in Veterans Administration Medical Centers. Some of these studies are complete; others are still in progress. The company is also considering analyzing the reasons for the product's steady use in homes for the retarded. The lactase enzyme is now being used among sick and malnourished children in certain areas such as Bangladesh.

Thorough evaluation of the enzyme's possible toxicity, utilizing LD_{50}, subacute, and subchronic techniques, has proven that it is innocuous. Given the enzyme's potential for enabling lactose-intolerant individuals to consume milk, the company has committed itself to expand its marketing of lactose-reduced milk and milk products. It is hoped that physicians, dieticians, and nutritionists will add lactose-reduced milk to the list of recommended nutritional options for patients suspected of or identified as being unable to digest lactose fully.

REFERENCES

Bureau of Nutritional Sciences, Department of National Health and Welfare: *Nutrition Canada.* Ottawa: Department of National Health and Welfare, 1973.

Keeney PG, Kroger M: Frozen dairy products. In *Fundamentals of Dairy Chemistry,* BH Webb, AH Johnson, JA Alford (eds). Westport, Conn.: AVI Publishing, 1974.

CHAPTER 25

REGULATORY PERSPECTIVE
ON LACTOSE INTOLERANCE

Joginder G. Chopra

The Food and Drug Administration (FDA) is a regulatory agency whose mission is consumer protection. Its goals are to ensure that (1) food is safe and wholesome; (2) drugs, biologic products, therapeutic devices, and diagnostic products are safe and effective; (3) cosmetics are safe; (4) the use of radiological products does not result in unnecessary exposure to radiation; (5) all products are labeled honestly; and (6) its action is understood both by the medical profession and by the industry.

It is often said that the FDA has ample authority to assure the nutritional quality of the country's food supply, but this remark is not necessarily justified. The federal Food, Drug and Cosmetic Act gives the FDA explicit authority to regulate toxic substances or filth in food but the agency's ability to regulate nutritional quality depends more upon implicit authority, and that authority may be much less extensive.

The concerns of consumers, regulatory agencies, and the Congress with respect to food have changed over the years. Initially, concern was with adulteration and contamination of food, and regulatory efforts were directed mainly towards protecting against fraud and against the sale of spoiled food. As food processing developed, a need was recognized for legislation to prohibit the inclusion in foods of substances that posed hazards. Subsequently, emphasis shifted towards assuring consistency in the ingredient composition and quality of

Views expressed are those of the author and not necessarily those of the U.S. Food and Drug Administration.

food products. These measures were designed as much to protect honest manufacturers as to insure consumers against fraud. As nutritional knowledge increased, concern about the nutritional quality of food products developed.

In the 1970s there have been significant new developments in food technology, developments that make possible fabricated food products that substitute for and resemble traditional foods, but that may not provide the same ingredients and nutritional value as the traditional foods. The FDA is concerned about finding ways to assure that the appearance of new fabricated (formulated) foods does not lead to significant degradation of the nutritional quality of the American food supply.

Currently, lactose-hydrolyzed products are not subject to any formal regulatory controls. The FDA's Bureau of Foods recognizes the need and therefore plans to develop regulation that will provide for classification and labeling of these products. Lactose and lactase derived from *Aspergillus niger* are considered GRAS substances but their GRAS status is based largely on the fact that they were in common use in foods long before 1958. GRAS affirmation of lactase derived from *Saccharomyces lactis* still is pending and presents problems due to inadequate toxicity data as well as lack of common use in foods prior to 1958.

EXISTING NUTRITION REGULATION PROGRAMS

The FDA currently has six nutrition regulation programs that might have significance with respect to new foods such as lactose-hydrolyzed products and has proposed a seventh. Standards of identity involving nutrition characteristics have existed for a long time for such basic food commodities as milk and bread. These regulations define the composition of many foods, state which optional ingredients may be used, and specify ingredients used that must be declared on the label. Required or mandatory ingredients used in such standardized foods are exempt by law from label declaration.

While the Food, Drug and Cosmetic Act gives the agency authority to standardize enriched foods, the FDA generally has not attempted to use its authority to prohibit the existence of unenriched food. The FDA has established standards of identity for such basic foods as milk and nonfat dried milk fortified with vitamins A and D, bread and enriched bread, and then has depended upon the marketplace for consumer selection of the enriched food rather than the unenriched food.

In 1973, the FDA published final regulations with respect to nutrition labeling of foods. The agency views nutrition labeling as the focal point for providing consumers with information about individual foods they purchase and eat. While nutrition labeling imposes no requirements with respect to nutritional quality of the food supply, the FDA believes as a result of such labeling, consumers will become more aware of the nutritional value of foods and more likely to consider nutritional factors in making purchasing selections.

A third approach is to establish common or usual name regulations that set minimum nutritional criteria to be met by certain types of nonstandardized foods. Fourth, the FDA has established nutritional quality guidelines for specific classes of foods. These guidelines prescribe the minimum level or a range of.nutrient composition (nutritional quality) appropriate for a given class of food (U.S., Office of Federal Register 1977).

Fifth, a food that substitutes for and resembles another food must be labeled imitation if it is nutritionally inferior to the other food. It need not be labeled imitation if (1) it is not nutritionally inferior to the food is resembles and for which it substitutes; (2) if it bears an appropriate name that accurately identifies or describes its basic nature (U.S., *Food Labeling* 1979).

Sixth, the agency encourages a regulatory climate designed to stimulate development of foods for special dietary use, and to offer protection from nutritional fraud and misleading labeling. The term *foods for special dietary use* encompasses any food intended as a sole item of the diet, as a supplementary source of nutrients, to increase total dietary intake of nutrients, or to supply special dietary needs that exist by reason of physical, physiological, pathological, or other conditions. Special dietary use regulations apply to foods such as dietary supplements, infant formulas, low sodium and hypoallergenic products, reduced and low calorie foods, and lactose-hydrolyzed products.

The FDA's Bureau of Foods also has the responsibility of ensuring that medical foods are safe, efficacious for the intended purpose, and properly labeled. Included in this category are all foods that are intended for use under medical supervision, to meet the nutritional requirements, because of special medical conditions. In addition, the bureau has responsibility to ensure that labeling of these products conforms to standards of accuracy and reliability. Currently, the bureau is developing regulations for labeling "medical foods." Lastly, the FDA has issued a final policy statement concerning nutrient fortification of foods. This statement is designed to promote the rational addition of nutrients to foods in order to preserve a balance of nutrients in the diet of American consumers (U.S. *Nutritional Quality of Foods* 1980).

NEW REGULATORY APPROACHES

To improve food labels as communication devices, the agency has undertaken a comprehensive review of food labeling and the laws and regulations that govern such labeling. The purpose is threefold: (1) to provide consumers with more complete information relating specifically to health; (2) to respond to consumer desires for better descriptions of ingredients in processed foods; and (3) to improve the manner in which information is presented to consumers.

Technological advances have produced changes at all steps in the food chain, from production, through processing, to preparation for serving. Concurrent with the increase in food production has been an increase in the amount of information available on nutrients and food products. To cope effectively with the volume of information on composition of foods, the FDA, in cooperation with the U.S. Department of Agriculture, the Canadian government, and the food industry, has developed a computerized Food Composition Data Bank for storage, retrieval, and summation of data by food groups. The information will be made available on request through the private sector.

To meet its responsibilities to individuals with intolerances to certain foods, the FDA will seek explicit authority from Congress to require the declaration of mandatory ingredients in standardized foods. Proposed laws would require listing of ingredients in all foods, whether standardized or not. This type of labeling would provide information for selecting well-balanced diets and for minimizing consumption of those foods that some consumers may wish to avoid for health and other reasons (Chopra 1979).

REGULATION OF LACTASE ENZYMES
AND LACTOSE-HYDROLYZED FOODS

Generally, products intended primarily to provide nutritional support should be regulated by the FDA's Bureau of Foods, even if the food is required by or intended for use by persons with specific diseases or disorders. Products intended for use in the "diagnosis, cure, mitigation, treatment or prevention of disease" should be considered to be within the jurisdiction of the FDA's Bureau of Drugs. Lactase enzymes and lactose-hydrolyzed foods could be regulated by the Bureau of Foods under the broad categories of safety and labeling in the Food, Drug and Cosmetic Act.

Since enzymes such as lactase become a component of food and affect the characteristics of food, they are considered food additives under the Food, Drug and Cosmetic Act. The Food Additives Amendment to the act requires that such additives be reviewed and regulated by the FDA before their use in food is permitted unless the ingredient specifically has been sanctioned for such use in food either by the USDA or by the FDA prior to 1958, or is Generally Recognized as Safe (GRAS).

GRAS status must be based upon either (1) information that the substance was in common use in food, or food manufacturing, in the United States prior to 1958; or (2) a petition containing the same quantity and quality of safety data as required for food additive approval, plus publication of these safety data so that general recognition of safety may be achieved by food safety scientists. Enzyme petitions are unusual in that petition data generally must demonstrate safety clearance not only for the enzyme but also for the final products of its action.

Forthcoming publication of affirmed GRAS enzymes, which includes new safety evaluations for enzymes that have been the subjects of previous FDA opinions (Select Committee on GRAS Substances 1977), should resolve the last outstanding ambiguities regarding the regulatory status of food use enzymes.

A number of microbial enzymes derived from *Aspergillus niger, Aspergillus flavus oryzae,* and *Bacillus subtilis* have been classified GRAS or sanctioned for use in foods under the broad classification of carbohydrases. Carbohydrases derived from *A. niger* refer to five enzymes: x-amylase, cellulase, glucomylase, lactase, and pectinase; those from *A. flavus oryzae* refer to amylase and amylglucosidase; and *B. subtilis* refers to amylase. Through GRAS review efforts, the FDA is searching the scientific literature for all available identity, use, and safety information on these enzymes. Once this information has been compiled and collated the GRAS affirmation status of the enzymes will be considered.

The FDA's GRAS review efforts also include enzymes from certain saccharomyces species of yeasts, and lactobacilli species commonly used in dairy products.

Lactase enzyme derived from *Saccharomyces fragilis* is GRAS. However, a petition seeking GRAS status for a lactase derived from another species of yeast, *Saccharomyces lactis,* currently is being reviewed. Although this enzyme is very closely related to *Saccharomyces fragilis,* both morphologically and physiologically, a 1968 FDA opinion indicated that lactase produced from *Saccharomyces lactis* was not considered GRAS based upon "common use in foods." GRAS affirmation for a list of microbial enzyme perparations including lactase derived from *Saccharomyces lactis* is still pending and presents problems due to inadequate toxicity studies as well as lack of common use in food for human consumption prior to 1958. Better identification of the enzymes and submission of the relevant data in the proper format can assist in faster processing of petitions. This in turn will result in a quicker introduction of newer and assured safe technology in the use of enzymes in food processing.

CONCLUSIONS

The agency believes that when it comes to issues of safety and health, there must be appropriate regulatory activity, but if the FDA works together with the industry this can be accomplished with minimal economic impact on the industry and hence, the consumer. With respect to other issues, regulation should occur only as justified by cost-benefit considerations. For example, the FDA and the industry both should be devoted to full and informative labeling of food products, but only after examining carefully the benefit derived for the cost imposed in each case.

As new knowledge is acquired concerning the relationship between food ingredients and the development and exacerbation of adverse reactions, the agency will move to ensure the integration of such knowledge into the prevention and treatment of the disease and nutrition education.

REFERENCES

Chopra JG: The role of Food and Drug Administration in food allergy. *Ann Allergy* 42: 1–4, 1979.

Select Committee on GRAS Substances: Evaluation of health aspects of GRAS food ingredients: Lessons learned and questions unanswered. Bethesda, Md.: Life Sciences Research Office, Federation of American Societies for Experimental Biology, 1977.

U.S., *Food Labeling: Tentative Positions of Agencies,* Federal Regulations 40, no. 247, Friday, 21 Dec. 1979.

U.S., *Nutritional Quality of Foods: Addition of Nutrients,* Federal Regulations 45, no. 18, Friday, 25 Jan. 1980.

U.S., Office of Federal Register, *Food Labeling,* Code of Federal Regulations Title 21, Food and Drugs Part 101.8, 1977.

CHAPTER 26

DAIRY COUNCIL PERSPECTIVE
ON LACTOSE INTOLERANCE

Robert S. Katz

Lactose intolerance and its accompanying symptomatology have been shown to be prevalent among many individuals around the world. Nevertheless, research has shown that many individuals labeled ''lactose intolerant'' based on a lactose tolerance test can safely consume recommended amounts of milk without discomfort. There is a paucity of data available concerning the effect of lactose intolerance on an individual's ability to utilize the nutrients in milk. Moreover, the data that are available do not suggest an adverse relationship. The nutrient contributions of milk are too important to eliminate this food from the diet casually, based on lactose intolerance, as has been suggested in numerous scientific and lay publications. The Protein Advisory Group of the United Nations, the Food and Nutrition Board, National Academy of Sciences, National Research Council, and the Committee on Nutrition of the American Academy of Pediatrics all have reviewed the situation and in general concur that the evidence to date does not warrant wholesale recommendations to restrict the intake of milk based on data concerned with primary lactose intolerance. For those individuals who are intolerant to an eight-ounce glass of milk, suitable alternatives include smaller quantities of milk consumed more frequently throughout the day, some cultured dairy products such as yogurt and some cheeses, and lactose-hydrolyzed milk. Research is being conducted concerning the efficacy of milk containing *Lactobacillus acidophilus* in overcoming the problem of lactose intolerance. Future research should focus on the nutritional consequences of lactose intolerance and on developing suitable methods for identifying those individuals who truly need be concerned. It must be realized that no food is perfect and the casual elimination of any food group from the diet of necessity increases the likelihood of nutrient deficiencies.

The milk group, excluding butter, supplies significant amounts of several nutrients to the American diet (table 26.1). In these times, with the concern about the relationship between diet and health, particularly obesity, the consumption of nutrient-dense foods such as those in the milk group plays an important role in assuring adequate nutrient intake without consuming excess calories. In addition, the milk group is for all practical purposes the sole source of lactose in the diet. A specific need for lactose has not been established, nevertheless a beneficial role for lactose regarding the utilization of several minerals in the diet has been observed (Armbrecht and Wasserman 1976).

The National Dairy Council is concerned about lactose intolerance for several reasons:

(1) The milk group is essentially the sole source of lactose in the diet.
(2) The erroneous generalization that lactose intolerance means milk intolerance may lead to undue avoidance of milk based on a lactose tolerance test.
(3) The erroneous generalization of milk intolerance to intolerance of all foods in the milk group may lead to unnecessary avoidance of all foods in this group.

Lactose intolerance has been defined as clinical symptoms (abdominal pain, diarrhea, bloating, flatulence) following a lactose tolerance test, ingestion of

TABLE 26.1
Contribution of dairy foods to the food supply, 1979

Nutrient	Percentage of total*
Food energy (calories)	10.7
Protein	21.7
Fat	11.8
Carbohydrate	6.3
Calcium	73.8
Phosphorus	34.7
Magnesium	21.2
Riboflavin	39.1
Vitamin B_{12}	20.7
Vitamin A value	13.2
Vitamin B_6	11.6
Thiamine	8.1
Niacin equiv. and Vitamin D	Significant amounts

Source: Marsten and Peterkin 1980, reprinted with permission.
*Nutrients contributed by diary foods, excluding butter, as a percentage of total nutrients available in U.S. diet.

lactose mixed in water in a standard dose (i.e., 50 g per m^2 or 2 g per kg or less) in a person with proven lactose malabsorption (Protein Advisory Group 1972). While three types of lactose intolerance have been described (Ransome-Kuti 1977, Garza and Scrimshaw 1976), primary lactose intolerance, due to an apparently normal developmental decrease in lactase activity, is the most common. It should be pointed out that 50 g lactose is that amount found in one quart of milk or four times the amount in an eight-ounce glass of milk—the usual recommended serving. Several investigators (Stephenson and Latham 1974, Bell et al. 1973, Reddy and Pershad 1972) have concluded, based on research evaluating the lactose tolerance test and lactose intolerance as practical means for assessing intolerance to milk, that such a large dose of lactose leads to a spuriously high estimate of intolerance to foods from the milk group and that lactose intolerance is not a reliable guide to assess milk intolerance.

MILK INTOLERANCE

Further confusion is generated by the nomenclature associated with lactose. Since milk is the primary source of lactose in the diet it often is referred to as "milk sugar" and many have concluded erroneously that lactose intolerance is synonymous with milk intolerance. It is imperative that these terms not be used interchangeably so as to avoid any confusion for the practicing physician and his or her patients.

While a clear definition of milk intolerance has not been utilized widely, it has been defined as the development of significant symptoms similar to those described for lactose intolerance following the consumption of usual amounts of milk (8 ounces) or products containing milk (Latham 1977). Most recently, researchers at the Massachusetts Institute of Technology (Haverberg et al. 1980, Kwon et al. 1980) have raised questions regarding the proper testing protocol to determine true milk intolerance. These researchers have concluded, using the double-blind procedure, that the true prevalence of milk intolerance due to lactose malabsorption cannot be determined in any other way except by double-blind studies. They stress the necessity of including a placebo (i.e., lactose-free milk) in such studies in order to determine the causal relationship that exists between lactose malabsorption and milk intolerance.

DIETARY IMPLICATIONS

While the debate goes on about the true prevalence of lactose intolerance or milk intolerance among various ethnic groups, these people should be identified and given proper dietary counseling. It seems reasonable that suitable alternatives for milk-intolerant individuals should provide the same nutrients as does milk. Lactose-hydrolyzed milk has been shown to be a suitable alternative in most cases (Payne-Bose et al. 1977, Mitchell et al. 1977, Jones et al. 1976,

Turner et al. 1976, Paige et al. 1975), however this may not always be the case (Nutritional significance of lactose intolerance 1978). In addition, other dairy foods such as cheese and fermented dairy products are tolerated well by the truly milk-intolerant individual (Baer 1970). Perhaps the first recommendations for these individuals should be to determine just how much milk they can tolerate. It has been shown (Bayless and Huang 1973) that many lactose-intolerant individuals could tolerate small quantities of milk with or without food, although ingestion of one cup of milk caused discomfort.

CLINICAL RELEVANCE

From a public health point of view, how important is the development of symptoms to the consumption of milk? Its importance is determined by the answers to two questions:

(1) Is the discomfort significant enough to cause the individual to avoid the food?
(2) Does the discomfort indicate that the individual is not receiving the full nutritional benefit of the food?

It is unreasonable to recommend consumption of a food if in fact such consumption is the cause of extreme discomfort. On the other hand it is just as unreasonable to recommend avoidance of foods that cause discomfort if, in the individual's judgment, this discomfort is inconsequential. Thus the first question can by answered only by the individual in question and studies assessing the prevalence of lactose intolerance in different populations and involving an investigator's assessment of symptomatology following consumption of milk add little to the practical situation in which recommendations must be made.

Unfortunately, there is a paucity of information addressing the question of bioavailability of milk's nutrients in the presence of lactose intolerance or milk intolerance. Future research should focus on this question, nevertheless present data suggest this is not a clinically important problem (Committee on Nutrition, American Academy of Pediatrics 1978).

The National Dairy Council bases its recommendations on the concept of a balanced diet in accord with scientific recommendations. The Protein Advisory Group of the United Nations (1972), the Food and Nutrition Board, National Research Council (1972), and the Committee on Nutrition, American Academy of Pediatrics (1974), all have issued statements dealing with the advisability of encouraging populations with a high rate of lactose intolerance to develop programs aimed at increasing milk consumption primarily among older infants and children, but also including pregnant and lactating women and adults. All three groups concluded it was inappropriate at that time to discourage the development of such programs based on milk intolerance. Recently the Committee on Nutrition of the American Academy of Pediatrics (1978) felt it was time to reexamine this question. The committee summarized its findings in part by stating "... intolerance to the consumption of 250 ml of milk apparently is rarely seen in preadolescents. Current research on the response of adolescents to hydrolyzed-lactose milk suggests that the symptoms observed in lactose-intolerant subjects after milk ingestion may be unrelated to lactose or mild enough to be of little practical significance. The effects of undigested lactose on nutrient absorption have received little attention, but preliminary data suggest this is not a problem, except perhaps when overall intakes are marginally adequate.''

JUDICIAL RULING

Even more recently, Daniel H. Hanscomb (1979), Federal Trade Commission (FTC) administrative law judge, dismissed FTC's complaint against the California Milk Advisory Board's use of an advertising slogan "Everybody needs milk" as not being "unfair, false, misleading and deceptive." The FTC's case was based primarily on the contention that a substantial number of individuals could not and should not drink milk because of milk allergy or symptomatic lactose intolerance. The judge heard 35 "expert" witnesses on these subjects, presenting the most recent experimental findings and opinions, and with respect to "symptomatic lactose intolerance," the judge found that "... the weight of the scientific and medical evidence established that milk in moderate amounts at a time was not detrimental but beneficial, even for people who could not digest lactose in milk. They benefited from all the other nutrients essential for a good diet."

The judge further stated in his 141-page decision that "Milk is one of the most nutritious foods in the nation's diet, and from the standpoint of the population as a whole, or even significant population groups, is literally 'essential, necessary and needed.' The withdrawal of milk from any major population group would amount to a nutritional disaster."

CONCLUSIONS

In conclusion, it must be recognized that no food is perfect and that all foods can contribute to a nutritionally balanced diet. However, the casual elimination of any food group from the diet of necessity increases the likelihood of nutrient deficiencies. To date, data regarding lactose intolerance and/or milk intolerance do not warrant altering recommendations for the inclusion of milk or other foods from the milk group in the diets of the general healthy United States population.

REFERENCES

Armbrecht HJ, Wasserman RH: Enhancement of Ca uptake by lactose in the rat small intestine. *J Nutr* 106: 1265–71, 1976.

Baer D: Lactase deficiency and yogurt. *Soc Biol* 17: 143, 1970.

Bayless TM, Huang SS: Recurrent abdominal pain due to milk and lactose intolerance in school-aged children. *Pediatrics* 47: 1029–32, 1973.

Bell RR, Draper HH, Bergan JG: Sucrose, lactose and glucose tolerance in northern Alaskan Eskimos. *Am J Clin Nutr* 26: 1185–90, 1973.

Committee on Nutrition, American Academy of Pediatrics: Should milk drinking by children be discouraged? *Pediatrics* 53: 576–82, 1974.

Committee on Nutrition, American Academy of Pediatrics: The practical significance of lactose intolerance in children. *Pediatrics* 62: 240–45, 1978.

Garza C, Scrimshaw NS: Relationship of lactose intolerance to milk intolerance in young children. *Am J Clin Nutr* 29: 192–96, 1976.

Hanscomb DH: In the matter of California Milk Producers Advisory Board an unincorporated association and Cunningham & Walsh, Inc. a corporation. Federal Trade Commission initial decision Docket no. 8988 (1979).

Haverberg L, Kwon PH Jr, Scrimshaw NS: Comparative tolerance of adolescents of differing ethnic backgrounds to lactose-containing and lactose-free dairy drinks: I. Initial experience with a double-blind procedure. *Am J Clin Nutr* 33: 17–21, 1980.

Jones DV, Latham MC, Kosikowski FV, Woodward G: Symptom response to lactose-reduced milk in lactose-intolerant adults. *Am J Clin Nutr* 29: 633–38, 1976.

Kwon PH Jr, Rorick MH, Scrimshaw NS: Comparative tolerance of adolescents of differing ethnic backgrounds to lactose-containing and lactose-free dairy drinks: II. Improvement of a double-blind test. *Am J Clin Nutr* 33: 22–26, 1980.

Latham MC: Public health importance of milk intolerance. *Nutr News* 40: 13, 16, 1977.

Marsten RM, Peterkin BB: Nutrient content of the national food supply. *Natl Food Rev, USDA,* Winter 1980.

Mitchell JD, Brand J, Halbisch J: Weight-gain inhibition by lactose in Australian aboriginal children: A controlled trial of normal and lactose hydrolyzed milk. *Lancet* 1: 500–502, 1977.

National Research Council: Background information on lactose and milk intolerance: A statement of the Food and Nutrition Board, Division of Biology and Agriculture, 1972.

Nutritional significance of lactose intolerance. *Nutr Rev* 36: 133–34, 1978.

Paige DM, Bayless TM, Huang SS, Wexler R: Lactose hydrolyzed milk. *Am J Clin Nutr* 28: 818–22, 1975.

Payne-Bose D, Welsh JD, Gearhart HL, Morrison RD: Milk and lactose-hydrolyzed milk. *Am J Clin Nutr* 30: 695–97, 1977.

Protein Advisory Group of the United Nations: PAG statement 17 on low lactase activity and milk intake. *PAG Bull* 2(2): 9–11, 1972.

Ransome-Kuti O: Lactose intolerance—a review. *Postgrad Med J* 53: 73–87, 1977.

Reddy V, Pershad J: Lactase deficiency in Indians. *Am J Clin Nutr* 25: 114–19, 1972.

Stephenson LS, Latham MC: Lactose intolerance and milk consumption: The relation of tolerance to symptoms. *Am J Clin Nutr* 27: 296–303, 1974.

Turner SJ, Daly T, Hourigan JA, Rand AG, Thayer WR: Utilization of low-lactose milk. *Am J Clin Nutr* 29: 739–44, 1976.

EPILOGUE

Robert H. Herman

The discovery and characterization of the small intestinal disaccharidases in general, and of lactase in particular, have generated a new dimension in the understanding of small intestinal function. These discoveries have provided new insights into gastrointestinal and nutritional problems. In this volume the disaccharidase lactase, which is contained in the brush border of the small intestinal epithelial cells, is considered in detail. Although lactase is just one of a number of disaccharidases, clinically it is of greater significance than the others. That an entire volume is devoted to lactose digestion and lactase is indicative of the importance of this enzyme.

A number of fundamental problems are discussed in the book, among them the importance of milk as a food for various population groups; the importance of lactose as a source of calories; the decrease in lactase levels after weaning in children as a *normal* physiological phenomenon; the delayed decrease in lactase activity in adults; the persistence of "normal" lactase activity in a minority of adults in the world; and the implications of lactose intolerance for the use of milk and milk products as food items in the United States and throughout the world.

Despite significant progress in enzyme research, we do not yet know why lactase activity declines at a given age in a majority of different ethnic groups and fails to decrease in a minority of other ethnic groups. Whatever the mechanism may be, at least there is general agreement that the change in lactase activity with age is genetically controlled.

The problem of the control of lactase activity is a special aspect of the general problem of control of gene expression, i.e., gene activation and inactivation. The concept has developed that certain genes function actively, while others are in a dormant or nonfunctioning state. The mechanism whereby certain genes remain permanently active and others permanently inactive is one of the major unsolved problems of molecular biology.

269

Certain genes can be activated or inactivated by a number of factors including substrates, metabolic products, hormones, and genetic preprogramming. Certain examples of gene activation and inactivation represent relatively permanent transitions from a state of active function to one of inactive function.

Little is known about the mechanisms that regulate disaccharidase biosynthesis. In contrast to lactase, there does not seem to be any loss of sucrase activity with age. Yet we do know that dietary carbohydrate can change the activity of sucrase but has little effect on lactase activity. Carbohydrates such as sucrose, maltose, and fructose cause an increase in the activity of sucrase and maltase in the human jejunum (Rosensweig and Herman 1968). Lactose, galactose, and maltose, on the other hand, do not have any appreciable effect on sucrase, maltase, or lactase activities (Rosensweig and Herman 1968). With very large doses of glucose it is possible to increase the activities of sucrase and maltase, but the response is much less than when equal amounts of fructose or sucrose are fed (Rosensweig and Herman 1970). It has been postulated that the ingested sugars affect the crypt cells and the disaccharidase responses become manifest only after the stimulated crypt cells have migrated into the villus (Rosensweig and Herman 1969). Progress in this area depends on a better understanding of the mechanisms that control disaccharidase biosynthesis.

It might be instructive to compare with lactose biosynthesis what we know about the control of hemoglobin biosynthesis, which is one of the best characterized systems concerning gene expression. In early fetal life, the embryonic globin chains are replaced by α-globin and two different fetal β-like globin chains by 8 weeks of age. During the transition period between embryonic and fetal development Hemoglobin Gower 2 ($\alpha_2\epsilon_2$) and Hemoglobin Portland ($\zeta_2\gamma_2$) are found (Kazazian 1974, Weatherall 1976, Proudfoot et al. 1980). The synthesis of the α chain continues throughout life. However ϵ-chain synthesis stops before the eighth week. The mechanism of the termination is unknown.

The synthesis of the β-chain starts at a low level in the eighth week, so that hemoglobin A ($\alpha_2\beta_2$) is present in an amount that is 8% to 10% of the total hemoglobin from the 8th to the 34th week of gestation. After the 34th week, β-chain synthesis increases, so that at birth, equal amounts of β and γ chains are synthesized. Three to four weeks after birth, β-chain synthesis is fully active, while γ-chain production persists only in a small population of erythropoietic cells. The nature of the γ- to β-chain switch is unknown. The γ-chain synthesis continues to decrease so that, at 1 year of age, hemoglobin F is less than 5% of the total hemoglobin. Hemoglobin F reaches the adult level of 1% at a variable age within the first few years of life.

Thus, there are two switches in the gene expression for the β-like genes: ϵ to γ from embryonic to fetal life, and γ to β from fetal to adult life. There is one switch in the gene expression for the α-like genes: ζ to α from embryonic to fetal and adult life. The arrangement of the β-like genes on the short arm of chromosome 11 (Lebo et al. 1979) is in the sequence of the developmental appearance of each of the β-like globin chains: ϵ, $^G\gamma$, $^A\gamma$, δ, β (Proudfoot et al. 1980). The arrangement of the α-like globin genes on chromosome 16 (Deisseroth et al. 1977) is also in the order of the developmental appearance of the α-globin genes: ζ_2, ζ_1, α_2, α_1 (Proudfoot et al. 1980).

How can this information be applied to the problem of lactase? It must be assumed that there are genes for each of the component parts of the lactase enzyme. In the genome there may be a set of DNA sequences (lactase regulatory sequences) that govern the switching off of lactase biosynthesis for one or more components of the complete lactase enzyme. These postulated DNA sequences also determine the age at which lactase activity will diminish. The decline in lactase activity resembles the decline in the production of the embryonic and fetal hemoglobins: the decline in the production of the ζ-, ϵ-, and γ-globin chains. The persistence of lactase activity indefinitely may resemble the hereditary persistence of fetal hemoglobin. The total deletion of the lactase regulatory DNA sequences would then lead to persistently "elevated" lactase levels (i.e., a failure of lactase production to decrease). The late decrease in lactase activity (in the third to fifth or later decades) would result from a partial deletion of the lactase regulatory DNA sequences roughly analogous to the partial deletion of the $\delta\beta$-gene seen in $\delta^0\beta^0$-thalassemia.

This analogy cannot be pushed too far, since data about human lactase deficiency are insufficient. How much residual lactase activity is present in the different ethnic groups with lactase deficiency? Is the decline due to the production of an enzyme inhibitor? Can lactase messenger ribonucleic acid be detected? Is there a failure of messenger RNA translation? Or, is the problem one of failure of messenger RNA transcription at the lactase gene level? Or, finally, is there a problem in the regulation of the lactase gene rather than a change in the lactase gene itself?

Obviously, to answer such questions will require investigation of the molecular genetics of the disaccharidases in general, and of lactase in particular. While awaiting answers to the questions posed, it is important to note how much progress has been made in our understanding of lactose absorption and its clinical and nutritional consequences. The current volume presents a comprehensive and authoritative discussion of knowledge to date on the subject of lactose. It both frames the progress made and raises the many theoretical questions yet to be studied.

REFERENCES

Deisseroth A, Nienhuis A, Turner P, Velez R, Anderson WF, Ruddle F, Lawrence J, Creagan R, Kucherlapati R: Localization of the human alpha-globin structural gene to chromosome 16 in somatic cell hybrids by molecular hybridization assay. *Cell* 12: 205–18, 1977.

Kazazian HH Jr: Regulation of fetal hemoglobin production. *Semin Hematol* 11: 525–48, 1974.

Lebo RV, Carrano AV, Burkhart-Schultz K, Dozy AM, Yu L-C, Kan YW: Assignment of human β-, γ-, and δ-globin genes to the short arm of chromosome 11 by chromosome sorting DNA restriction enzyme analysis. *Proc Natl Acad Sci USA* 76: 5804–08, 1979.

Proudfoot NJ, Shander MHM, Manley JL, Gefter ML, Maniatis T: Structure and in vitro transcription of human globin genes. *Science* 209: 1329-36, 1980.

Rosensweig NS, Herman RH: Control of jejunal sucrase and maltase activity by dietary sucrose or fructose in man: A model for the study of enzyme regulation in man. *J Clin Invest* 47: 2253-62, 1968.

Rosensweig NS, Herman RH: Time response of jejunal sucrase and maltase activity to a high sucrose diet in normal man. *Gastroenterology* 56: 500-505, 1969.

Rosensweig NS, Herman RH: Dose response of jejunal sucrase and maltase activities to isocaloric high and low carbohydrate diets in man. *Am J Clin Nutr* 23: 1373-77, 1970.

Weatherall DJ: Fetal haemoglobin synthesis. In *Congenital Disorders of Erythropoiesis,* Ciba Foundation Symp. 37 (new series). Amsterdam: Elsevier, 1976, pp 307-28.

INDEX

Abdominal pain, 126, 165, 214, 215. *See also* Cramps; Recurrent abdominal pain
Absorption, lactose, 17–18, 59, 80, 227, 228, passim
  in adults, 12, 29, 135–37, 138
  in Africa, 31
  as autosomal dominant trait, 18
  in children, 152, 163
  in India, 31
  and lactase levels, 105
  measurement of, 53, 55, 81–84, 163–64, 179
  in Northern Europe, 3, 17, 30, 31
  nutritional advantage of, 30–32
Absorption
  monosaccharide, 58, 59, 80, 92
  of other nutrients. *See* Colonic salvage; Nutrient bioavailability
Acquired carbohydrate intolerance. *See* Intolerance, carbohydrate
Adaptive (induction) hypothesis, 4, 13, 14–15, 20
Afghanistanis, 36
Africa, sub-Saharan, 38–43
Age, and intolerance, 129, 152–53, 158, 195, 207–8, 254. *See also* Intolerance, lactose; Lactase activity
Alactasia. *See* Isolated low lactase
Alcohol
  beverages, from whey, 237–38
  and lactase deficiency, 75
  in tolerance testing. *See* Galactose, plasma levels of
Allergy, and carbohydrate intolerance, 187–88
Amino acids, in nutritional products, 251
Animal protein, in nutritional products, 251
Antibiotics
  effect on hydrogen breath test, 104, 208–9
  and symptom onset, 179

Aqueous lactose
  compared to other lactose sources, 129
  dosage and symptoms, 135, 138–39
  with gelatin, 144
  in tolerance testing, 94–95, 102–3, 119, 127, 142, 265
Arabs, 12, 30, 37–38
Aryans, 32
Ascorbic acid, 144–45, 147
Aspergillus flavus oryzae, 261
Aspergillus niger (Lactase LP, Lactase N), 220, 222, 225, 231, 258, 261
Australian aboriginal children, 166
Autosomal dominant trait. *See* Genetic control, of lactase activity

Baboon (*Papio papio*), 72
Bacillus subtilis, 261
Bacterial flora. *See* Intestinal flora
Bacterial metabolism, 86, 87, 121, 184, 187. *See also* Hydrolysis
Bangladeshi children, 33, 195–201, 255
Bantu, 39, 41, 140–41
Barium sulfate, 94
Bedouins, 31, 37–38
Beta-galactosidase, 219, 223, 231, 244, 252
Biffidus factor, 189
Bile acids, 63–64, 187
Blacks (American)
  age and lactase activity in, 13, 70–71, 175
  prevalence of malabsorption, adults, 15–16
  prevalence of malabsorption, children, 151, 152–53, 163, 164, 176
Blenderized hospital diet, 249
Bloating, 119, 134, 135, 136, 139, 153, 228
Blood tests, 94–95. *See also* Galactose, plasma levels; Glucose, plasma levels
Bowel sounds, computer assessment of, 97